Here are your

1992 WORLD BOOK HEALTH & MEDICAL ANNUAL Cross-Reference Tabs

For insertion in your WORLD BOOK set

The Cross-Reference Tab System is designed to help link THE WORLD BOOK HEALTH & MEDICAL ANNUAL's major articles to related WORLD BOOK articles. When you later look up some topic in your WORLD BOOK and find a Tab by the article, you will know that one of your HEALTH & MEDICAL ANNUALS has newer or more detailed information.

How to use these Tabs

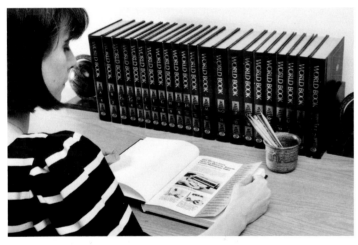

First, remove this page from THE HEALTH & MEDICAL ANNUAL.

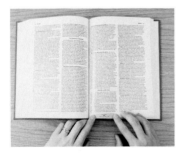

Begin with the first tab, **AIDS.** Take the A volume of your WORLD BOOK set and find the **AIDS** article. Moisten the **AIDS** Tab and affix it to that page by the article.

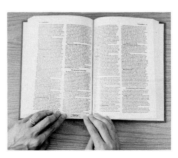

Go on to glue all the other Tabs in the appropriate WORLD BOOK volumes. Your set's *H* volume may not have an article on **Hospices.** If it doesn't, put the **HOSPICE** Tab in its correct alphabetical location in that volume —near the article **Hospital.**

Special Report
AIDS
1992 Health & Medical Annual, p. 12

Special Report
BOTULISM
1992 Health & Medical Annual, p. 196

Special Report
CANCER
1992 Health & Medical Annual, p. 68

Special Report
CHILD
1992 Health & Medical Annual, p. 182

Special Report
DRUG ADDICTION
1992 Health & Medical Annual, p. 110

Health Studies
DRUG
1992 Health & Medical Annual, p. 368

Special Report
GALL BLADDER
1992 Health & Medical Annual, p. 40

Close-Up Article
GENETIC ENGINEERING
1992 Health & Medical Annual, p. 286

People in Health Care
HOSPICE
1992 Health & Medical Annual, p. 354

Special Report
MEASLES
1992 Health & Medical Annual, p. 28

People in Health Care
MEDICINE (Careers)
1992 Health & Medical Annual, p. 340

Special Report
MENSTRUATION
1992 Health & Medical Annual, p. 124

Special Report
PARKINSON'S DISEASE
1992 Health & Medical Annual, p.138

Special Report
PLAGUE
1992 Health & Medical Annual, p. 166

Special Report
PNEUMONIA
1992 Health & Medical Annual, p. 82

Special Report
PREGNANCY
1992 Health & Medical Annual, p. 96

Special Report
SCHIZOPHRENIA
1992 Health & Medical Annual, p. 152

Close-Up Article
THYROID GLAND
1992 Health & Medical Annual, p. 291

Special Report
VENEREAL DISEASE
1992 Health & Medical Annual, p. 210

Close-Up Article
WEIGHT CONTROL
1992 Health & Medical Annual, p. 336

The World Book Health & Medical Annual

1992

World Book, Inc./Chicago • London • Sydney • Toronto
a Scott Fetzer company

The Year's Major Health Stories

From the dawning of the age of genetic medicine to the devastation of a cholera epidemic in South America, it was an eventful year in medicine. On these two pages are stories that *Health & Medical Annual* editors selected as among the most important, the most memorable, or the most promising of the year, along with details about where to find them in the book.

The Editors

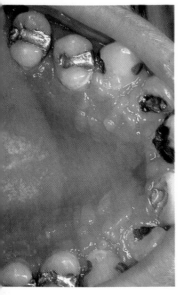

"Silver" Filling Safety
New evidence from animal studies reported in August 1990 prompted a debate in 1991 about whether dental amalgam fillings release enough toxic mercury to present a health risk. In the Health & Medical News Update section, see DENTISTRY.

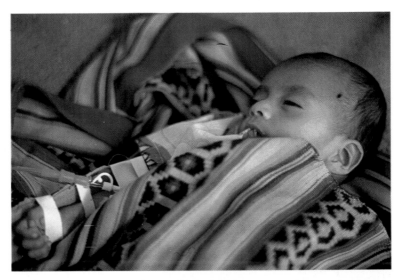

Cholera Epidemic
A cholera epidemic spread through Peru and neighboring countries in South America during 1991, afflicting nearly 300,000 people by August. In the Health & Medical News Update section, see INFECTIOUS DISEASES (Close-Up).

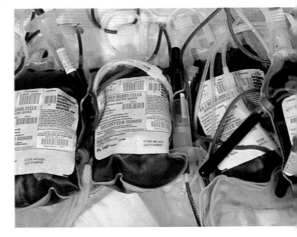

Making the Blood Supply Safer
American Red Cross in May 1991 announced new blood collecting, processing, and distributing procedures in response to criticisms about problems with its former methods. In the Health & Medical News Update section, see BLOOD.

World Book, Inc.
525 West Monroe
Chicago, IL 60661

ISBN 0-7166-1192-9
ISSN 0890-4480
Library of Congress Catalog Card Number: 87-648075
Printed in the United States of America

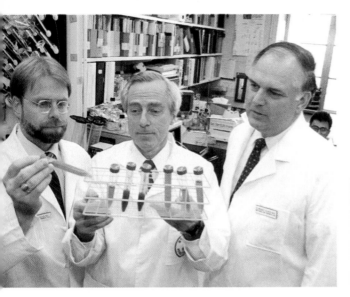

Dawn of Gene Therapy
Medical researchers in September 1990 began the first federally approved human trial of gene therapy, an approach that involves giving a patient new genes to correct a genetic defect or treat a disease. In the Health & Medical News Update section, see GENETICS (Close-Up).

First Portable Heart Pump
Surgeons in May 1991 implanted the first fully portable mechanical device to help the failing heart of a patient awaiting a heart transplant. In the Health & Medical News Update section, see HEART AND BLOOD VESSELS.

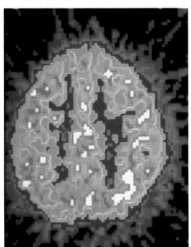

Hyperactivity and the Brain
Scientists reported in November 1990 that specific abnormalities in the brain may play a role in hyperactivity and problems involving attention span. In the Health & Medical News Update section, see MENTAL HEALTH.

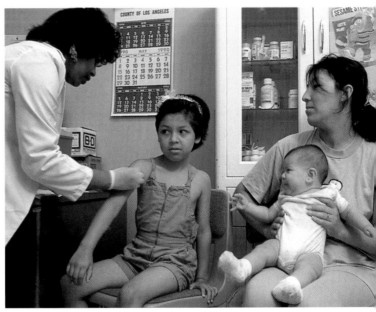

Measles Outbreaks
Measles cases in the United States soared during 1990 and 1991—even though there has long been an effective vaccine against the disease. In the Special Reports section, see MEASLES ON THE RISE.

Contents

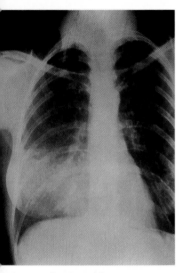

See page 82.

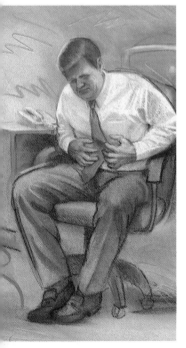

See page 41.

The Year's Major Health Stories   2
A review of the top health stories in the news and where
to find information about them in this edition of *The World
Book Health & Medical Annual.*

Special Reports   10

Fifteen articles present in-depth information about topics of
current importance in the fields of health and medicine.

The Specter of AIDS   12
by Richard Trubo

Measles on the Rise   28
by Rebecca Voelker

New Options for Treating Gallstones   40
by Thomas H. Maugh II

Healthy Skepticism   54
by Patricia Thomas

Combating Prostate Cancer   68
by William H. Allen

Pneumonia Still Can Be a Killer   82
by Beverly Merz

Healthy Mothers, Healthy Babies   96
by Cristine Russell

Defeating Drug Dependency   110
by Dianne Hales

The Puzzle of PMS   124
by Sally Squires

Closing in on Parkinson's Disease   138
by Michael Woods

Learning to Treat Schizophrenia   152
by Bruce Bower

Apocalypse Then: A History of Plague   166
by Robin Netherton

What's Behind Shyness?   182
by Richard Saltus

Poison on a Plate   196
by Yvonne Baskin

Sexually Transmitted Danger   210
by Joseph Wallace

Health & Medical News Update   226

Forty-one alphabetically arranged articles report on the year's major developments in health and medicine, from "Aging" and "AIDS" to "Veterinary Medicine" and "Weight Control." In addition, six Close-Up articles focus on noteworthy developments:

Few Answers for Chronic Fatigue Sufferers [Allergies and Immunology]   238

Gene Therapy: A New Era in Medicine [Genetics]   286

A Medical Mystery at the White House   291

The Legacy of Nancy Cruzan   296

Cholera Strikes a Continent [Infectious Diseases]   304

The New Way to Weigh In [Weight Control]   336

People in Health Care   338

Two articles spotlight people who contribute to health care.

Medicine at the Front   340
by Marc S. Micozzi

Caring for the Terminally Ill   354
by Paul Galloway

Health Studies   366

The World Book Health & Medical Annual takes a wide-ranging, in-depth look at an important area of medicine today.

Prescription Drugs and Human Health   368
by Ricki Lewis

Index   385

A cumulative index of topics covered in the 1992, 1991, and 1990 issues of *The World Book Health & Medical Annual.*

Cross-Reference Tabs

A tear-out page of cross-reference tabs for insertion in *The World Book Encyclopedia* appears before page 1.

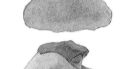
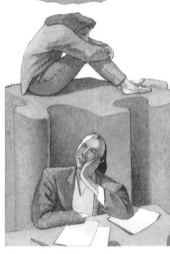

See page 128.

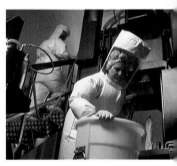

See page 344.

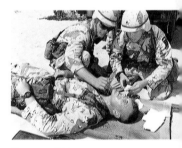

See page 380.

Staff

Editorial Advisory Board

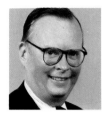
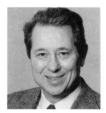
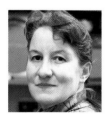
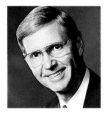

Contributors

Allen, William H.,
B.S., M.A., M.S.J.
Science Writer,
St. Louis Post-Dispatch.
[Special Report, *Combating Prostate Cancer; Diabetes; Smoking; Weight Control* (Close-Up)]

Arndt, Kenneth A., M.D.
Professor of Dermatology,
Harvard Medical School.
[*Skin*]

Balk, Robert A., M.D.
Director of Medical Intensive
Care Unit and Director of
Respiratory Therapy,
Rush-Presbyterian-St. Luke's
Medical Center.
[*Respiratory System*]

Barone, Jeanine, M.S.
Nutritionist and Exercise
Physiologist,
American Health Foundation.
[*Nutrition*]

Baskin, Yvonne, B.A.
Free-lance Science Writer.
[Special Report, *Poison on a Plate; Genetics* (Close-Up)]

Baum, John, M.D.
Professor of Medicine and
Pediatrics and of Preventive
Family and Rehabilitation
Medicine, University of
Rochester School of Medicine.
[*Arthritis and Connective Tissue Disorders*]

Birnbaum, Gary, M.D.
Professor of Neurology,
University of Minnesota.
[*Brain and Nervous System*]

Bower, Bruce, B.A., M.A.
Behavioral Sciences Editor,
Science News.
[Special Report, *Learning to Treat Schizophrenia; Child Development; Mental and Behavioral Disorders*]

Bowers, Kathryn E., M.D.
Clinical Instructor, Dermatology,
Beth Israel Hospital.
[*Skin*]

Cates, Willard, Jr., M.D., M.P.H.
Director, Division of Sexually
Transmitted Diseases/
HIV Prevention,
Centers for Disease Control.
[*Sexually Transmitted Diseases*]

Crawford, Michael H., M.D.
Chief, Division of Cardiology,
University of New Mexico
School of Medicine.
[*Heart and Blood Vessels*]

Franklin, James L., M.D.
Associate Professor,
Rush-Presbyterian-St. Luke's
Medical Center.
[*Digestive System*]

Friedman, Emily, B.A.
Contributing Editor,
Medical World News.
[*Financing Medical Care; Health-Care Facilities; Health Policy; Health Policy* (Close-Up)]

Galloway, Paul
Writer and Reporter,
Chicago Tribune.
[Special Report, *Caring for the Terminally Ill*]

Gartland, John J., M.D.
Chairman Emeritus,
Orthopaedic Surgery,
Jefferson Medical College.
[*Bone Disorders*]

Goldstein, Robert, M.D., Ph.D.
Director, Division of Allergy, Immunology and Transplantation,
National Institute of Allergy and
Infectious Diseases.
[*Allergies and Immunology*]

Hales, Dianne
Free-lance Writer.
[Special Report, *Defeating Drug Dependency*]

Hamilton, Gayle R., Ph.D.
President, Drug Abuse Training Associates; Associate Research Professor, George Mason University.
[*Alcohol and Drug Abuse*]

Harman, Denham, M.D., Ph.D.
Emeritus Professor of Medicine,
University of Nebraska
College of Medicine.
[*Aging*]

Hussar, Daniel A., B.S., Ph.D.
Remington Professor of Pharmacy,
Philadelphia College of Pharmacy
and Science.
[*Drugs*]

Jubiz, William, M.D.
Director, Medical Service,
Department of Veterans Affairs.
[*Glands and Hormones*]

Lake, Laura, B.A., M.A., Ph.D.
Adjunct Assistant Professor of
Environmental Science and
Engineering, School of Public
Health, University of California
at Los Angeles.
[*Environmental Health*]

Lane, Thomas J., B.S., D.V.M.
Associate Professor,
University of Florida.
[*Veterinary Medicine*]

Lewis, Ricki, Ph.D.
Adjunct Assistant Professor of
Biology, State University of
New York at Albany.
[Special Report, *Prescription Drugs
and Human Health; Weight
Control*]

Maugh, Thomas H., II, Ph.D.
Science Writer,
Los Angeles Times.
[Special Report, *New Options for
Treating Gallstones*]

McInerney, Joseph D.,
B.S. M.S., M.A.
Director, Biological Sciences
Curriculum Study,
The Colorado College.
[*Genetics*]

Merz, Beverly, A.B.
National Editor, Science
and Technology, *American
Medical News.*
[Special Report, *Pneumonia Still
Can Be a Killer; Ear and Hearing;
Eye and Vision; Stroke; Glands and
Hormones* (Close-Up)]

Micozzi, Marc S., M.D., Ph.D.
Director, National Museum of
Health and Medicine, Armed Forces
Institute of Pathology.
[Special Report, *Medicine at the
Front*]

Moore, Margaret,
A.M.L.S., M.P.H.
Head, Information Management
Education Services, Library of the
Health Sciences, University of
North Carolina at Chapel Hill.
[*Books of Health and Medicine*]

Netherton, Robin, B.J.
Free-lance Editor and Writer.
[Special Report, *Apocalypse Then:
A History of Plague*]

Newman-Horm, Patricia A.,
B.A.
Chief, Press Office,
National Cancer Institute.
[*Cancer*]

Pessis, Dennis A., M.D.
Associate Attending and
Assistant Professor of Urology,
Rush-Presbyterian-St. Luke's
Medical Center.
[*Urology*]

Powers, Robert D., M.D.
Director, Emergency Medical
Services, University of Virginia
Health Sciences Center.
[*Emergency Medicine*]

Roodman, G. David, M.D., Ph.D.
Professor of Medicine,
University of Texas
Health Science Center.
[*Blood*]

Russell, Cristine, B.A.
Free-lance Medical Writer,
The Washington Post.
[Special Report, *Healthy Mothers,
Healthy Babies; Pregnancy*]

Saltus, Richard, B.A.
Science Writer,
Boston Globe.
[Special Report, *What's Behind
Shyness?*]

Siscovick, David, M.D., M.P.H.
Associate Professor of Medicine
and Epidemiology,
University of Washington.
[*Exercise and Fitness*]

Squires, Sally, M.S.
Staff Writer,
The Washington Post.
[Special Report, *The Puzzle
of PMS*]

Thomas, Patricia, B.A., M.A.
Correspondent,
Medical World News.
[Special Report: *Healthy
Skepticism*]

Thompson, Jeffrey R., M.D.
Assistant Professor of Medicine,
University of Texas, Southwestern.
[*Kidney*]

Trubo, Richard, B.A., M.A.
Contributing Editor,
Medical World News.
[Special Report, *The Specter of
AIDS; AIDS; Infectious Diseases*
(Close-Up)]

Voelker, Rebecca, B.A., M.S.J.
Associate Editor,
American Medical News.
[Special Report, *Measles on the
Rise*]

Wallace, Joseph, B.A.
Free-lance Writer.
[Special Report, *Sexually
Transmitted Danger*]

Woods, Michael, B.S.
Science Editor,
The Toledo Blade.
[Special Report, *Closing in on
Parkinson's Disease; Dentistry;
Infectious Diseases; Safety;
Infectious Diseases* (Close-Up)]

Special Reports

Fifteen articles present in-depth information about
topics of current importance in health and medicine.

The Specter of AIDS   12
by Richard Trubo
AIDS has claimed thousands of lives during its brief history. As the number
continues to soar, scientists search for ways to battle the disease.

Measles on the Rise   28
by Rebecca Voelker
Although a vaccine had almost eliminated measles in the United States by
1983, the disease is again on the rise. Here's a look at who is at risk—and why.

New Options for Treating Gallstones   40
by Thomas Maugh II
New treatments can relieve the painful symptoms of gallstones without the
discomfort and lengthy recuperation time of traditional surgery.

Healthy Skepticism   54
by Patricia Thomas
Confused by the news media's seemingly contradictory reports about the
findings of medical studies? Here are some tips on how to read between the
lines and become a critical consumer of medical news.

Combating Prostate Cancer   68
by William H. Allen
Prostate cancer kills about 32,000 men each year in the United States.
With early detection, many of those lives could be saved.

Pneumonia Still Can Be a Killer   82
by Beverly Merz
Most people no longer think of pneumonia as a life-threatening illness. But
the ailment still ranks as the sixth leading cause of death in the United States.

Healthy Mothers, Healthy Babies   96
by Cristine Russell
By taking care of their own health and seeking prenatal care, women today
have far greater opportunities than ever before to have a healthy baby.

See page 51.

See page 89.

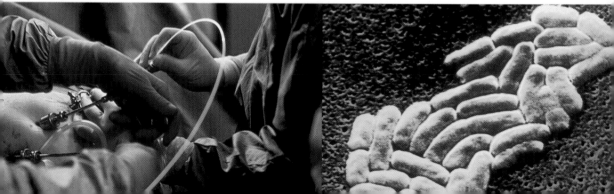

Defeating Drug Dependency   110
by Dianne Hales
Breaking the devastating habit of drug abuse can be a daunting challenge.
But for many people, the right treatment program can make the difference.

The Puzzle of PMS   124
by Sally Squires
Although researchers have not yet identified the cause of premenstrual syndrome, many women have found effective ways of coping with this condition.

Closing in on Parkinson's Disease   138
by Michael Woods
Scientists believe they are close to finding the cause or causes of Parkinson's
disease, a brain disorder that results in a loss of muscle control.

Learning to Treat Schizophrenia   152
by Bruce Bower
Schizophrenia's symptoms bring anguish to patients and their families.
But there is hope for recovery.

Apocalypse Then: A History of Plague   166
by Robin Netherton
During the 1300's, a mysterious and deadly disease wiped out a third of
Europe—roughly 20 million people.

What's Behind Shyness?   182
by Richard Saltus
Psychologists say that some people are born with a tendency to be shy.
Many learn to cope with their shyness, and parents can help shy children.

Poison on a Plate   196
by Yvonne Baskin
What caused Canada's largest outbreak of botulism, a deadly form of food
poisoning? A team of "disease detectives" turned up an unlikely suspect.

Sexually Transmitted Danger   210
by Joseph Wallace
Rising at epidemic rates, sexually transmitted diseases rank among the
most serious public health problems in the United States.

See page 96.   See page 138.   See page 196.

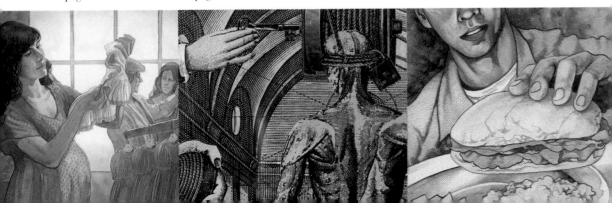

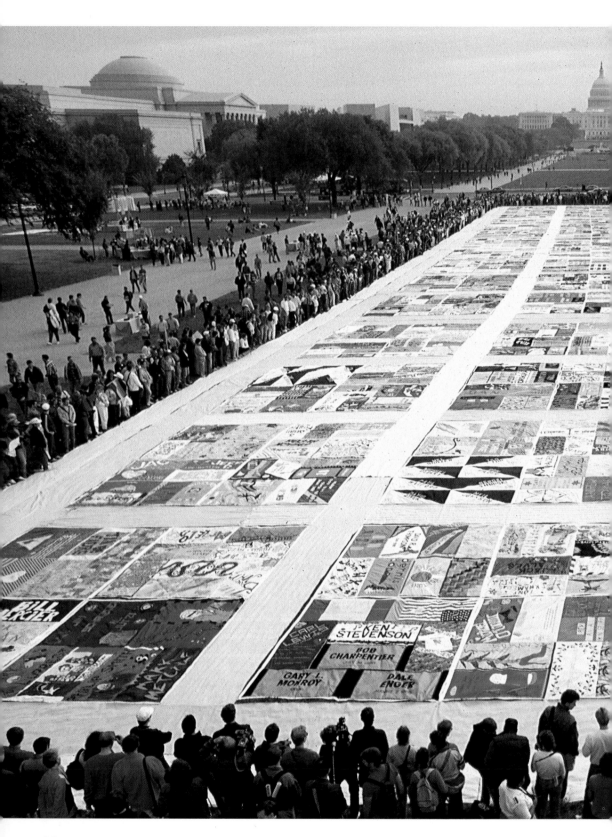

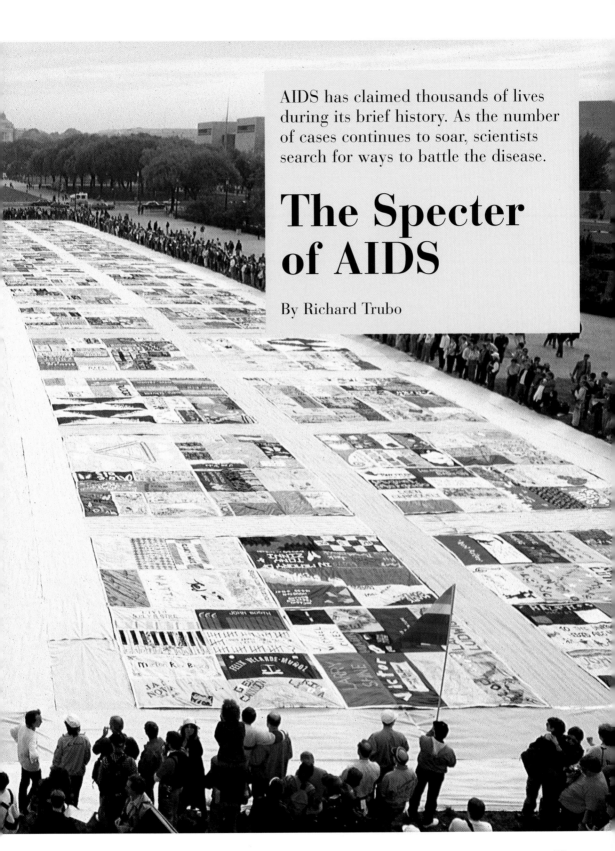

AIDS has claimed thousands of lives during its brief history. As the number of cases continues to soar, scientists search for ways to battle the disease.

The Specter of AIDS

By Richard Trubo

Previous pages: The AIDS quilt—thousands of quilted panels commemorating people who have died of AIDS—on display in Washington, D.C.

The author:

Richard Trubo is a contributing editor for *Medical World News*.

Many people can barely remember a time when AIDS was not one of the world's most ominous health threats. The media report news of the disease almost every day. Yet when the 1980's began, AIDS was not even an identified disease.

The first cases were reported in the United States in June 1981, when five young men were diagnosed with an extremely rare, serious infection—*Pneumocystis carinii* pneumonia (PCP), an illness that occurs in people with impaired immune systems. The men, all homosexuals, shared other symptoms, too, such as fatigue, night sweats, and *thrush*—a fungal infection of the mouth. Doctors were baffled as they tried to diagnose this mysterious combination of symptoms.

Since then, researchers have learned a lot about AIDS. By 1982, doctors had identified the constellation of symptoms as a new *syndrome* (a group of signs and symptoms that together indicate a particular disease). They named the syndrome *acquired immune deficiency syndrome* (AIDS), in recognition of the crippling effects the disease has on the body's infection-fighting immune system.

Other advances followed swiftly. In late 1983 and early 1984, French and American researchers isolated the virus that causes AIDS—the *human immunodeficiency virus* (HIV). By spring 1985, researchers had created a blood test to detect *antibodies* (disease-fighting proteins) made by the body in response to HIV infection. The presence of HIV antibodies in a person's blood (which doctors describe as "HIV-positive") strongly suggests that the virus is present, too. Researchers also discovered that HIV destroys specific white blood cells, called T-helper cells, that are essential for the routine functioning of the immune system. And in March 1987, the United States Food and Drug Administration (FDA) approved the first drug to combat the AIDS virus itself—zidovudine (AZT), which has modestly extended the life span of some patients.

Scientists in the 1980's also determined that HIV is contracted in four basic ways: intimate sexual contact, sharing of contaminated needles, transfusion of contaminated blood or blood products, and transmission from infected mothers to their offspring during pregnancy or at delivery. Armed with this knowledge, public health officials began to distribute educational materials through clinics and other means in an attempt to control the spread of the infection.

Despite such accumulation of knowledge about AIDS, no cure yet exists nor is there a vaccine that can prevent HIV infection. The virus can remain 10 years or more in a person without causing any symptoms. But once the person develops one of the key AIDS-related illnesses, such as PCP or *Kaposi's sarcoma*, a rare skin cancer, doctors diagnose the patient as having AIDS. Statistics indicate that, once diagnosed, an AIDS patient probably will die, usually within two to three years.

AIDS: A global problem

Most AIDS cases have been reported in the United States, though experts note that countries with less accurate record keeping than the United States may have more cases than they report. Africa had the second highest number of cases in 1990 and 1991. The World Health Organization estimates that the number of new cases in the United States and Europe may begin to level off in 1995, but will continue to rise in Asia and Africa beyond the year 2000.

AIDS around the world

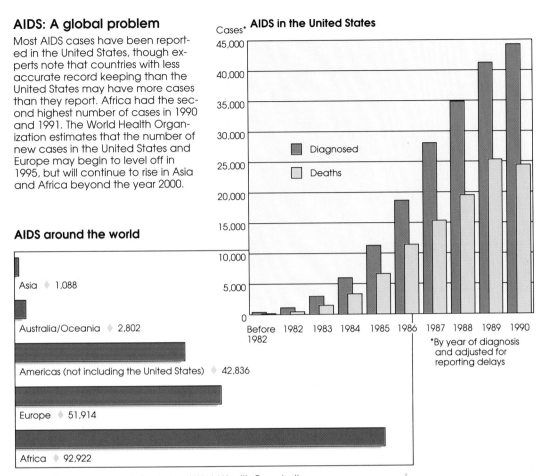

AIDS in the United States

Cases*

Diagnosed
Deaths

Before 1982 1982 1983 1984 1985 1986 1987 1988 1989 1990

*By year of diagnosis and adjusted for reporting delays

Asia ◆ 1,088

Australia/Oceania ◆ 2,802

Americas (not including the United States) ◆ 42,836

Europe ◆ 51,914

Africa ◆ 92,922

Source: Centers for Disease Control and World Health Organization.

A growing epidemic

The magnitude of the AIDS crisis is staggering. As of June 31, 1991, the Centers for Disease Control (CDC) in Atlanta, Ga., reported nearly 183,000 men, women, and children in the United States were diagnosed since 1981 as having AIDS, and more than 114,000 of these individuals had died. The worldwide statistics for AIDS are even more grim. Jonathan M. Mann, former director of the World Health Organization (WHO) Global AIDS Program, has labeled AIDS a *pandemic* (a widespread epidemic). WHO estimated that there were more than 1.3 million AIDS cases globally at the end of 1990 and about 8 million to 10 million people worldwide were infected with the AIDS virus.

Moreover, the epidemic is gaining momentum dramatically, and many experts are predicting that the worldwide epidemic will become much worse before it is effectively managed. Nearly 64,000 people died from AIDS in the United States in the three years from 1988 through 1990, exceeding the total number of

In the United States, AIDS is most prevalent in major metropolitan areas. As of June 30, 1991, the 10 hardest-hit U.S. cities had reported a total of more than 88,000 AIDS cases to the Centers for Disease Control, *above.*

U.S. deaths in the first seven years of the epidemic. The U.S. Public Health Service projects that by the end of 1993, the cumulative death toll in the United States could be as high as 340,000. By the year 2000, WHO estimates that 6 million people worldwide could have AIDS, and as many as 40 million people could be infected by the virus.

No region in the world has a more devastating AIDS crisis than Africa. More than half of the HIV-infected people worldwide live on this continent, experts say. The disease is infecting men and women alike, and it is striking people of all economic levels. In some cities in central Africa, an estimated 20 to 40 per cent of women of childbearing age are HIV-infected. In a 1990 study of corpses in morgues in Abidjan, the capital of Ivory Coast, 41 per cent of males and 32 per cent of females were infected with the virus. AIDS in many parts of Africa is spreading from urban areas to the rural areas where most Africans live.

In Latin America, the Pan American Health Organization estimates the number of HIV-infected people at nearly 1 million. The organization also reports that the infection rate is rising steeply, particularly among the people of Caribbean nations, such as Haiti. But Brazil is the country with the second highest number of recorded AIDS cases in the Western Hemisphere, after the United States, according to a July 1991 report. Health experts predict that this South American country's 18,000 AIDS cases will escalate to 250,000 cases by the year 2000. The port city of Santos has Brazil's highest infection rate, with an estimated 3 per cent of the city's 520,000 people already infected with HIV. According to public health specialists in Santos, the AIDS virus is transmitted mainly through intravenous drug use. They say that about half of the city's AIDS cases were infected via injection of drugs.

Asia, especially Thailand, is also showing staggering increases in AIDS cases, according to reports given at the Seventh International Conference on AIDS held in Florence, Italy, in June 1991. James Chin, who tracks and forecasts the global AIDS epidemic for WHO, said that HIV has infected 400,000 Thais. He also reported that, based on the results of a study of 20,000 to 30,000 Thai soldiers, at least 6 per cent of the Thai military are infected with HIV.

The rising cost of care

The medical costs for AIDS patients are soaring with the epidemic. Nearly half of WHO's $90-million global AIDS program went to Africa in 1990, an amount the organization acknowledged as inadequate. In the United States, according to a study conducted jointly by the Health Insurance Association of America and the American Council of Life Insurance, private insurers estimated in 1989 that they paid more than $1 billion for AIDS-

AIDS in the United States

When the AIDS virus was first identified in 1984, fewer than 5,000 people in the United States were diagnosed with the disease. In 1990 and early 1991, more than 3,000 cases were reported each month to health authorities.

The pattern of U.S. AIDS cases

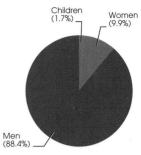

More than 88 per cent of the AIDS cases reported in the United States from 1981 through May 1991 have been men, *right,* with far fewer cases among women and children. But experts predict that the number of women and children with AIDS will grow substantially during the 1990's.

Children (1.7%)
Women (9.9%)
Men (88.4%)

How AIDS is transmitted in men

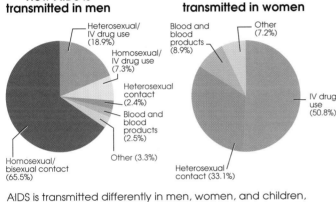

Heterosexual/IV drug use (18.9%)
Homosexual/IV drug use (7.3%)
Heterosexual contact (2.4%)
Blood and blood products (2.5%)
Other (3.3%)
Homosexual/bisexual contact (65.5%)

How AIDS is transmitted in women

Blood and blood products (8.9%)
Other (7.2%)
IV drug use (50.8%)
Heterosexual contact (33.1%)

How AIDS is transmitted in children

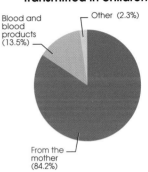

Blood and blood products (13.5%)
Other (2.3%)
From the mother (84.2%)

Source: Centers for Disease Control.

AIDS is transmitted differently in men, women, and children, *above.* Most men diagnosed with AIDS are homosexuals, bisexuals, or intravenous drug users. The largest percentages of women with AIDS are intravenous drug users or women who contracted AIDS through sexual contact with an HIV-infected man. The vast majority of children with AIDS were infected by their mothers, either before or during delivery.

The rise of AIDS in women

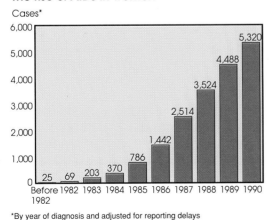

Cases*

6,000 — 5,320
5,000 — 4,488
4,000 — 3,524
3,000 — 2,514
2,000 — 1,442
1,000 — 786
25 69 203 370

Before 1982 1982 1983 1984 1985 1986 1987 1988 1989 1990

*By year of diagnosis and adjusted for reporting delays
Source: Centers for Disease Control.

The rise of AIDS in children

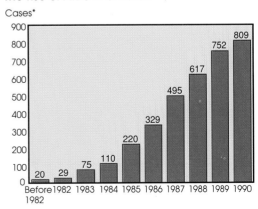

Cases*

900 — 809
800 — 752
700 — 617
600 — 495
500 — 329
400 — 220
300 — 110
200 — 75
100 — 20 29

Before 1982 1982 1983 1984 1985 1986 1987 1988 1989 1990

*By year of diagnosis and adjusted for reporting delays
Source: Centers for Disease Control.

More than 75 per cent of women reported with AIDS since 1981, *above left,* were in the childbearing age range of 20 to 44 years at the time of diagnosis. As more HIV-infected women have children, the number of babies who develop AIDS also rises, *above right.*

related claims for health and life insurance, a 71 per cent increase over 1988. Yet, the U.S. National Center for Health Statistics reports that private insurers' share for AIDS care is dropping and public financing is rising.

Many AIDS patients have no private insurance because they cannot afford it or have lost coverage provided by their employers when they became too sick to work. Some U.S. public hospitals are now teetering on the brink of bankruptcy by trying to care for such patients, and state Medicaid systems are experiencing severe financial stress. New York City, with the most reported AIDS cases of any U.S. city, is particularly hard hit. Medical services are already strained caring for 11,000 AIDS cases, and city health officials say that at least half of the 220,000 HIV-infected New Yorkers need immediate treatment.

Whether publicly or privately financed, care for AIDS patients is very expensive. Studies have shown that in the United States, the lifetime medical costs of treating each AIDS patient average from $40,000 to $75,000.

The shifting epidemic: Who is infected?

In the early years of the epidemic, most people with AIDS in the United States were homosexual and bisexual men. (In Africa, AIDS has been primarily a heterosexually transmitted disease, afflicting both women and men.) Other U.S. groups at risk then were intravenous (IV) drug users who shared HIV-infected needles and people who received HIV-contaminated blood transfusions. People with *hemophilia* (a disorder in which the blood fails to clot properly) were vulnerable because their clotting medications, made from blood, might contain the AIDS virus.

Various measures have succeeded in stemming the spread of AIDS for some of these high-risk groups. Education programs, including those promoting the use of condoms and other "safer sex" measures, have significantly slowed further spread of the AIDS virus among homosexual and bisexual men. This group, however, still accounts for more than half of the cumulative AIDS cases. Thanks to the introduction in 1985 of tests to screen donated blood for HIV, transfusion-related cases declined dramatically. The American Red Cross in 1989 estimated that with the widespread use of these tests only 1 of 153,000 units of transfused blood now contains HIV. More conservatively, the CDC estimates that as many as 1 in 36,000 units of blood may be infected. And new ways of manufacturing blood-clotting preparations has virtually eliminated this one source of risk for people who have hemophilia.

As the 1980's progressed, AIDS began to increase in other groups in the United States besides homosexual and bisexual men. By mid-1991, IV drug users of both sexes numbered almost 40,000 cases, or 22 per cent of the total reported. And

AIDS among heterosexual men and women has risen to more than 10,000 cases, or 6 per cent of the total reported. WHO predicts that heterosexual transmission globally will predominate in most industrial countries—as it now does in Africa—by the year 2000.

The growing incidence of AIDS among women in the United States is due primarily to IV drug use or sexual intercourse with HIV-infected men. Most of these men are IV drug users or bisexuals. Studies show that during unprotected heterosexual contact, an uninfected woman is more likely to contract AIDS from an HIV-infected man than is an uninfected man from an infected woman. Women (classed as females 13 years and older) with AIDS increased from 6 per cent of total cases in 1982 (69 cases) to about 10 per cent by mid-1991 (18,201 cases reported through June 1991).

Children with AIDS

A woman with AIDS can pass the disease to her unborn child, and statistics show that the number of children diagnosed with AIDS is increasing as more women become infected with HIV. Of the more than 3,100 cases of pediatric AIDS diagnosed through June 1991, 84 per cent contracted the disease from their mothers, mostly before or at birth. Less commonly, young children acquired HIV after birth through contaminated blood and blood-clotting preparations, particularly in the years before blood-screening tests and other safety measures were available. The number of pediatric AIDS cases in the United States grew 41 per cent from 1989 to 1990, according to the American Academy of Pediatrics, and WHO estimates that there may be another 20,000 infants in the United States who are HIV-infected but not yet diagnosed. In April 1991, CDC experts predicted that 1,800 to 2,000 infants born in the United States during 1991 would be infected with HIV at birth.

AIDS is also becoming more prevalent among sexually active teen-agers, through both heterosexual and homosexual contact. Studies have shown a link between certain sexually transmitted diseases and an increased risk for contracting HIV infections, though AIDS transmission can occur independent of other sexually transmitted diseases. Given the CDC's estimates that there are about 2.5 million cases of sexually transmitted diseases every year among American teen-agers, the threat of AIDS to this age group is tremendous. About 1 in 500 university students is already infected with HIV, according to a CDC study published in November 1990. The study concluded that the use of alcohol and other drugs on college campuses impairs judgment and may lead to unsafe sexual behavior and increased risk of sexual transmission of AIDS. For information on sexually transmitted diseases, see SEXUALLY TRANSMITTED DANGER on page 210.

Questions about AIDS

What causes AIDS?
AIDS (acquired immune deficiency syndrome) is caused by the human immunodeficiency virus, or HIV.

What is the difference between being HIV-infected and having AIDS?
People who are HIV-infected may have no symptoms for many years or may develop a wide range of complaints, such as fatigue, fever, night sweats, weight loss, and enlarged lymph nodes. People are diagnosed with AIDS after they develop one or more of the key AIDS-related illnesses, which occur because the immune system is compromised.

What are the key illnesses of AIDS?
People with AIDS have infections that usually only strike people with impaired immune systems, particularly *Pneumocystis carinii pneumonia* and a type of cancer called *Kaposi's sarcoma*, in which purple tumors appear on the skin. *Cryptococcal meningitis*, an infection of the membranes surrounding the brain and spinal cord, is also common in AIDS patients.

How is the AIDS virus transmitted?
Most people with AIDS contracted the disease through intimate sexual contact with an HIV-infected person or by injecting illegal drugs using needles and syringes contaminated with the AIDS virus. Blood transfusions and blood products contaminated with HIV also can transmit AIDS. Pregnant women infected with HIV can pass the virus to their fetuses, or, very rarely, through their milk during breast-feeding.

Who is at greatest risk for getting AIDS?
Most people with AIDS are homosexual or bisexual men who became infected through sexual contact. The second largest group with AIDS consists of heterosexual men who became infected by injecting drugs. Homosexual or bisexual men who also inject drugs make up the third largest group. And the fourth largest group consists of women who inject drugs.

Are women more susceptible to getting AIDS than men?
The vast majority of AIDS cases in the United States are among men. But the number of women with AIDS is on the rise, due primarily to intravenous (IV) drug use and to sexual intercourse with men who are HIV-infected. As for heterosexual transmission, research suggests that a woman is more likely to get AIDS from an HIV-infected man than is an uninfected man to get AIDS from an infected woman.

Can children catch AIDS from a classmate with the disease?
There is strong evidence that HIV cannot be transmitted by casual contact. For example, AIDS cannot be "caught" by hugging an infected individual, by sharing toys or other objects, or by using the same drinking glass or utensils. The virus cannot be passed from person to person by sneezing or coughing, nor can it be transmitted through bites of mosquitoes or other insects.

How is an HIV infection diagnosed?
Blood tests—called the ELISA (Enzyme-Linked Immunosorbent Assay) and the Western Blot—can detect antibodies the body has formed in reaction to the AIDS virus. The ELISA is usually the first test performed.

How accurate are these tests?
Although these tests are extremely accurate, they can, under some circumstances, produce misleading results. Some people infected with HIV may get negative ELISA results (indicating no infection) if they are tested in the first few weeks after exposure to HIV, *before* the body has formed antibodies to the virus. There is a small incidence of false positive ELISA tests, which means people who have a positive test result do not actually have the infection. If an ELISA test is positive, it must be repeated for confirmation. All positive ELISA tests must also be confirmed by a Western Blot test to make a definitive diagnosis of HIV.

What should a person do if he or she tests positive for HIV?
Anyone who tests positive for the AIDS virus should seek medical care immediately. The doctor will advise the patient about how to prevent spreading the virus to others.

How can one avoid becoming HIV-infected?
Avoid illegal IV drugs and the sharing of contaminated needles. To avoid sexual transmission of AIDS, either abstain from sexual activity or enter into a mutually faithful, monogamous relationship with an uninfected partner. (The greater the number of sexual partners, the greater the risk of contracting AIDS.) For those who are sexually active, public health officials recommend using a condom and a virus-killing spermicide.

A growing problem for small communities

Just as the prevalence of AIDS among different groups has changed since the early 1980's, so the geographical distribution of the disease has broadened since the epidemic first surfaced. Cities with large populations of male homosexuals and IV drug users—particularly Los Angeles, New York, and San Francisco—already are burdened by large numbers of AIDS cases. But as the 1980's drew to a close, there was a surge in the incidence of AIDS in communities with populations under 100,000. According to the CDC, these areas reported nearly 2,100 cases of AIDS in 1988 and about 2,800 cases in 1989, an increase of more than 35 per cent. To compound the problem, many small communities are ill-equipped to treat AIDS, having inadequate health-care services and human support for patients. In a 1990 report, the National Commission on AIDS urged federal assistance for many small-town clinics that are overwhelmed by trying to treat HIV-infected individuals.

Probing the AIDS virus

As AIDS grew from a few isolated cases to a burgeoning epidemic, doctors struggled to find its cause. By early 1984, scientists had identified the AIDS virus and learned to culture it in the laboratory. Initially, U.S. researchers called the virus *HTLV-III* (human T-lymphotrophic virus type 3); French scientists labeled it *LAV* (lymphadenopathy-associated virus). Eventually, an international commission agreed upon a single name—HIV.

Viruses are extremely small organisms—visible only with a powerful electron microscope—yet, they can create havoc within the human body. In AIDS patients, HIV destroys a specific type of white blood cell—called T-helper or CD4 cells—that are essential for the routine functioning of the immune system. With inadequate numbers of T-helper cells, the immune system literally turns off, leaving the individual susceptible to a form of cancer called Kaposi's sarcoma and to many *opportunistic infections*, including such respiratory infections as PCP, a sight-threatening eye infection called *cytomegalovirus retinitis*, and *cryptococcal meningitis* (a brain and nervous system inflammation). These infections are called opportunistic because HIV weakens the immune system, making a person with AIDS vulnerable to these illnesses, which a person with a normal immune system would easily fight off.

HIV seems to stay in the body indefinitely. The disease, however, progresses at different rates in different people. According to the CDC, about 50 per cent of the people die within 12 months of being diagnosed with AIDS. One study found that about 3 per cent of AIDS patients lived for five years. In the mid-1980's, some researchers estimated that only a fraction of individuals infected with HIV would ultimately develop AIDS.

The search for an effective vaccine

A scientist, *right,* examines an experimental vaccine that will be tested for its safety and effectiveness against the AIDS virus, *below.* But by mid-1991, no safe and effective vaccine was on the horizon, despite the efforts of dozens of federal and private laboratories engaged in vaccine research.

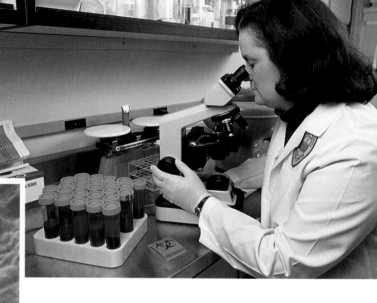

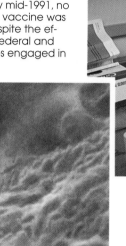

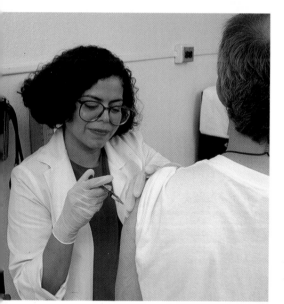

A volunteer receives an injection of an experimental vaccine during a test trial, *above.* At least six vaccines were undergoing human testing in the United States by the end of 1990.

In 1989, however, a report from the CDC suggested that as many as 99 per cent of the people infected with HIV could eventually develop the disease.

A second AIDS virus, which scientists are calling HIV-2, was discovered and reported in 1985 in west Africa, where it is now quite prevalent. HIV-2 causes symptoms and infections similar to those of HIV-1. In the United States, the first confirmed case of HIV-2 infection was detected in 1987, but U.S. cases are still quite rare. Most cases are found among west Africans who have emigrated to the United States or who are traveling in America. The blood tests developed to detect HIV infection can identify some, but not all, cases of HIV-2 infection. Thus, scientists developed an antibody test for HIV-2, which was approved for use in the United States in 1990. Other, as yet undiscovered AIDS viruses might exist as well, which could complicate testing and blood screening.

Treating AIDS

Researchers hope that by learning more about HIV, and how it attacks the body, such knowledge will enable them to develop more effective therapies. For example, biologists report that they have identified 13 steps in the life cycle of the AIDS virus—each step providing a possible target where drugs could block viral activity. Nevertheless, scientists acknowledge that it may take many years to develop such treatments. As of June 1991, AZT was still the only drug approved by the FDA to fight the AIDS virus itself. However, in July 1991, a FDA panel recommended approval of dideoxyinosine (DDI) to treat children and adults with AIDS who cannot tolerate AZT or who do not improve with AZT. In clinical studies of DDI, volunteer patients showed a slight increase in the number of T-helper cells and reduced HIV levels in their blood. Although the recommendation to approve DDI is not binding on the FDA, the agency was expected to approve its use by the autumn of 1991. About 8,000 AIDS patients are already taking the drug under special dispensation.

AZT combats AIDS by interfering with replication of HIV inside T-helper cells, but it does not eliminate the virus from the body. While researchers always have emphasized that AZT does not cure AIDS, it does modestly increase the life span of patients. The San Francisco Department of Public Health reported in January 1990 that patients the department studied who were taking AZT had a median life expectancy of about 21 months after diagnosis, compared with 14 months for those not taking the drug. AZT also improves T-helper cell counts and decreases the number and frequency of opportunistic infections.

In March 1990, the FDA approved AZT for people who are HIV-positive and who have T-helper cell counts of 500 per cubic millimeter of blood or less—even if they are symptom-free. Before then, the drug was FDA-approved only for patients with AIDS symptoms and T-helper cell counts of 200 or less or for those patients who had developed PCP. The normal T-helper cell range for people is 800 to 1,200. A lower count indicates a deteriorating immune system. Children age 13 years down to 3 months who show signs of impaired immune systems also may receive AZT. The FDA approved the drug's use for this group in May 1990.

Treating AIDS-related illnesses

Since AZT's introduction in 1987, researchers have been concerned about its side effects, including its interference with the production of red blood cells, which are needed to transport oxygen throughout the body. Many AIDS patients must have blood transfusions to combat this AZT-caused anemia. In January 1990, the FDA approved a reduction in the recommended long-term AZT dosage from 1,200 milligrams to 600 milligrams daily. Then a study by several research groups reported in October 1990 that even lower daily doses of the drug (as little as 300 milligrams a day) proved just as effective as higher doses of up to 1,500 milligrams a day. Patients also experienced significantly fewer side effects at these lower levels. So most AIDS patients now take reduced AZT doses. And on Jan. 2, 1991, the FDA approved the administration of erythropoietin, a substance that fights anemia brought on by AZT—further extending AZT's usefulness.

Doctors prescribe a number of other drugs to treat opportunistic infections and cancers that frequently kill people with AIDS:

- Pentamidine, prescribed in aerosol form to prevent the onset of PCP and in injectable form to treat patients already infected.
- Corticosteroids, used with pentamidine to treat PCP.
- Alpha interferon, a hormonelike protein, used to treat Kaposi's sarcoma.
- Ganciclovir, prescribed for treating cytomegalovirus retinitis.
- Fluconazole, used to treat cryptococcal meningitis and *candidiasis*, a fungal infection of the mouth and esophagus.

These drugs have enabled some AIDS patients to live months and sometimes years longer than they otherwise might have. With these increased life spans, however, individuals sometimes fall prey to other diseases not commonly seen in the earlier years of the epidemic, such as non-Hodgkin's lymphoma, a cancer of the *lymphatic system* (a network of vessels and nodes that carry a fluid, lymph, that bathes the body's tissues). The National Cancer Institute estimates that nearly half the people with AIDS taking AZT for three years probably will develop this cancer. The institute based its estimate on a study of patients who were among the first to receive AZT, between 1985 and 1987. Researchers are trying to discover if AZT causes the cancer directly or if the increased life spans of patients with weakened immune systems allows more time for tumors to develop.

Search for an AIDS vaccine

Although drugs may someday provide much more effective therapies for AIDS, researchers are also trying to create a vaccine against HIV. A vaccine stimulates the body's immune system to produce antibodies against a particular infectious disease without causing the disease. Vaccines can consist of dead bacteria or viruses or weakened live ones. Vaccines have been developed successfully for other viral illnesses, such as measles and polio.

In the early days of the AIDS epidemic, many scientists were pessimistic about the prospect of ever developing an AIDS vaccine. They pointed out that HIV differs in important ways from viruses against which researchers had developed effective vaccines. HIV places a copy of its genetic material inside a cell's own genetic material, thus hiding from attack by antibodies. HIV also *mutates* (changes its chemical structure) quickly so that a single vaccine might not be able to protect the body

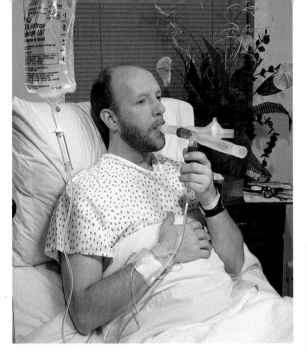

AIDS treatment

A patient inhales the drug pentamidine, *left,* to prevent the onset of the respiratory infection called *Pneumocystis carinii pneumonia.* This type of pneumonia is one of a number of *opportunistic infections* that frequently kill AIDS patients. Such infections tend to occur in people with impaired immune systems, such as people with AIDS.

against the virus in all of its forms.

As of 1991, no safe and effective vaccine was on the immediate horizon. But, by the end of 1990, at least six vaccines were in various stages of human testing in the United States. Most researchers concentrated on developing vaccines using the virus's "envelope" (outer cover) of proteins. Other scientists were working to develop vaccines using other HIV proteins that approximate the whole virus. Still others were at work on preparations based on the whole, killed virus.

Results from the first experimental AIDS vaccine to enter human testing were reported in January 1991. Volunteers had received up to four doses of the vaccine, which was developed from virus envelope proteins, over a period of 18 months. The most sensitive blood tests found that 30 of 33 healthy volunteers experienced some degree of immune response after inoculation with the vaccines. Scientists say that perhaps the most important result of this study is that it demonstrates the possibility of recruiting appropriate volunteers for AIDS vaccine trials. Researchers had to find volunteers (who were not infected with HIV) willing to develop antibodies that would falsely suggest HIV infection on subsequent medical examinations. The volunteers received special cards identifying them as trial participants.

AIDS drug research

Scientists are examining dozens of experimental drugs that might block the AIDS virus from infecting human cells or eliminate the virus once it has invaded the body. But the testing and approval process for drugs in the United States can take up to 10 years. In response to critics charging that this process is too slow, the United States Food and Drug Administration in May 1987 devised a program that allows people with AIDS to obtain experimental drugs while researchers continue tests to determine the safety and effectiveness of the drug.

Another criticism of the drug-testing process is that women, children, and racial minorities are underrepresented in studies. Their exclusion means these groups may not have the opportunity to obtain some health-care services available to others.

Some experimental drugs show promise against AIDS. Dideoxycytidine (DDC) may be able to slow the progress of HIV infection. It could be an alternative for patients who cannot tolerate the approved drug, AZT. Another experimental medication, called soluble CD4, may be able to attach to the AIDS virus and prevent it from entering white blood cells. Although preliminary studies indicate that this drug may be safe, its effectiveness is still under investigation by researchers.

Another experimental substance, compound Q, has been widely publicized, partly because of an unauthorized study conducted by an AIDS activist group. Although activists claimed that 8 of 46 patients improved, health experts criticized the underground nature of the study. Studies of compound Q (also called trichosanthin or GLQ-223) are now underway at medical research centers.

Education to prevent AIDS

Most health experts agree that until a cure is found, education is the best preventive measure against AIDS. The facts about AIDS are taught in sex education classes across the United States, such as in New York City, *below.* The poster, *right,* is one of many the U.S. Public Health Service distributed to inform the public of the danger of AIDS.

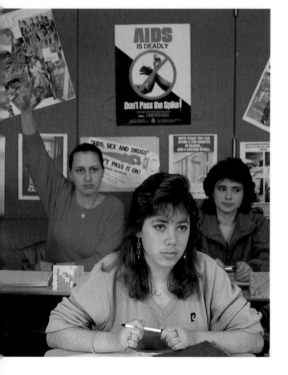

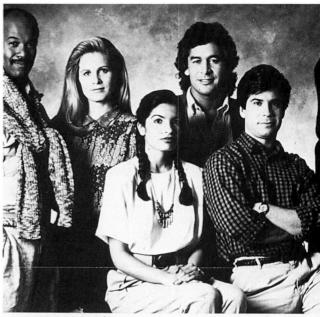

They show all the signs of having HIV.

There aren't any you can see. You just can't tell from outward appearance who is infected with HIV, the virus that causes AIDS. To determine your risk for HIV and AIDS, call your State or local AIDS hotline. Or call the National AIDS Hotline at 1-800-342-AIDS. Call 1-800-243-7889 (TTY) for deaf access.

AMERICA
RESPONDS
TO AIDS

HIV is the virus that causes AIDS.

AIDS education efforts

Until a successful vaccine is developed, the best preventive measure against AIDS is education. Early in the epidemic, critics charged that the federal government was not providing the public with explicit information on AIDS prevention through such measures as "safer sex" practices and not sharing needles—or better yet through avoiding sexual contact and IV drug use altogether. In response, the U.S. Public Health Service spent about $60 million in fiscal 1984 on AIDS—including scientific research, surveillance programs, and prevention campaigns— and by 1990, that figure exceeded $1 billion a year. The federal government mailed brochures called *Understanding AIDS* to 114 million households in the United States during 1988.

Private educational efforts proved very effective in the homosexual communities in large cities. Studies indicate that high-risk behaviors, such as unprotected anal intercourse and multiple sex partners, have decreased dramatically in these groups.

Over the next decade at least, the widening AIDS epidemic will produce even more of a national and international health crisis than is occurring now. With no treatment or cure in hand, health experts advise that abstinence or a mutually faithful relationship, such as marriage, between two uninfected individuals is the best way to prevent the sexual transmission of HIV. Short of that, health experts recommend limiting the number of sexual partners and using condoms in both heterosexual and homosexual intercourse.

Meanwhile, scientists continue to search for the elusive breakthrough to halt the epidemic. "We have learned more about the AIDS virus than any other virus that affects humans," says pathologist William Haseltine, an AIDS researcher at the Dana Farber Cancer Institute at Harvard University in Boston. He notes that only poliovirus has been studied in such similar detail—but thorough knowledge of that virus took 40 years to accumulate. Research on the AIDS virus has been compressed into just a fraction of that time, since HIV was discovered. Nevertheless, a magic bullet against this disease cannot arrive fast enough for those already under siege by HIV and AIDS.

For more information:
The National AIDS Hotline
(1-800-342-AIDS) for English speakers.
(1-800-344-SIDA) for Spanish speakers.
(1-800-AIDS-TTY) for the hearing impaired.

For further reading:
The National AIDS Information Clearinghouse, P.O. Box 6003, Rockville, MD 20850 (1-800-458-5231) offers numerous government and nongovernment publications, many of them free. Titles include *Understanding AIDS, How You Won't Get AIDS*, and *HIV Infection and AIDS: Are You At Risk?*

Although a vaccine had almost eliminated measles in the United States by 1983, the disease is again on the rise. Here's a look at who is at risk—and why.

Measles on the Rise

By Rebecca Voelker

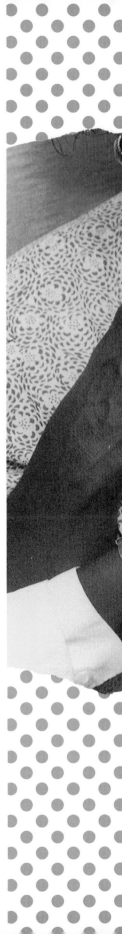

During 1990, a highly infectious disease considered routine and under control in the early 1980's soared to more than 27,000 cases and took more than 90 lives in the United States. The infection's explosive rise, which had begun in 1989, continued into 1991, particularly in the nation's major cities. In New York City, for example, during the first 12 weeks of 1991, health authorities reported about 2,000 cases of the disease—nearly double the number of cases the city had recorded for all of 1990. Public health experts in Los Angeles, San Diego, and Dallas were hoping that their epidemics, among the largest outbreaks of 1990, had already peaked. But health authorities predicted that 1991 was going to be a bad year for the infection.

The identity of the old disease that was prompting new concerns: measles. In 1990, the number of measles cases reported to the Centers for Disease Control (CDC) in Atlanta, Ga., a federal health agency, was the highest since 1983's record low of 1,497. But what is more distressing is that the disease is preventable. A measles vaccine had been licensed in the United States in 1963 and had nearly stamped out the disease by 1983.

In fact, the major reason for the spiraling number of cases

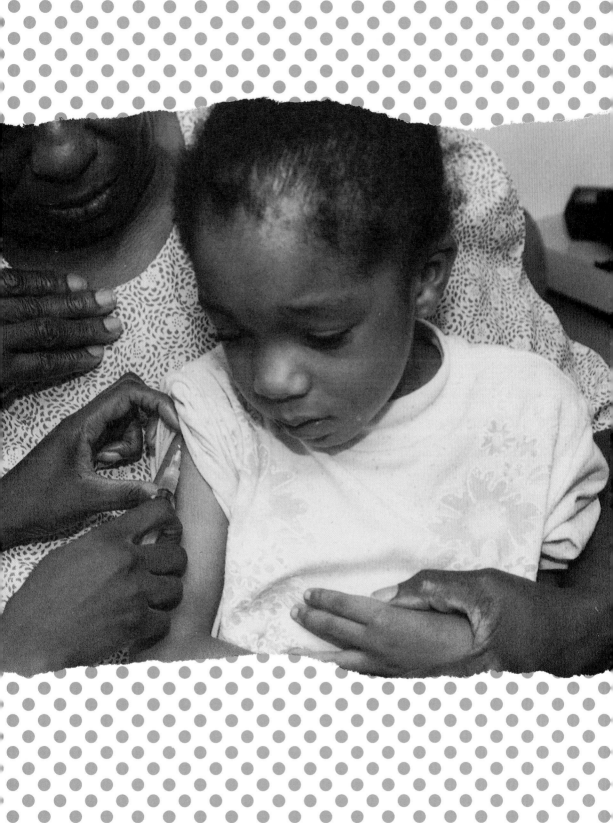

since 1983 was inadequate vaccination. In the prevaccine era, it was generally expected that measles would strike nearly every American at some time in his or her lifetime, and hundreds of thousands of cases were reported each year. But the measles vaccine proved so successful that people seemed to believe that measles had disappeared all by itself, rather than as a result of aggressive immunization programs in the United States and other industrialized nations. As a result, fewer people were vaccinated, and measles has reappeared. In many developing countries, where the vaccine is not readily available, measles remains a principal cause of death among children.

Causes and symptoms of measles

Measles is one of the most contagious of all diseases. It is caused by a virus that circulates through the body in the bloodstream and infects and grows in the tissues that line the respiratory tract. Although the measles virus can live for only a few hours outside of the body, it spreads easily when an uninfected person inhales tiny droplets expelled by a cough or sneeze from an infected person. Another factor that makes measles such a troublesome disease is that it is most contagious during its long *incubation period*—the time it takes a person to develop symptoms of a disease once he or she has been infected with the microorganism that causes it. The measles incubation period is 9 to 11 days, which means a person infected with the virus can pass measles on to others for nearly two weeks before knowing he or she has the disease.

An Arabian writer first described measles as a serious illness in the 900's. However, written records indicate that in those earlier times, it was often confused with *scarlet fever* and *smallpox*—contagious diseases that, like measles, are spread by nasal droplets in the air and are characterized by rashes. It was Thomas Sydenham, a British physician, who classified measles as a separate disease, after he observed symptoms of an epidemic raging throughout London about 1670. The disease now is often called *red measles*, or *rubeola*, to distinguish it from *rubella*, or German measles—a much milder illness, but one that also produces a fever and a skin rash.

Measles begins with symptoms similar to those of a cold or influenza—coughing, runny nose, inflamed eyes, sensitivity of the eyes to light, and fever. Within two to four days after infection, tiny red spots with blue-white centers called *Koplik's spots* often appear in the mouth. The spots usually fade a day or two later, when measles' characteristic blotchy, red rash appears on the forehead and spreads downward to the face, neck, trunk, and limbs over the next 2 to 13 days. This rash can last up to a week, and the fever can rise as high as 105 °F. Measles sufferers are often sensitive to light, because the measles virus can cause

The author:

Rebecca Voelker is an associate editor for *Medical World News*.

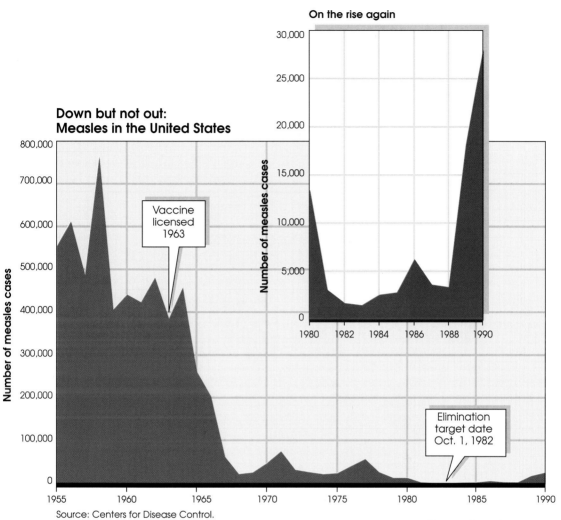

On the rise again

**Down but not out:
Measles in the United States**

Vaccine
licensed
1963

Elimination
target date
Oct. 1, 1982

Source: Centers for Disease Control.

The number of measles cases in the United States fell dramatically once a vaccine became available in 1963, and 1982 was targeted as the year for eliminating the disease altogether. Instead, measles cases rose dramatically, beginning in 1988, *inset.* Nevertheless, measles cases remain far below prevaccine levels.

conjunctivitis, an inflammation of the membrane covering the eye that does not affect vision. When the rash peaks, the fever usually falls, indicating that the disease has run its course.

Most measles patients recover quickly, often feeling well before the rash disappears. However, at least 5 per cent of measles sufferers are hospitalized for conditions that result from measles. (In 1990 outbreaks, more than 21 per cent of reported measles cases were hospitalized.) About 4 per cent of measles cases develop respiratory complications, including pneumonia, and about 5 per cent develop middle-ear infections. About 0.1 per cent develop *encephalitis,* an inflammation of the brain, which can lead to hyperactivity, learning disabilities, mental retardation, paralysis, and sometimes death. Another uncommon though serious complication, signaled by a dark purple skin rash, is bleeding due to a loss of *platelets* (disklike structures that help the blood clot). If contracted by a pregnant woman, measles can cause premature labor, miscarriage, or low birth weight in the infant. About 1 in 1,000 individuals die from complications associated with measles. However, in the 1990 outbreaks, the death rate was 3.2 per 1,000 cases.

There is no cure for measles. Once a person has contracted the virus, progression of the infection cannot be interrupted. Doctors advise taking steps to reduce the patient's fever, such as offering plenty of liquids, and make the patient as comfortable as possible—care similar to that given for a cold or the flu. Measles is contagious from approximately four days before until five days after the rash appears. During this period, the ill person should not come in contact with anyone who might be susceptible to measles, such as a child or young adult who has not been vaccinated against measles. Fortunately, once a person recovers from the infection, he or she usually has lifelong immunity against measles.

Development of a measles vaccine

Because there is no cure for measles, the most effective way to combat the disease is through vaccination to prevent infection by the virus. A vaccine mimics a real disease-causing organism—such as the measles virus—and so prompts the body to defend itself by producing disease-fighting proteins called antibodies. Later, if the body is infected with the real measles virus, it is able to defend itself.

Some vaccines are made from killed or inactivated viruses or bacteria; others contain live strains, weakened so that they cannot cause disease. The first measles vaccines were licensed in the United States in 1963, and for three years—1963 to 1966—physicians and public health officials used a measles vaccine made from dead measles virus. Its use was discontinued, however, because it was unreliable and caused complications, such as fever and aches, in individuals who later were exposed to the live virus. The preferred vaccine, however, was made from live, weakened virus.

Until 1967, the live-virus vaccine was often given along with immune globulin, which contains antibodies from the blood of someone who has been exposed to a specific disease-producing organism—in this case, the measles virus. Immune globulin was used to lessen reactions from the measles vaccine, but sometimes it actually prevented the vaccine from "taking." An improved live-virus vaccine, licensed in 1968, remains the only vaccine in use in the United States. Manufacturers began adding a stabilizing agent to this vaccine in 1980 to reduce the effect of light and temperature variations on stored supplies. This agent was added because CDC officials believed that some high school and college students immunized before 1980 became infected

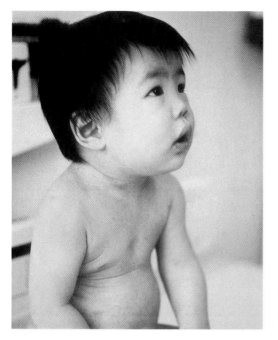

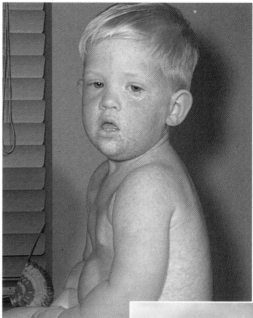

because they received vaccine inactivated by improper storage.

Measles vaccine is given by injection and often is combined in one dose with the vaccines for mumps and rubella. Complications from the vaccine are rare, but they can occur anywhere from 5 to 14 days after the vaccine is administered. About 15 per cent of those who receive the vaccine will develop a slight fever; in about 5 per cent, a mild skin rash appears. In some—usually adult women—arthritis may result, but usually this joint inflammation lasts no longer than about 10 days. Encephalitis has been reported in 1 of every 1 million vaccinations, but such vaccine-related cases usually cause no lasting problems.

There are only a few groups for which the vaccine is not recommended. These include pregnant women, individuals who are severely allergic to eggs (the vaccine is prepared in a culture containing chicken embryo cells), individuals who are sensitive to neomycin (a component of the vaccine), and those whose immune systems have been weakened, for example, by illness or drug therapy.

Measles symptoms
Both measles (*rubeola*) and German measles (*rubella*) cause rashes, but they differ in appearance. A rash of small pink and red spots characterizes rubella, *top left.* A measles rash, *top right,* consists of red blotches that develop about two days after small red spots with blue-white centers called Koplik's spots (indicated by arrows) appear on the tongue and inside the cheeks, *above.*

Measles almost conquered

For the first five years after the measles vaccine was licensed in 1963, the vaccine's effectiveness was reflected in the declining number of measles cases. In 1963, the CDC reported 385,156 cases of measles resulting in 364 deaths; in 1968 it reported 22,231 cases and 24 deaths. Then the steady decline ended. During the 1970's, the annual number of reported cases fluctu-

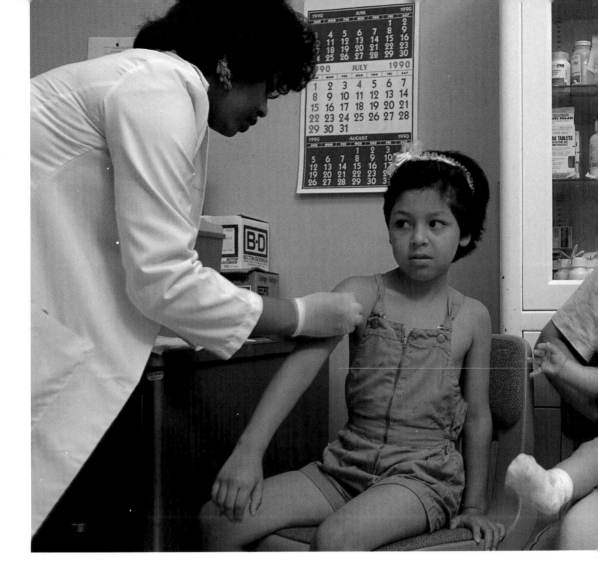

ated from about 22,000 cases to more than 75,000 cases.

Although the federal government restored some funding for measles vaccine and issued reminders to the public that vaccination was essential to control the disease, reported measles cases jumped to more than 57,000 in 1977. The CDC feared that up to 20 million American children under the age of 15 might not be properly vaccinated. So they launched a program called the Childhood Immunization Initiative in the spring of 1977 to address the problem. The program had two goals: to immunize at least 90 per cent of such children against a number of diseases for which vaccines were available, including diphtheria, pertussis, and polio, and to develop a permanent system to maintain that level of protection.

The immunization initiative focused on schoolchildren, because viruses are easily transmitted within the confines of a classroom. Federal officials surveyed the school records of more than 28 million young students to identify those lacking the

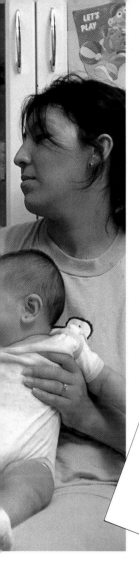

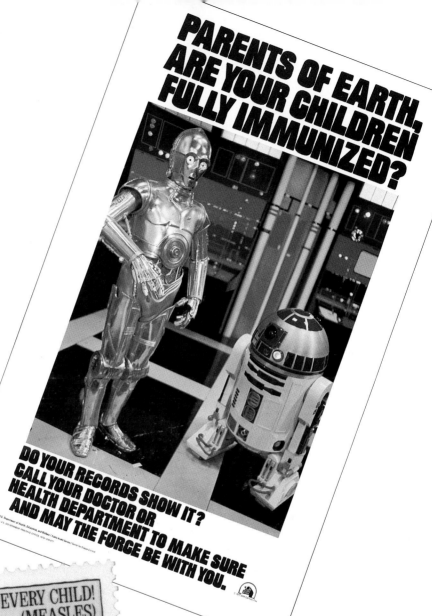

PARENTS OF EARTH, ARE YOUR CHILDREN FULLY IMMUNIZED?

DO YOUR RECORDS SHOW IT? CALL YOUR DOCTOR OR HEALTH DEPARTMENT TO MAKE SURE AND MAY THE FORCE BE WITH YOU.

U.S. Department of Health, Education, and Welfare / Public Health Service / Center for Disease Control

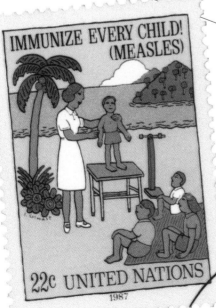

IMMUNIZE EVERY CHILD! (MEASLES)

22¢ UNITED NATIONS

1987

Preventing measles

A health-care worker in a Los Angeles clinic immunizes children with the measles vaccine, *top left*, the most effective protection against the measles virus. Worldwide efforts to inform the public about the importance of immunization against measles range from a U.S. Public Health Service poster, *above*, to a United Nations stamp, *left*.

Recommendations for measles vaccination

- **In most areas of the United States:** Children should receive two doses of vaccine—the first at age 15 months and the second at between ages 4 to 6 years.

- **In high-risk counties, such as those with large inner-city populations:** Children should receive two doses of vaccine—the first at age 12 months and the second at between ages 4 to 6 years.

Recommendations for proof of measles immunity

- **Colleges and other institutions of higher education:** Institutions should require documentation that the student has received two doses of measles vaccine after the first birthday, or has natural immunity acquired by a physician-diagnosed measles infection, or was born before 1957.

- **Medical personnel beginning employment:** New employees should be required to show proof of two doses of measles vaccine after the first birthday or other evidence of measles immunity.

Recommendations for controlling measles outbreaks

- **Outbreaks in preschool-age children:** Vaccinate children as young as 6 months of age in outbreak area if cases are occurring in children younger than 12 months of age.

- **Outbreaks in day-care centers, elementary and high schools, colleges, and other institutions:** Vaccinate people who do not have documentation of immunity to measles, including students, their siblings, and school personnel born during or after 1957.

- **Outbreaks in medical facilities:** Vaccinate all medical workers born during or after 1957 who have direct patient contact and who do not have proof of immunity to measles. In addition, susceptible workers who have been exposed to people with measles should be relieved from direct patient contact from the 5th to the 21st day after exposure. If they become ill, these workers should avoid patient contact for 7 days after they develop a rash.

Source: Centers for Disease Control.

proper vaccinations. State governments also responded. By July 1979, all states and the District of Columbia required proof that a child had received all available vaccines as a condition for a student to enter school for the first time; 30 states required proof of immunization for all students, from kindergarten through grade 12. By 1980, 91 per cent of students from kindergarten through the 12th grade had presented their schools with proof of either having had natural measles or the measles vaccination.

At first, this immunization initiative was so successful that the government thought a victory over measles was inevitable. In autumn 1978, Joseph A. Califano, Jr., then U.S. secretary of health, education, and welfare, announced a target date of Oct. 1, 1982, for the elimination of measles in the United States.

Meeting that eradication goal hinged on several factors. The most fundamental one was making sure that large numbers of children and young adults were immunized, and that those high levels were maintained. In addition, health officials realized the need for effective monitoring of locations where measles cases were reported and for aggressive measures to control outbreaks. School officials helped curb outbreaks by establishing clinics where children could voluntarily come to be immunized when reports of measles surfaced in their districts.

With extensive control measures in place through monitoring

and immunization programs in elementary and secondary schools, colleges, and even some day-care centers, federal officials were guardedly optimistic that the eradication goal could be met. National surveys showed that 96 per cent of students entering school for the 1981-1982 school year were vaccinated against measles. By the end of 1981, reported measles cases nationwide had plummeted to 3,124—a significant drop from the nearly 27,000 cases reported in 1978, the year the eradication goal was announced. Although the 1982 target date quietly passed, with 1,714 measles cases reported to the CDC, the goal still appeared attainable. Reported measles cases fell even further the following year, to a record low of 1,497.

Vaccinations down, measles up

Health officials recognized that measles could be eradicated only with a concerted and sustained effort from state and local health departments, physicians, and the general public. Official optimism began to wane, however, as reported measles cases fluctuated, always above the 1983 level. Then, the number of measles cases exploded, leaping from nearly 3,400 cases in 1988 to more than 18,000 cases in 1989. Although the number of reported cases was rising sharply, the total still was far below the half-million cases annually reported up until the mid-1960's.

Measles cases in the late 1980's occurred mainly in major cities. In 1989, outbreaks among unvaccinated preschool children in just three cities—Chicago, Houston, and Los Angeles—accounted for nearly 25 per cent of all measles cases nationwide. State laws requiring vaccination for school entry had reduced measles infection among school-age children. And infants younger than six months were not considered at extremely high risk for measles since they possess antibodies passed on by their mothers that give temporary protection against the disease. But, unlike older and younger children, unvaccinated preschoolers fell through the medical and natural safety nets.

In the vulnerable preschool population, minority inner-city children appear to be at the highest risk for contracting measles. During a measles epidemic in Chicago in 1989, city public health officials reported that 75 per cent of the 2,232 cases reported were in children age 4 or younger. City officials also reviewed the immunization records of schoolchildren to determine where vaccination deficiencies existed. They found that nearly 80 per cent of students entering schools attended predominantly by white children had been properly vaccinated by age 2. However, only about half of the children entering schools attended predominantly by black and Hispanic children had received adequate vaccinations. Health officials in other cities where outbreaks had been concentrated saw similar patterns.

Some vaccinated teen-agers and young adults were also vulnerable to measles. From 1985 to 1989, 80 per cent of measles cases in vaccinated children were in those over age 12. One reason for this vulnerability was the vaccine's failure rate of 2 to 5 per cent; some health officials say that rate could be as high as 10 per cent. Vaccine failure means immunity never was established, or the immune response faded over time. Another reason for vaccine failure stems from the age of the child at time of vaccination. Many children, especially in outbreak areas, were vaccinated at the age of 12 to 14 months old, an age when maternal antibodies to measles could still be present and interfere with a child's own response to the vaccine. As these children grew older, their risk for contracting measles increased.

During 1989, students on college campuses also accounted for a substantial number of reported measles cases—1,638, or 9 per cent of all cases reported that year. However, almost half of the individuals who contracted measles on a college campus from 1986 through 1989 had never received a measles vaccination. During the first six months of 1990, measles outbreaks were reported in at least 17 colleges and universities in 14 states. As a result, several colleges started massive vaccination programs, administering more than 80,000 doses of vaccine.

Because measles rates had dipped so low in the early 1980's, many young physicians entering the medical profession during this period had never diagnosed a case of the illness. Word spread quickly through the medical community: Each young patient being treated for a minor illness or injury should be vaccinated against measles.

New vaccination guidelines

The CDC and the American Academy of Pediatrics in 1989 issued new vaccination guidelines. In addition to an initial measles vaccination at the age of 15 months, the new guidelines say that children should be given a second dose between ages 4 and 6 years—the usual age for entering school. The second dose is intended to provide immunity to the 5 to 10 per cent of children in whom the first vaccine fails. Also, the guidelines call for giving susceptible adults born after 1957 a second dose of vaccine. Adults born before 1957 are not considered at risk because they probably have either survived a bout with measles or built up natural immunity after contact with infected people.

Students entering colleges and other programs following high school should show proof of two vaccinations or evidence of immunity—a physician's diagnosis of measles or a blood test showing the presence of antibodies to the measles virus. Because health-care settings, especially hospital emergency rooms, are considered high-risk areas for the transmission of measles, new health-care employees also should show proof of immunity.

Most at risk are unvaccinated or ineffectively vaccinated:

- Infants and preschoolers.
- College students.
- Health-care workers.
- International travelers.
- Anyone age 19 to 33 who has not had measles.
- Anyone who is exposed to measles and is unsure whether he or she is immune.

The revised CDC guidelines recommended additional strategies for areas where measles outbreaks were already underway. In these regions, the CDC advised vaccinating children as young as 6 months if measles was reported among youngsters less than a year old. In the event of outbreaks in day-care centers, elementary and high schools, and colleges, the guidelines recommended revaccinating any school personnel, students, and brothers and sisters of students who do not have proof of immunity. The same recommendation applied to health-care workers who come in direct contact with patients.

Can measles be eradicated?

CDC officials say measles could be eliminated among school-age children and college students—if the guidelines are followed. They also believe that adherence to the guidelines could prevent up to 40 per cent of measles cases attributed to vaccine failure in children over the age of 5 years. Nevertheless, it will take several years for vaccination efforts to reduce the amount of virus circulating in communities across the country.

Moreover, many experts believe that measles is likely to be around for the foreseeable future because certain segments of the population, such as the urban poor, are having difficulty obtaining vaccinations due to cuts in federal funding for immunizations. In a January 1991 report, the National Vaccine Advisory Committee cited instances in which parents waited for months to get appointments for their children in public clinics. Once there, the report added, families waited for hours in crowded clinics and paid for vaccinations that once were provided by these public clinics without charge.

The advisory committee asked the government to boost its budget for immunizations by 20 per cent. The committee also said insurance coverage of immunizations should be mandatory. As of January 1991, less than half of the private insurance companies paid for immunizations, while about two-thirds of health maintenance organizations did so. The committee also asked for a revision of immunization practices in clinics so that children could be immunized without first having a comprehensive medical examination. And the committee suggested that immunizations be required for entry to day-care programs and that social welfare programs provide measles vaccinations.

The CDC estimates that, through 1990, measles vaccine has prevented nearly 75 million cases of the infection, 24,200 cases of measles-related mental retardation, and 7,450 deaths. The number of measles cases since 1989 is still only a fraction of the cases reported before a vaccine was available. But these cases, too, were preventable. Many health experts believe that with the cooperation of public health officials, physicians, and the public, measles could be eradicated from the United States.

New treatments can relieve the painful
symptoms of gallstones without the
discomfort and lengthy recuperation
time of traditional surgery.

New Options
for Treating
Gallstones

By Thomas H. Maugh II

Because I spend a lot of time in front of a computer, backaches
are not unusual. But the stabbing back pains that struck last
fall were incapacitating. I could do nothing more than lie mo-
tionless on a mattress on the floor for two and a half days. By
the end of that time, the pain had shifted from my back to the
front of my chest. I assumed that I had somehow bruised my
chest by lying on the floor.

But after the pain finally subsided, I began to have second
thoughts. Perhaps the new pain wasn't related to the back pain.
Maybe I had suffered a minor heart attack. Although I was feeling better, I made an appointment with my doctor—better safe
than sorry, I told myself. Besides, I had been having some other
minor problems that could stand to be checked. For several
months, I had been gulping antacid tablets for indigestion. Perhaps I had the beginnings of an ulcer caused by stress. And every now and then, I recalled uneasily, I got a sharp pain in my
right shoulder. More symptoms of a heart attack.

My physician listened as I described my symptoms, then hit
me with a completely unexpected diagnosis: a gall bladder
problem. Although my symptoms were a bit unusual for a gall

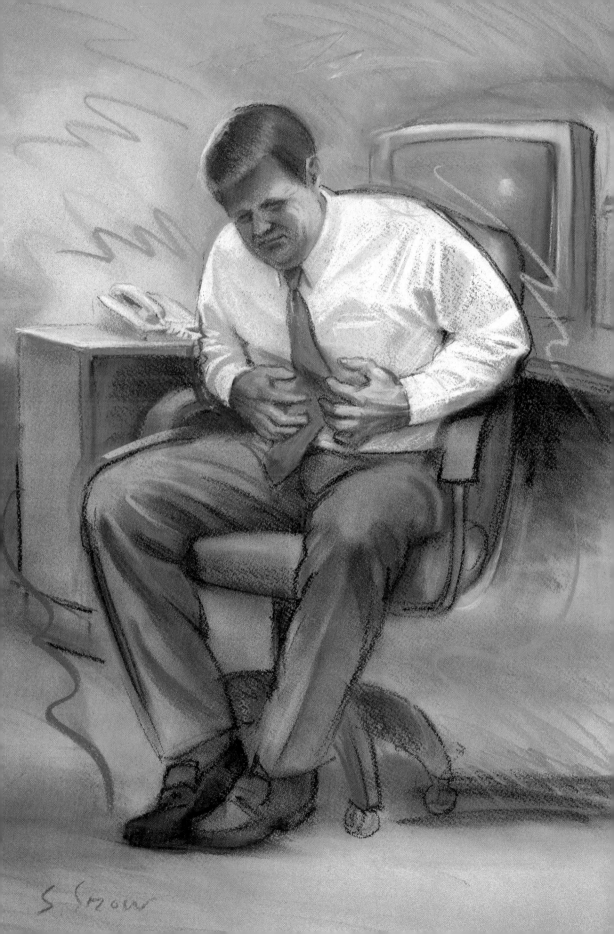

The author:

Thomas H. Maugh II is a science writer for the *Los Angeles Times*.

bladder disorder—gall bladder pain more commonly starts in the upper abdomen—he thought that it was the most likely source of my misery. Surprisingly, this possibility had never crossed my mind, even though my 82-year-old father had undergone gall bladder surgery not five months earlier.

To make sure there were no obvious heart problems, my physician ran a few tests. When they turned up nothing, it seemed likely that I would become one of 700,000 Americans who have their gall bladders removed each year. According to the National Institutes of Health in Bethesda, Md., gall bladder surgery is the second most common major operation in the United States, surpassed only by the Caesarean section, in which a baby is delivered through an incision in the mother's abdomen and uterus.

It was after this doctor's appointment that I learned about a remarkable new surgical technique, which literally sucks the gall bladder out through a tiny incision in the patient's navel. This procedure spares gall bladder patients most of the pain of traditional surgery, which involves a much larger incision through the nerves and muscles of the abdominal wall.

The new surgical technique also cuts hospitalization to an overnight stay, as compared with nearly a week for traditional surgery, and reduces recuperation from nearly five weeks to one. Although performed in the United States only since 1988, the "bellybutton surgery" now accounts for almost half of all gall bladder operations. Many medical experts expect it will soon become the standard method for treating gall bladder disorders.

The gall bladder: what, where, and why?

The gall bladder is a pear-shaped, muscular organ, about 3 inches (7.5 centimeters) long and 1 inch (2.5 centimeters) wide at its thickest point. It sits on the underside of the liver just below the lower ribs and is connected to the liver and the small intestine by *ducts* (narrow tubes). The gall bladder functions chiefly as a reservoir for *bile*, a fluid manufactured in the liver. Bile promotes the digestion and absorption of fats in the diet. After a person eats a meal, the gall bladder contracts and sends the bile through a duct into the intestine. Bile is rich in a fatty substance called *cholesterol*. It also contains large amounts of *bile salts*, which the liver produces from cholesterol, and *bilirubin*, a reddish pigment that results from the breakdown in the liver of red blood cells.

What can go wrong: gallstones

The most common problem that arises in the gall bladder is the formation of *gallstones*, hard masses that can be smaller than a pea or as large as a small pear. Autopsy studies have shown that

20 to 25 per cent of women and 10 per cent of men in the United States develop gallstones to some degree by the time they die. The longer people live, the greater their chances of developing gallstones.

Gallstones typically form from cholesterol, though some are composed of calcium and bilirubin. If these substances become too highly concentrated in bile, they may no longer remain completely dissolved. Tiny, solid particles form instead. These gallstones gradually grow as more material attaches to them.

But no one knows precisely what triggers this process or why some people are more likely to develop gallstones than others. Physicians do know, however, that the groups at highest risk for gallstones include people with diabetes, Native Americans, and women—especially women who are overweight or who have had multiple pregnancies. A family history of gallstones also increases the likelihood that an individual will develop gallstones.

Gallstones sometimes remain unnoticed in the gall bladder or pass painlessly into the intestine. They cause severe pain, however, if they block the flow of bile from the gall bladder. The pain occurs when the gall bladder contracts but cannot empty. It subsides when the obstructing gallstone falls back into the gall bladder or moves into the intestine.

Other gall bladder problems

An inflammation of the gall bladder, known as *cholecystitis*, may accompany gallstones. (The word *colecyst*, a synonym for *gall bladder*, comes from combining the Greek words for *bile* and *cyst*.) The inflammation usually results when bile cannot leave the obstructed gall bladder. The trapped bile may then become highly concentrated and irritate the lining of the gall bladder. Moreover, if the gall bladder does not empty properly and the bile stagnates, a bacterial infection can develop, complicating cholecystitis. In rare cases, an untreated infection causes the gall bladder to swell and eventually burst, leading to a life-threatening inflammation of the lining of the abdomen called *peritonitis*.

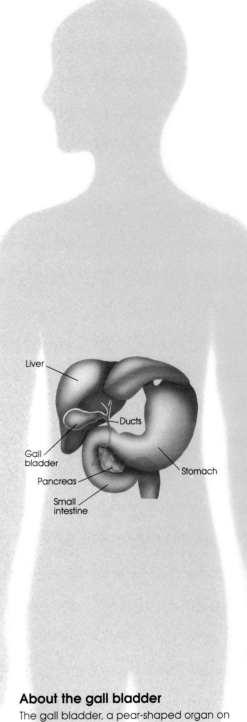

Liver

Ducts

Gall bladder

Pancreas

Small intestine

Stomach

About the gall bladder

The gall bladder, a pear-shaped organ on the underside of the liver, is connected to the liver and intestine by tubes called *ducts*. The gall bladder serves chiefly to store *bile*, a digestive fluid produced in the liver. After a person eats a meal, the gall bladder contracts and sends the bile through a duct into the intestine. If the gall bladder is removed, the bile flows through a duct directly from the liver to the intestine.

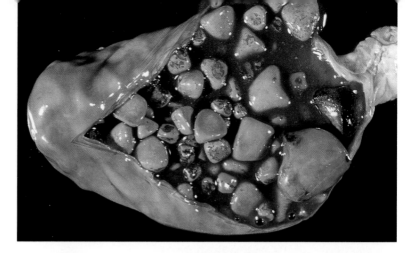

Gallstones: a common disorder

The most common problem that arises in the gall bladder is the formation of *gallstones,* hard masses that can be smaller than a pea or as large as a small pear, *top right.* Physicians do not know exactly what triggers the formation of gallstones or why some people are more likely to develop them than others. But they do know that gallstones typically form from excess *cholesterol* (a fatty substance) and calcium in the bile. Gallstones can cause severe pain, especially if they become trapped in the neck of the gall bladder or in a duct leading from it, thereby blocking the flow of bile, *bottom right.*

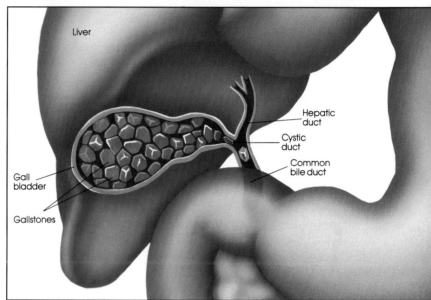

Liver

Hepatic duct

Cystic duct

Common bile duct

Gall bladder

Gallstones

Symptoms of gallstones

Many gallstones remain "silent" and produce no symptoms. When symptoms do occur, people may experience the following:

- Severe pain in the upper right part of the abdomen, sometimes extending back to the right shoulder blade. The pain usually strikes a few hours after a meal. Although the pain may subside after several hours, soreness may persist for days.

- Nausea and vomiting accompanying the pain.

- Jaundice, a yellowing of the skin and eyes, develops in a few cases where a trapped gallstone blocks the flow of bile through the duct leading to the intestine.

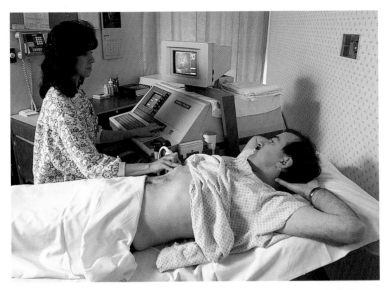

Gallstones are typically diagnosed by ultrasound or X-ray examination. In an ultrasound examination, *left,* high-frequency sound waves, emitted by the device the technician is guiding, bounce off tissues in the patient's abdomen. A computer uses the reflected sound waves to produce an image of the gall bladder. In an X ray, *below,* gallstones show up as spots after the gall bladder absorbs a dye that causes it to appear as a dense mass.

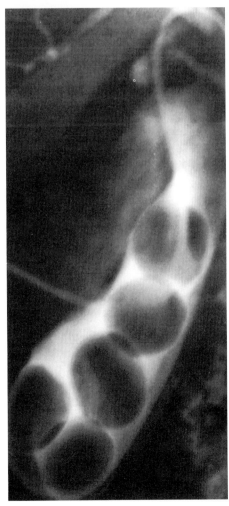

A far less common gall bladder disorder is the growth of a cancerous tumor. Only about 3,000 to 4,000 people in the United States develop cancer of the gall bladder each year, a tiny fraction of the millions of Americans with gallstones. But chronic inflammation of the gall bladder or a gallstone more than 1 inch (2.5 centimeters) in diameter may increase the risk of developing gall bladder cancer.

Diagnosing the problem

The most common signs of gall bladder disease are pain and tenderness in the upper right quarter of the abdomen. The pain may extend to the ribcage and the shoulder. Some patients also experience fever, nausea, and vomiting. Occasionally, a yellowish discoloration of the skin, called *jaundice,* develops from a blockage of the duct leading into the intestine, which causes bilirubin to build up in the body.

Tipped off by these clues, a physician normally orders an examination by *ultrasound*—sound waves with a frequency too high for human hearing. In the examination, a technician runs a wand, which emits a beam of ultrasound, over the patient's abdomen. As the sound waves encounter tissues inside the abdomen, they are reflected back to the wand at intensities that vary with the density and depth

Gall bladder surgery: the traditional way

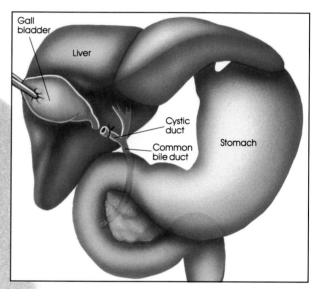

Gall bladder

Liver

Cystic duct

Common bile duct

Stomach

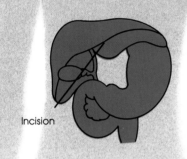

Incision

Traditional gall bladder surgery requires an incision 6 to 8 inches (15 to 20 centimeters) long through the abdominal wall. Working through the incision, the surgeon seals off the duct and blood vessels leading to and from the gall bladder. The gall bladder is then cut free and removed. Recovery following the surgery takes four to five weeks.

of the tissue. A computer connected to the wand uses the information from these echoes to form a visual image called a *sonogram*. The gall bladder, like other internal organs, appears in outline on the sonogram, and gallstones typically show up as small spots inside it.

But ultrasound does not work for everyone. If the patient is somewhat overweight, for example, the image will be blurred because the reflected sound waves must pass through extra layers of fat. The sonogram might also be unclear if the stones are very tiny or if they form a kind of sludge that does not reflect the ultrasound beam.

Without a definitive diagnosis from ultrasound, physicians may fall back on an X-ray examination called an *oral cholecystogram*. The patient usually goes on a fat-free diet a day or two before the exam. The night before, the patient takes pills containing an iodine compound. If the gall bladder is functioning normally, the iodine will concentrate inside it. Iodine blocks X rays, causing the gall bladder to show up as a dense area in X-ray images of the abdomen. The stones, which do not absorb the iodine, appear as spots inside the gall bladder.

After a technician takes an X ray, the patient eats a snack, which should cause the gall bladder to contract and empty. About 15 minutes later, a second X ray is made. If the gall bladder appears less dense in this X ray, it has gotten rid of most of the iodine and is functioning normally.

But the gall bladder may not take up the iodine and so will not show up well in the first X ray. This can happen if the gall bladder is inflamed or if a gallstone blocks the duct leading from the liver. The pills sometimes cause diarrhea, which prevents the iodine from being absorbed by the body and reaching the liver. Intestinal disorders that impair digestion can have the same effect. If an X ray does not show the gall bladder clearly, the physician turns to a procedure called a *nuclear scan*.

Before the scan, a technician injects a compound containing a tiny amount of radioactive material directly into the patient's vein. An X-ray machine or similar scanning device picks up the radiation emitted by the radioactive chemicals as they travel through the body. By tracing this movement in images made over a two-hour period, the scanning machine measures how well the gall bladder is working. If the gall bladder is diseased, the radioactive material bypasses it and moves directly through the ducts from the liver to the intestines.

Treatment options

Once gall bladder disease is diagnosed, patients have three options. They can decide to live with the condition. They can choose treatment with drugs that dissolve the stones or with machines that crush them. Or they can have the gall bladder surgically removed.

The first option is usually considered only for patients whose gallstones have caused little or no pain. In an effort to control symptoms, some physicians advise their patients to eat smaller amounts at meals, eat at regular intervals, and limit their consumption of fats. Other physicians question how much these measures actually help.

For many people, however, recurrent pain makes living with their gallstones an unrealistic option. Studies have shown that from 2 to 6 per cent of people whose gallstones have not yet caused problems will experience moderate to severe symptoms within one year. Over five years, that number will grow to between 7 and 27 per cent, according to varying estimates derived from follow-up studies.

Dissolution or destruction of the gallstones represents an alternative for individuals who cannot undergo surgery or do not wish to. The drawback to nonsurgical therapies is that they can be used only on small gallstones formed of cholesterol. Moreover, they may not eliminate the problem: Gallstones frequently recur and require further treatment.

Dissolving gallstones

Nearly two decades ago, Mayo Clinic researchers in Rochester, Minn., reported that *chenodiol* (a cholesterol-dissolving acid that occurs naturally in bile) could dissolve gallstones when administered for several months. But in 1981, a follow-up study at several large U.S. medical centers showed that only 13 per cent of the patients treated with the bile acid were completely free of gallstones after 24 months. Because of the low success rate, this bile acid therapy fell into disfavor.

Researchers have also experimented with a drug called *methyl tertiary-butyl ether* to dissolve gallstones. To inject the drug, the physician inserts a *catheter* (thin tube) through an incision in the wall of the abdomen and into the gall bladder. Within hours after injection, the ether dissolves the gallstones, and the stones and the ether can be drawn out through the catheter. The procedure is fairly risky, however, because the ether can be *toxic* (poisonous) if it accidentally passes from the gall bladder into the intestine. For this reason, the procedure is currently performed only by experienced physicians at a few medical centers.

Smashing gallstones

A technique called *lithotripsy* attracted much excitement in the late 1980's by offering the possibility of a safe and effective alternative to gall bladder surgery. The goal of lithotripsy is to smash the gallstones into fragments that are small enough to pass out of the gall bladder without causing discomfort.

During lithotripsy, a machine called a *lithotripter* generates a series of *shock waves*—sudden, sharp pulses of pressure. With the aid of ultrasound images, these brief bursts of pressure can be focused on the gallstones, thereby shattering them. In early trials, patients sat in a water bath, which transmitted the shock waves generated by the lithotripter to the gall bladder. Newer machines transmit the shock waves through a water-filled cushion placed over the abdomen while the patient lies on a padded table. Before the treatment, patients are given a *sedative*, a drug that relaxes them.

Lithotripsy has proved very successful in breaking up stones that form in the kidney. In 1986, researchers at the University of Munich in Germany reported that lithotripsy could also successfully destroy gallstones. Two years later, the researchers reported that they had fragmented stones in 78 per cent of those treated by lithotripsy in combination with a stone-dissolving drug. But they considered fewer than 3 out of every 10 gallstone patients to be promising candidates for lithotripsy. The team excluded patients with more than three stones, obstructed ducts, and calcium-containing stones that had hardened.

In a major follow-up trial to evaluate lithotripsy, 600 patients with no more than three small gallstones were treated at 10 U.S.

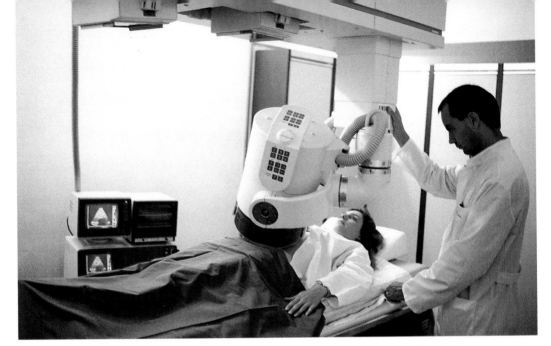

Shock-wave treatment

In a procedure called *lithotripsy*, shock waves are used to shatter gallstones into fragments small enough to pass from the gall bladder. Guided by an ultrasound image, a physician positions the machine that produces the shock waves, *above*. Lithotripsy is used only on an experimental basis in treating gallstones in the United States.

medical centers. Some of the patients also received a gallstone-dissolving drug called *ursodiol*. The only significant side effect the physicians observed from the drug was diarrhea, and it was not a major problem.

But the researchers reported in November 1990 that gallstones were still present in many of the patients. After six months, only 21 per cent of the patients treated by lithotripsy and ursodiol, and 9 per cent of those treated by lithotripsy alone, were free of gallstones. People with only one gallstone fared somewhat better, though stones recurred in a majority of these patients as well.

Noting the high recurrence rate among lithotripsy patients—and the cost of the ursodiol pills ($4 to $6 per day)—surgeon Lawrence W. Way of the University of California at San Francisco questioned the value of the therapy. "The patient treated by lithotripsy and dissolution essentially remains a patient for life," Way wrote in an editorial in the *New England Journal of Medicine*. He concluded that patients who wish to be cured of their symptoms and get on with their life would find the treatment undesirable.

A few physicians have experimented with another method of destroying gallstones, *percutaneous cholecystolithotomy*. In this procedure, the surgeon inserts a catheter through the abdomen and into the gall bladder and then threads a device—a flexible tube with a cutting device that looks like a miniature kitchen blender—through the catheter. When activated, the device draws in the stones and chips them into tiny pieces that can be suctioned out through the catheter. This experimental procedure, like lithotripsy, leaves the gall bladder in place, providing the opportunity for more stones to form.

Surgical removal: the traditional way

The majority of gall bladder patients thus choose surgery as the most effective way of ending their gallstone problem. Traditional gall bladder surgery, known as *cholecystectomy*, begins with a vertical incision 6 to 8 inches (15 to 20 centimeters) long on the right side of the abdomen. Working through the incision, the surgeon seals off the duct that leads from the gall bladder as well as the artery and vein that circulate blood through it. The gall bladder can then be cut free and removed. Before stitching up the incision, the surgeon usually checks the duct leading to the intestine to make sure no gallstones are lodged there. Cholecystectomy can take as little as 45 minutes, but the average time is about one hour.

Despite the short time it takes, gall bladder surgery is a serious operation that requires the surgeon to cut through muscles and nerves in the abdominal wall. Recuperation in the hospital typically takes four to six days and recovery at home another three or four weeks. Many patients suffer significant discomfort in the first few days following the surgery.

Surprisingly, the human body works almost as well without the gall bladder as with it. With the gall bladder gone, bile flows through a duct directly from the liver to the intestine, which receives a continuous trickle of bile rather than a periodic spurt. For this reason, the intestine sometimes contains more bile than it needs for digestion. At other times, it has so little bile that some fats pass through undigested. In the first weeks after the surgery, this imbalance often leads to diarrhea, which usually disappears as the body adjusts. *Flatulence* (excessive gas in the intestines) is also common after gall bladder surgery, but it too subsides with time. Most patients return to their normal diets soon after the surgery, though some physicians put their patients on a low-fat diet for a while.

Removal of the gall bladder does not always end the gallstone problem, however. In fewer than 5 per cent of patients, a gallstone forms in the ducts that have been left behind to transport bile. Such patients usually undergo surgery once again to remove the offending stone.

Surgical removal: a new way

The new bellybutton gall bladder surgery, performed in the United States since the late 1980's, sharply reduces the pain and the recuperation time of traditional surgery. The procedure, known medically as *laparoscopic cholecystectomy*, is made possible by a periscopelike instrument called a *laparoscope*, which enables surgeons to view the inside of the abdomen and perform surgery through only four tiny incisions.

After the patient is anesthetized, the surgeon makes a half-inch (1.25-centimeters) cut in the navel and three more small

A new operation for gall bladder removal

Laparoscopic surgery, introduced in the United States in 1988, spares patients most of the pain and recovery time of traditional surgery. The procedure involves pulling the gall bladder out through a tiny incision in the navel. Patients are typically hospitalized overnight and can return to work in a few days.

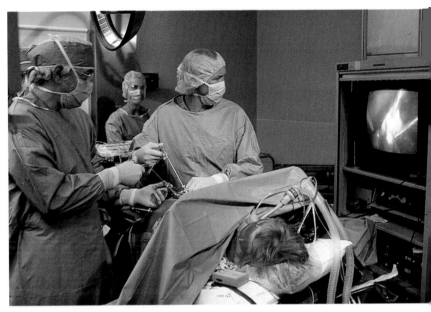

While viewing the surgical area on a television screen, *right,* surgeons guide a *laparoscope* (a device equipped with a television camera) within the abdomen and use another instrument to push aside tissues near the gall bladder. To sever the gall bladder from the liver, the surgeons may use a light-amplifying device called a *laser, below.* Light-transmitting fibers, shown in green, transmit the laser light.

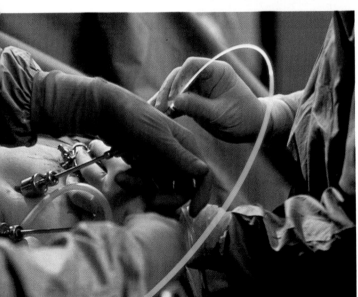

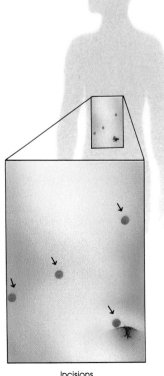

Laparoscopic surgery involves four tiny abdominal incisions, *right,* each about 0.5 inch (1.25 centimeters) long, eliminating the need for a long incision through the abdominal wall. Through the incisions, the surgeons insert miniaturized instruments and the laparoscope.

Incisions

slits above the navel on the right side of the abdomen. These incisions are made with sharp-edged, hollow tubes called *trocars*. Through the trocar in the navel, an assisting surgeon inserts the laparoscope, a flexible tube with a tiny television camera at the end that goes into the abdomen. Light-transmitting strands called *optical fibers* run through the tube, linking the camera to a light source and a television screen in the operating room. The optical fibers carry light into the area near the TV camera and transmit the camera's view of the abdomen to the screen.

The operating surgeon inserts miniaturized surgical instruments through two of the abdominal openings and guides the instruments to the gall bladder by watching the TV screen. Carbon dioxide gas injected into the fourth opening inflates the abdominal cavity, giving the surgeons more room to work.

The basic procedure is similar to a conventional gall bladder removal. The surgeon manipulates the miniature instruments to seal off the duct and blood vessels leading to and from the gall bladder. Then, grasping the gall bladder, the doctor uses either a *laser* (light-amplifying device) or an electric current to sever it from the main bile duct. To make it easier to slide the gall bladder out of the body, the surgeon may drain most of the bile from it and cut up the larger stones with a scissorlike instrument. Finally, the surgeons use suction to draw the gall bladder through the tube in the navel, and they close the small incisions with a few stitches. The entire procedure can be performed in an hour, but more commonly it takes 75 to 90 minutes.

Laparoscopic cholecystectomy was invented in France in 1988 and has since been popularized in the United States by surgeons Eddie Joe Reddick and Douglas O. Olsen of West Side Hospital in Nashville, Tenn. Several hundred thousand people throughout the United States have already had their gall bladders removed by this revolutionary technique, and more and more surgeons are adopting it.

Pros and cons of "bellybutton surgery"

The major advantage of laparoscopic surgery is that it eliminates the need to cut through the abdominal muscles, substantially reducing postoperative pain and recovery time. The surgery is occasionally done on an outpatient basis, but usually the patient stays in the hospital overnight. Most patients can return to work in four to six days.

Laparoscopic cholecystectomy is not without risk, however. According to Reddick, at least 15 of the first 10,000 patients suffered major complications from the procedure. Although this is a small number, fewer patients suffer complications from conventional surgery. The greatest risk is that the surgeons will puncture blood vessels or the intestines while making the incisions or that they will damage tissue while working in the tightly packed area near the gall bladder. One patient died after a trocar punctured a major artery. But physicians note that any new procedure is riskiest while physicians are perfecting it.

A panel of experts reported in March 1991 that surgeons who perform the new technique should be thoroughly trained to meet strict qualifying guidelines. Thus, in considering laparoscopic cholecystectomy, it's important to look for a surgeon who has experience with the procedure.

When traditional surgery must be used

Laparoscopic surgery cannot be used on everyone. If the patient is substantially overweight, for example, the instruments will not reach the internal organs and the physicians will not have sufficient room to work. Scar tissue and *adhesions* (joined tissues) from previous surgery also interfere with the operation. In addition, surgeons do not like to perform the operation if the gall bladder is severely inflamed or if the nearby pancreas or kidney have also become inflamed.

In 5 to 10 per cent of cases, surgeons begin the laparoscopy and find that they cannot finish it. In my case, the surgeon found my gall bladder too tightly attached to my liver to be safely removed with the laparoscopic procedure's miniature instruments. Loops of intestine also were in the way. As a result, the surgeon had to make a larger incision and remove my gall bladder the conventional way. Nevertheless, I was back at work five weeks after the operation, troubled no longer by indigestion and mysterious pain.

Although surgery remains the most effective method of permanently eliminating the symptoms of gall bladder disease, researchers continue to look for ways to improve such nonsurgical options as drugs and lithotripsy for patients who cannot undergo an operation. And many experts predict that someday, most patients who can tolerate surgery will benefit from the substantially reduced pain and recovery time of the new laparoscopic operation. For the million Americans who develop gall bladder disease each year, that is welcome news indeed.

For further reading:

Lewis, Ricki. "The Gallbladder: An Organ You Can Live Without." *FDA Consumer*, May 1991.

"About Cholecystectomy," a booklet explaining traditional gall bladder surgery, is available from the American College of Surgeons, 55 E. Erie Street, Chicago, IL 60611.

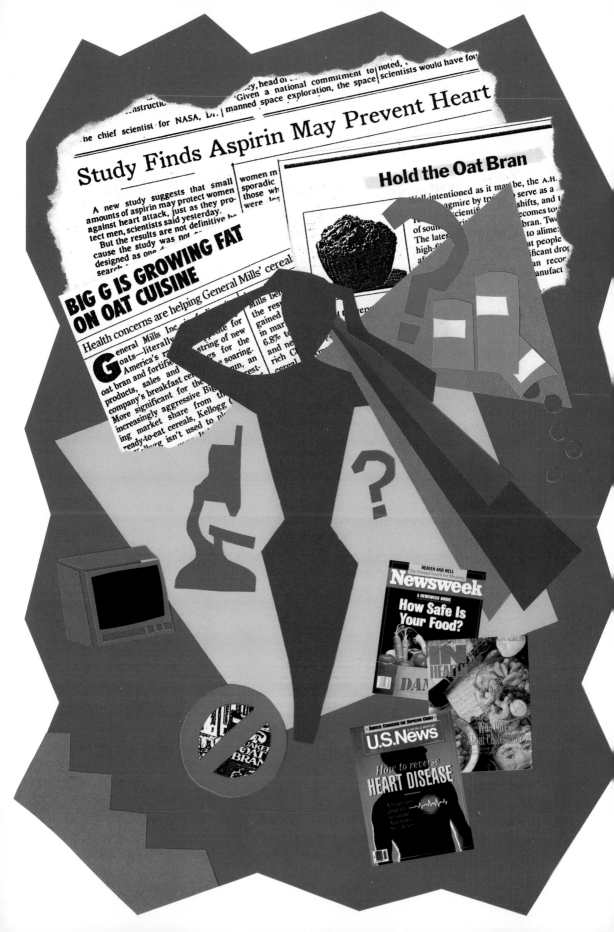

Seemingly contradictory reports about the findings of medical studies make it difficult to know what is good or bad for your health. Here are some tips on how to read between the lines and become a critical consumer of medical news.

Healthy Skepticism

By Patricia Thomas

Consider these headlines:

"Scientists see a link between alcoholism and a specific gene" (*The New York Times*, April 18, 1990)

"Researchers cannot confirm a genetic link to alcoholism" (*The New York Times*, Dec. 26, 1990)

No wonder news stories on medical research leave many people confused. Does a report on a new test for cancer mean you should rush to the doctor? Should a headline about cholesterol in eggs cause you to swear off omelets forever?

In most cases there's no reason to panic. But that can be hard to figure out if you don't understand just what medical studies prove—or don't prove.

As a reporter and editor specializing in medicine, I size up thousands of medical studies every year. My colleagues and I hear scientists talk about their work at conferences, and we read their reports in medical journals. When we think a study might interest our readers and viewers, we try to explain its significance in an article or a broadcast. Sometimes the explanation can get complicated. Or, perhaps worse, it can get too simple.

The author:

Patricia Thomas is editor of the *Harvard Health Letter.*

So how can a reader or listener know what to believe about medical reports and what to do in response? The best way is to learn a little about how scientific research is done. By knowing the key points to look for and how to weigh their effects, you will have a better idea of what a study's findings mean to you.

We can all understand the basic questions that underlie medical research—questions that range from "What causes disease, and how can we cure it?" to "Why do we age?" or "How does life begin?" The questions that scientists address in individual studies, however, are far more specific. A researcher might carry out a study to find out, for instance, how a new drug affects the level of a specific blood chemical in people with a particular medical condition.

The result of such a study, by itself, might not be of much use to most patients and their doctors. But taken in the context of many other studies, it could contribute to scientists' understanding of how the body works.

In other words, all medical studies—the few we hear about in the news as well as the thousands of others done every year—are pieces of an enormous puzzle scientists are trying to assemble. Sometimes enough pieces fit together to allow researchers to see part of the picture. That's when their work is most likely to become news.

That's also when confusion tends to arise. When reporters talk to scientists or read their reports, they may miss some details. Sometimes a scientist, accustomed to working with other specialists, forgets that reporters do not necessarily make the same assumptions in interpreting a study. Sometimes a reporter fails to recognize some small but crucial element that limits the significance of a study's results.

Misunderstandings also occur when the media present news to the public. A news report might not have the time or space to explain a study sufficiently. Or the reader or viewer might not understand the meaning of some point, reaching conclusions that the journalist—and the scientists—never intended.

It isn't that scientists or journalists want to make mistakes or mislead anyone. It is just that there is ample room for ambiguity in both science and journalism. And because scientists, journalists, and the public all speak different languages, it's easy to lose something in the translation.

To make sense of a scientific study, you need to know that all studies conform to a generally accepted format that guides how the study is set up, carried out, and reported. Analyzing a study without knowing this format is like watching a football game without knowing the rules. Medical studies, in particular, come in two forms—epidemiologic and experimental studies.

Epidemiologic studies determine where and how often a par-

A look at risk factors

Some scientists specialize in calculating the likelihood that particular groups of people will develop—and possibly die from—one disease or another. They speak of this likelihood as risk. A risk factor is a behavior or exposure that is statistically likely to contribute to disease.

Based on research, scientists can say, for example, that men aged 45 to 64 have more than three times the risk for heart attack than do women of the same age. They can also note that while the risk for developing Alzheimer's disease is extremely small in middle age, it rises to about 1-in-20 after age 65. And they can state confidently that the risk for sickle cell anemia exists almost exclusively among blacks.

These types of risk—based on sex, age, or race—are beyond our control. But we do have the power to reduce other risks. More than 40 years of research has established that cigarette smoking increases the risk of having a heart attack or stroke and for developing lung cancer or emphysema. Clearly we can lower our risk for those diseases by not smoking.

Similarly, scientists have shown that obesity increases the risk of such health problems as heart disease, diabetes, gallstones, and back pain. We have at least some control over our weight—and thus our risk.

Some risks should be taken more seriously than others. Suppose you read "Eating five bananas a week doubles risk for cancer death." Before swearing off bananas, you should certainly check with an authoritative source such as the American Cancer Society (ACS).

You may also be able to put the claim in perspective by looking critically at the study that produced it. Suppose this fictional study focused on cancer of the larynx. According to the ACS, the risk of dying from cancer of the larynx is 2.6 per 100,000 for men and less than 1 per 100,000 for women. In other words, this cancer is so rare that even if bananas did double your risk, the overall threat would still be almost nonexistent.

On the other hand, if solid evidence surfaced that eating five bananas a week doubled the risk of dying from breast cancer, which claims 10 times as many lives as cancer of the larynx, the increase would indeed be sizable. If that were the case, then banana lovers might want to rethink their eating habits.

Of course, rarely should you change your behavior on the basis of a single study. It's generally wise to wait until subsequent research bears the claim out—especially if the finding sounds as preposterous as this one!   [P. T.]

A calculated risk

If a new study says that a certain behavior in combination with other factors doubles or triples a health risk, should you alter that behavior? That depends on how great the initial risk is.

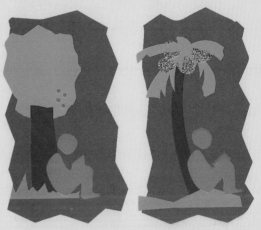

In considering the possibility of personal injury, most people would regard sitting under a cherry tree as being a very low risk behavior —even in the unlikely event that a soft, little cherry falls and strikes the sitter. On the other hand, the risk of injury is much greater for a person sitting under a coconut tree in the event that a coconut might fall and strike the sitter. Being clobbered by a big, hard coconut could cause serious bodily harm.

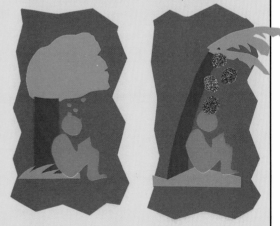

If a stiff wind starts to blow, this increases the likelihood that fruit might fall from a tree. The person sitting under the cherry tree is still in little danger, because the initial risk (getting hurt by a cherry) was negligible. In contrast, the person under the coconut tree is in much greater danger of suffering injury, because the initial risk (getting hurt by a coconut) was fairly high.

ticular medical condition occurs in a population. Epidemiologists might analyze data from hospitals, government agencies, or other standard sources, or they might gather new data themselves. This allows them to document a problem's extent, compare it with other medical conditions, and identify risk factors and trends.

For example, since 1973, the National Cancer Institute (NCI) in Bethesda, Md., has been tracking cancer cases and deaths in 11 metropolitan areas. From these data, NCI researchers can estimate cancer rates nationwide with a high degree of certainty. They can also compare data on different types of cancer and monitor rates of survival and cure.

Results of such studies often influence public policy. For example, epidemiologic studies found that lung cancer rates are much higher among smokers. This along with other findings about health hazards of cigarette smoke has led to laws banning smoking in many public places and requiring health warnings on cigarette packs and advertisements. Similarly, governments at all levels rely on epidemiologic studies for guidance when deciding how to allocate limited funds for health services.

Experimental studies are those in which scientists apply a test, administer a treatment, or take some other specific action in order to measure that action's effects. In medical research, the procedure generally involves a carefully chosen group of cells, animals, or people. For instance, researchers studying a disease-causing bacterium might see what happens when they expose it to various substances in test tubes. And sometimes the only way to learn how an important human disease can be treated is to test drugs first in animals who have the disease.

More elaborate experimental studies, called *clinical trials*, use groups of human volunteers. Clinical trials let researchers see how specific procedures or treatments actually work in people. Findings from clinical trials help doctors decide what drugs, tests, and therapies to give to their patients. Such studies are also used in the drug-approval process; the United States Food and Drug Administration, the government agency that monitors drug safety and effectiveness, approves only medications that have been tested in elaborate clinical trials.

When scientists plan a study, they make many choices, such as the number of volunteers to include in a clinical trial and how many days, months, or years the study will last. Such choices influence not only how the study is done but how the results can be applied. For example, to date, studies have found no link between use of birth control pills and an increased risk of breast cancer—but experts point out that those studies cannot tell us whether the pill raises the lifetime breast cancer risk for women. Because breast cancer is most likely to occur after *menopause*

Safety in (large) numbers

In general, the greater the number of subjects in a study, the more comprehensive the results. A larger sample acts as a magnifying glass. Even relatively uncommon events (such as inheriting a gene for red hair or having an unusual side effect from a drug) are more likely to show up in a large sample than a small one.

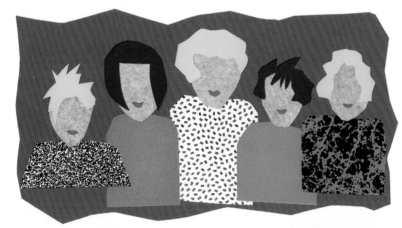

If scientists were studying hair color in women, for example, a small sample size of just a few women might lead them to conclude that all women are blondes or brunettes. This is, of course, not true.

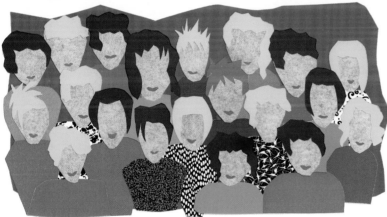

If the scientists did the same study with a larger sample size, they would discover that, in addition to the women with blond or brunette hair, a few women have red hair.

(the time of life when menstruation ceases), and the earliest users of the pill are only now reaching this stage of life, epidemiologic studies will not be able to prove or disprove this relationship for another 10 years.

Studies that look at very specific problems in limited circumstances might be able to provide information quickly and accurately. In turn, however, there's no guarantee that this information will apply under any conditions other than the particular ones used in the studies. These limitations do not mean that a study is bad. But it does mean that it may be useful only to other researchers. Although studies of this sort rarely make the news, they are often essential in guiding later, larger studies.

Limitations are not the same as errors. Like all of us, scientists sometimes make mistakes. If a researcher bases a study on a misconception or gathers data improperly, the study's findings

Who is in the study?

The makeup of a sample (the people being studied) is an important consideration in medical research. A sample that has only subjects who have specific characteristics, such as white, middle-class men with sedentary jobs, may reveal details about how a certain habit affects health in people with those same traits. If researchers want to see if such results apply to the population as a whole, they need to do studies using samples that represent a spectrum—such as men and women of different races, ages, and backgrounds.

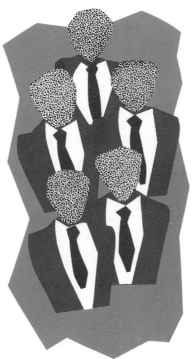

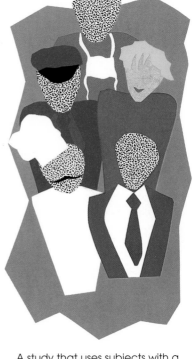

A study that uses subjects who share common traits—such as white, middle-aged men with sedentary office jobs—can reveal information that applies to other people with those same traits. But that information may not be valid for the population as a whole.

A study that uses subjects with a range of characteristics may reveal information that can be generalized to the population as a whole. But such a varied sample would be less useful for studying a condition that only affects certain types of people.

will be useless. But even well-designed and well-conducted studies involve some uncertainty. Uncertainty is impossible to eliminate in medical research, partly because living organisms are such complicated and varied entities. The "best" studies, then, are those that keep uncertainty to a minimum. Six elements of a study's design play particularly important roles in determining just how accurate and applicable a study is:

Sample size. A study sample is the group of people, animals, cell cultures, or other subjects that are analyzed or acted upon. The sample must be large enough that various responses will show up in measurable proportions. If the sample is too small, there's no way of knowing if an unusual finding is a true (if rare) effect or simply an unrelated coincidence.

Statisticians use formulas to calculate the number of subjects needed to achieve a valid conclusion. In general, the larger the sample, the more valid and reliable the results. A large sample acts as a magnifying glass. Because even small differences will appear in a larger quantity, they are easier to see. This is particularly important in testing new drugs, because unusual side effects are more likely to turn up in a large sample.

Sample composition. The nature of the subjects in a sample determines how broadly any findings might be applied. Researchers who want to apply their findings to many kinds of people strive for a sample that represents a highly varied population. For example, to study a disease that affects many Americans, a researcher would ideally choose a sample that included men and women of many races and ages, in proportions reflecting the U.S. population. Of course, such a sample would also have to be very large to be useful.

On the other hand, in looking at a disease that occurs in highly limited circumstances, a researcher might deliberately choose subjects of the type most likely to be affected—for example, diabetic women of childbearing age. The findings, in turn, would only apply to people of this type.

Controls. A control group is a second sample used for comparison purposes. Researchers do not give this group the experimental procedure or drug. Instead, they usually give controls a *placebo*—an inactive substance (such as a sugar pill) or a "pretend" procedure that resembles the treatment under study. The aim of having a control group is to see what happens to subjects who don't receive the treatment. Without controls, it would be impossible to tell whether a response is due to the drug or procedure or whether it would have happened anyway. Studies that are well designed ensure that the control and experimental groups are as much alike as possible.

Duration. Some research questions can be answered in days, others take years. This difference is especially important in cancer research, when scientists want to know whether a certain factor, such as exposure to radiation or industrial chemicals, increases long-term risk for cancer. Cancer biologists now think that many cancers occur as a result of a process that takes 20 or 30 years or more. If researchers follow people exposed to a toxic chemical for only five years, they could mistakenly conclude that the substance is harmless.

Bias. This term refers to any irrelevant factor that can lead to inaccurate results—especially someone's conscious or unconscious expectations of what the study will prove. Careful researchers use several strategies to minimize the chance of bias affecting their work.

For instance, in a clinical trial testing a new drug, patients must be randomly assigned to the experimental group or the control group. If the researchers do not use an impartial method, such as a coin toss, to determine who gets the drug, it's possible that the researchers—intentionally or unintentionally—may give the drug to the patients they think will do best.

Similarly, because patients' expectations can influence their physical and emotional reactions, the subjects should not know who is receiving the drug. For this purpose, researchers give the control group members a placebo that looks like the real drug. This arrangement ensures that any difference in the groups' responses is due to the drug itself, not the patients' assumptions about what the drug might do.

In addition, the patients must be assessed by researchers who don't know which patients received the drug. Otherwise, if the doctors believe that the drug is effective, they might look more closely for changes in those who are getting it. When neither patients nor doctors know who is getting the drug or the placebo, the study is said to be double-blinded.

Measurement. Because most studies focus on identifying differences, they must have accurate means of measurement. Asking people if a treatment caused them to feel less pain is a fuzzy way to measure change. A more precise way might be to measure levels of certain pain-associated substances in the blood before and after treatment.

Of course, one must know how valid and reliable the laboratory test is. A valid test is one with a nearly 100 per cent chance of correctly identifying a condition in people who actually have it, and an equally high chance of ruling out that condition in those without it. A reliable test is one that produces the same results for the same conditions even if the test is done by another technician at another time or place—a situation that often arises in large clinical trials involving patients at several locations.

After researchers collect and summarize the data from a study, they must decide what it all means. Scientists agree that interpreting results is a tricky business, even when they're writing for other scientists who have the same background. When reporters get into the act, they must translate the research findings into language the public can understand. That second layer of interpretation further complicates matters.

Nevertheless, it's still possible for nonscientists to sense when someone has leaped to an unjustified conclusion. Here are a few questions to ask when you read or hear about a new study:

How strong are the claims? Words like "breakthrough" or "cure" should arouse skepticism. As *Washington Post* science writer Victor Cohn notes, "breakthroughs" occur mainly in headlines. Careful editors and reporters won't make these leaps, but not everyone involved in the media understands that medical news rarely provides definitive answers.

Be cautious, too, about claims that one study "proves" something. Scientific truths are the sum of dozens of studies; they rarely burst on the scene in a single report. Also, any finding is subject to corroboration by additional studies. Responsible journalists and scientists know that today's best guesses may change with tomorrow's new research.

Who sponsored the research? Reporters may misjudge the significance of new research after interviewing someone with a hidden agenda. For example, the importance of a finding may be exaggerated by a corporation hoping to turn the discovery into a high-profit drug or medical device. Similarly, a researcher who is paid by an organization to do a study may feel pressured to produce results that will support the organization. To help identify possible bias, many research institutions and medical journals ask researchers to reveal their sources of funding and any personal involvements (such as investments or consulting work) that may relate to their research topic.

How broadly can the findings be generalized? The conclusions drawn from data on one sample do not necessarily apply to the larger population. Caught up in the excitement of new in-

The importance of a control group

When researchers design a study to test a new treatment, they usually include at least two comparable groups: an *experimental group* (which is given the treatment) and a *control group* (to provide a standard for comparison). The only difference between the groups is the factor being tested.

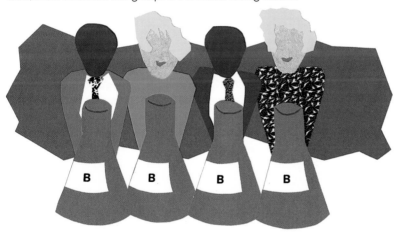

Subjects in the experimental group receive the treatment that researchers want to learn more about—a pill or liquid containing a new drug for high blood pressure, for example.

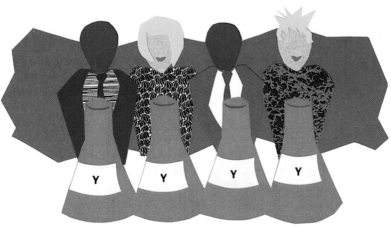

A similar group of people, the control group, receives a *placebo* (a pill or liquid that does not contain the new blood pressure drug—or a solution containing the conventional drug for high blood pressure). By comparing the results of the two groups, researchers can gauge the effectiveness of the new drug.

sights, researchers may fail to make clear—or reporters may fail to recognize—that they don't know whether a treatment works for people who differ from the study population in sex, age, race, or other characteristics.

In the late 1980's, for example, some scientists, legislators, and citizens began to question whether results obtained by studying men can legitimately be applied to women. In particular, these people noted, studies of heart disease have typically focused on men or male animals. But the few studies that have looked at women suggest that women respond differently to both the disease and to standard treatments—and thus might require different medical approaches. Similar questions have emerged about some medications, originally tested on whites, that have since been shown to have stronger or weaker effects in blacks, Hispanics, or Asians.

Is the conclusion logical? When a study links an action and a result, it's easy to assume one causes the other. For example, news reports highlighted a 1990 study showing that children who watch more than two hours of television daily have higher levels of cholesterol in their blood than children who watch less. Does this mean that TV watching raises cholesterol?

Of course not—and the researchers, from the University of California at Irvine, made that clear. They proposed a different explanation: that cholesterol levels are higher among TV watchers because these young "couch potatoes" exercise less and eat more high-calorie snacks than their peers. Diet and exercise have a well-established connection to cholesterol levels.

Similarly, studies published early in the 1980's found that people who ate large quantities of oat bran also showed a drop in levels of harmful cholesterol in their blood. These results gave rise to the widespread conviction that the particular kind of dietary fiber found in oat bran caused the improvement—and the grain turned up in everything from bagels to beer.

In January 1990, this belief in oat bran's powers was shaken by a small study that put 20 healthy volunteers on diets high in either oat bran or low-fiber refined wheat products. Both diets lowered blood cholesterol levels by roughly the same amount, and neither did so by very much, according to researchers at Brigham and Women's Hospital in Boston.

The researchers acknowledged criticism that the study sample was small and consisted of people whose cholesterol was at normal levels to start with. But they also suggested a common-sense explanation for both the earlier oat-bran findings and the later ones: People who fill up on complex carbohydrates—of which oat bran is only one example—simply won't have as much room for unhealthy fat- and cholesterol-laden foods. Still, as with so many medical issues, only additional research will

What is a blinded study?

Many experiments that test new treatments are *blinded*, which means that neither the subjects nor the researchers knows which group receives the treatment and which one does not. This feature helps prevent unconscious expectations of the researchers or the patients from influencing the results. For example, patients might feel better just knowing they are receiving an experimental treatment.

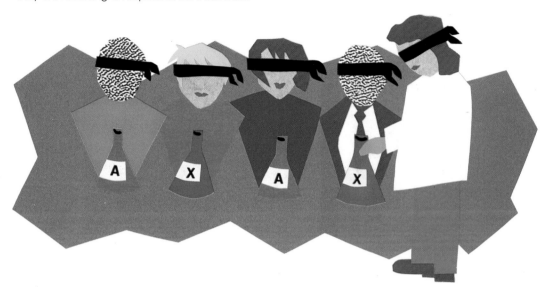

When researchers test a new drug, for example, neither the physicians who administer the drug nor the people participating in the study know which subjects are receiving the new drug and which subjects are receiving the placebo or an established drug. Typically, the drugs are dispensed to the subjects in coded containers.

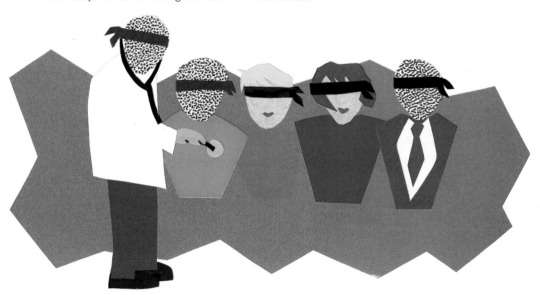

In a well-designed study, the researchers who evaluate the subjects' condition before and after treatment are also "blinded"—that is, they do not know which patients received the new drug and which ones were given a placebo. After such evaluations are complete, the researchers decode the samples and analyze their findings.

clarify the question of oat bran's role in lowering cholesterol.

Taking all these factors into account, let's look at the stories behind the two conflicting headlines that appear at the beginning of this article. How could these studies have achieved such different results?

Both of the newspaper articles referred to studies published in *The Journal of the American Medical Association* (*JAMA*). In the first study, researchers at the University of California in Los Angeles and the University of Texas Health Science Center in San Antonio reported that people with a specific gene were more likely to develop severe alcoholism than were other people. They estimated that within five years, doctors would be able to use a test for this gene to identify potential alcoholics.

The researchers identified their alcoholism gene by testing brain tissue from 35 people who had died of various causes ascribed to alcoholism. They also tested the brains of 35 people whose relatives and medical records indicated they were not alcoholics. The person who performed the genetic tests did not know which brains belonged to which group.

The researchers looked for several genes that earlier studies had suggested might play a role in alcoholism. They found one of the genes in 69 per cent of the alcoholics' tissues and 20 per cent of the tissues from the control group.

The first question we should ask is, did the researchers test enough brains? For a study trying to pin down causes of such a complicated disease as alcoholism, this would be considered a small sample in statistical terms. It might not be reasonable to examine 70 brains and draw conclusions about the entire U.S. population of 250 million people.

Did the sample reflect the population from which it was drawn? The researchers did include men and women, blacks and whites. But too few (10) of the 70 brains were from women, and too many (24) from blacks, to be representative of the national population. That doesn't automatically invalidate the findings, but it does reduce the confidence with which they can be generalized.

Was the control group appropriate? Medical records and family interviews may well have been the best sources available for confirming that the control group members were not alcoholics. But alcoholism is often denied by relatives and not officially noted by doctors. The possibility that the control group included some hidden alcoholics adds some uncertainty.

Did they use an appropriate test? This question is worth asking because genetic tests vary widely in their validity and reliability. As an editorial accompanying the published report in *JAMA* noted, the test used by these researchers is most often used to track the recurrence of a gene throughout a family—not to study unrelated individuals such as those in this study.

Given these and other issues, which were raised by scientists and nonscientists alike, the researchers' conclusions might have gone somewhat further than their data warranted. In addition, other alcoholism researchers noted that attributing so much influence to one gene challenged scientific common sense, based on earlier evidence about the ways alcoholism might be inherited. But the paper certainly raised valid questions. Obviously, the matter deserved additional study.

So scientists at the National Institute on Alcohol Abuse and Alcoholism in Bethesda, Md., used a different test to look for the suspected gene in blood samples from 40 alcoholic patients and 127 nonalcoholics. They also tested 14 members of two families with widespread alcoholism to see whether the gene showed up consistently in people with the problem.

This study had its own set of limitations. But it found no evidence that the proposed "gene for alcoholism" showed up any more frequently in alcoholics than in nonalcoholics.

Fortunately, it's rare to find two studies that flatly contradict each other. But unwarranted conclusions can be drawn from well-designed studies, and poorly conceived research can mislead scientists—and the rest of us. Still, by understanding where the conclusions come from, we can often distinguish the good, the bad, and the ambiguous.

We can also seek expert advice. Local chapters of national groups such as the American Heart Association or the American Cancer Society can often clarify new findings or suggest people or publications that can answer additional questions.

Meanwhile, most scientists and reporters alike would probably advise people not to start or stop taking a medication or change any significant health behavior on the strength of a news report about a medical study. Rather, an individual's own physician is in the best position to judge how relevant a new finding is to his or her health.

But doctors, just like everyone else, need time to think about what a new study means—so they may not have all the answers immediately after a newspaper or TV report. If the news sounds too good to be true, it probably is. But if it seems to make a logical contribution in the context of what is already known, then it may well be a small but important step in the continuing search for medical knowledge.

For further reading:
Cohn, Victor. *News and Numbers*. Iowa State University Press, 1989.

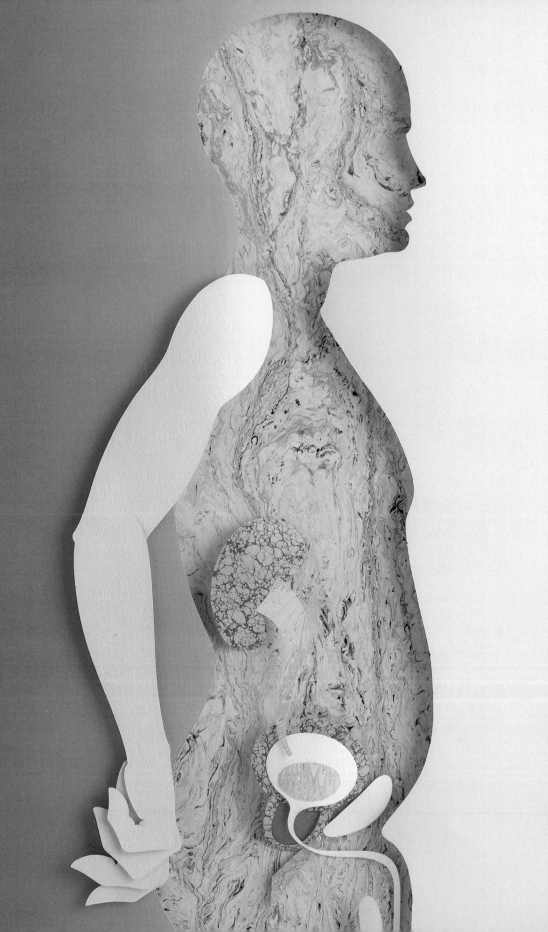

Prostate cancer kills about 32,000
men each year in the United States.
With early detection, many of those
lives could be saved.

Combating Prostate Cancer

By William H. Allen

An urgent need to urinate broke into John's sleep. Groggily, he shuffled to the bathroom for the third time that night. Even after urinating, his bladder did not feel completely empty—a puzzling occurrence he had noticed almost nightly of late.

For thousands of men each year, such a scenario is the first sign of a potentially serious health problem that requires a visit to the doctor—without delay. These symptoms most likely mean trouble with the *prostate*, a gland that only men have.

Determining the exact cause of such urinary problems usually requires the expertise of a *urologist* (a physician specializing in the urinary and genital organs). In most cases, the cause may be an infection or the gradual enlargement of the prostate that normally occurs with increasing age. But difficulty with urination may also indicate something much more serious: prostate cancer, the second leading cause of cancer deaths in American men. Prostate cancer need not mean death, however. As with many other cancers, early detection offers the best chance for a cure.

More than 120,000 cases of prostate cancer were reported in 1990. About 1 in every 11 American men will develop the disease during his lifetime, almost always in late middle or old age.

Benign prostatic hyperplasia, also called benign prostatic hypertrophy (BPH): Abnormal but noncancerous enlargement of the prostate.

Biopsy: The removal and examination of a sample of tissue for diagnosis.

Grade: A numerical rating of how abnormal and how aggressive prostate cancer cells are.

Prostate: A gland in males encircling the urethra, the tube that carries urine from the bladder.

Prostatectomy: The surgical removal of the prostate gland.

Prostatitis: Inflammation of the prostate gland, usually caused by infection.

Stage: A letter score indicating how much a patient's cancer has spread.

Transurethral resection of the prostate (TURP): Surgical removal of all or part of the prostate gland by an instrument inserted through the urethra.

Urologist: A physician specializing in the urinary and genital organs.

The author:

William H. Allen is a science writer for the *St. Louis Post-Dispatch.*

According to the American Cancer Society, prostate cancer kills 32,000 men a year in the United States. Most of these deaths could be prevented—if the cancer is detected and treated before it has a chance to spread. Physicians agree that a routine procedure, a digital rectal examination, is the best means of screening for prostate cancer, as well as cancer of the rectum. For this reason, the American Cancer Society recommends that all men over 40 have an annual rectal exam.

A troublesome gland

The prostate gland lies just below a man's bladder, encircling the *urethra*, the tube that carries urine from the bladder. At birth, the prostate is the size of a pea. It grows steadily until a man reaches his 20's, when it resembles a large walnut and weighs less than 1 ounce (28 grams). The prostate produces a milky, white fluid that forms part of *semen* (the liquid that transports sperm cells).

Despite the prostate's small size, the organ can be troublsome. It causes, according to urologist Stephen N. Rous of Dartmouth Medical School in Hanover, N.H., "more grief for more men than just about any other structure in the body." More than 1 million men develop some kind of prostate disorder each year. One common prostate problem is *prostatitis*, an inflammation of the prostate often caused by bacterial infection. In such cases, physicians usually prescribe antibiotics to cure the infection.

Another common disorder is *benign enlargement*, which usually begins as men pass into middle age. This is a noncancerous growth, but doctors may recommend surgery or other treatments if it causes troublesome symptoms. See BENIGN ENLARGED PROSTATE, page 78.

Prostate cancer

The most serious disorder that affects the prostate gland is cancer. Prostate cancer usually occurs in older men, with the vast majority of cases discovered in patients over the age of 50. The average age at which the disease is diagnosed is about 73. The incidence of prostate cancer rises with age more rapidly than any other cancer.

Before 1900, when life expectancy was much shorter—about 47 years compared with about 75 years today—prostate cancer was rare. But as the century progressed, medical science conquered many ailments, particularly many major infectious diseases. Life expectancy rose and so did the incidence of prostate cancer. In other words, men are now living long enough to develop prostate cancer.

Prostate cancer develops in such a way that it may go undetected for years. Unlike benign enlargement, which starts near

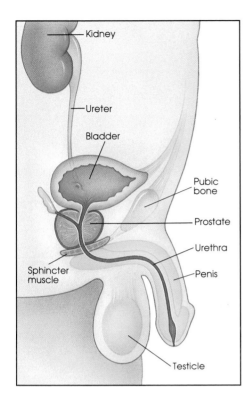

Major kinds of cancer affecting men in the United States		
Primary body site	New cases each year	Deaths each year
Prostate	122,000	32,000
Lung	101,000	92,000
Colon & rectum	79,000	30,000
Bladder	37,000	6,400
Lymph tissues	23,800	10,600

Source: American Cancer Society; 1991 estimates.

Prostate cancer is the most common type of malignancy affecting American men. It ranks second only to lung cancer as a cause of male cancer death in the United States.

The prostate gland, which only men have, lies just below the bladder, encircling the *urethra*, the tube that carries urine from the bladder through the penis. A normal prostate is about the size of a large walnut.

the center of the prostate gland, cancer of the prostate usually begins on the outer edge. The malignancy grows silently for many years, causing no symptoms or apparent complications. The cancer must move to the center of the gland before it puts enough pressure on the urethra to cause symptoms, mainly urinary difficulties.

Eventually, the cancer may spread beyond the prostate gland. The main route by which the disease spreads is through the *lymphatic system*. This network of vessels and tissue masses throughout the body plays an important role in the immune system. At this stage, the cancer may cause additional symptoms such as blood in the urine, pain in the lower back or pelvic region, weakness in the legs, weight loss, and fatigue.

Once the cancer has *metastasized* (spread to other parts of the body), there is little chance that the patient can be cured. For this reason, it is crucial to discover prostate cancer before it spreads.

The digital rectal exam

The most common method for diagnosing prostate cancer is the digital rectal examination, which is performed by a physician as part of a regular physical checkup, especially for older men. During a rectal exam, the doctor inserts a finger, covered with a

71

When to see a doctor

Any of the following symptoms may mean prostate trouble and require a visit to the doctor—without delay:

- Frequent or urgent need to urinate, especially at night.
- Discomfort or pain during urination.
- Inability to urinate, or difficulty beginning urination.
- A feeling that the bladder does not empty completely during urination.
- Pain in the pelvic or rectal area.
- A decrease in force or volume of the stream of urine.
- Inability to stop urinating without dribbling.
- Blood in the urine.

The rectal exam
A simple procedure called a digital rectal examination is the best means of detecting prostate cancer. During the procedure, a doctor inserts a finger, covered with a lubricated glove, into the rectum. With a fingertip, the doctor probes for bumps or hardened areas on the prostate, which may indicate cancer. The American Cancer Society recommends that all men over 40 have the exam annually.

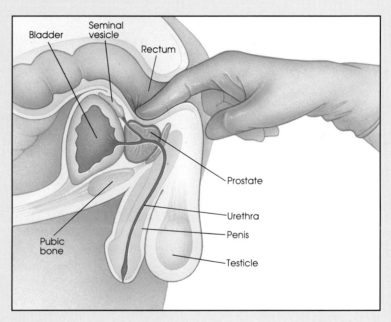

lubricated glove, into the rectum. With a fingertip, the physician searches for bumps or hard areas on the surface of the prostate, which may indicate a tumor. A normal prostate has a smooth surface and a uniformly soft consistency. Less than half of all abnormal growths or hardened areas discovered during rectal exams prove to be cancerous.

Many men dread rectal exams because they find the procedure embarrassing. According to one survey, only about a third of men over 50 get an annual rectal exam. But cancer experts stress that the exam is the best way of finding the disease before symptoms become apparent—when the chances for a cure are still good.

Other diagnostic methods

A digital rectal exam cannot find cancer if the tumor is growing deep within the prostate or in an area of the gland that lies out of reach. Although digital exams are still the standard method of detection, two other techniques also help in diagnosing prostate cancer. In one of these, known as *transrectal ultrasound,* a probe inserted into the rectum transmits high-frequency sound waves through the pelvic region and detects the echoes created as the sound waves encounter objects within the body—such as normal and cancerous tissue. A computer converts the echoes into images displayed on a video screen. Most urologists use transrectal ultrasound to locate small cancers within the prostate and to guide them in obtaining samples of tissue to examine for the presence of cancer.

Extremely promising as a means of screening for prostate cancer is a blood test that measures levels of a substance called *prostate-specific antigen* (PSA). Elevated levels of PSA in the blood may indicate an enlarged or infected prostate, and still higher levels of PSA may signal prostate cancer.

A study published in April 1991 indicated that the PSA test may be more accurate than rectal exams in detecting prostate cancer. Study director William J. Catalona, chief of urological surgery at Washington University School of Medicine in St. Louis, Mo., recommended that the blood test be made part of checkups for all men over age 50. Other doctors disagree, believing the blood test yields too many false readings to be suitable for screening.

Even doctors who question the accuracy of the PSA test at its present stage of development agree that a simple and effective blood test would save lives. They believe men will find a blood test more acceptable than a rectal exam, and therefore more men will get a regular prostate cancer screening. The end result could be a drastic reduction in the number of deaths due to the disease.

When cancer is suspected

If a rectal exam reveals suspicious growths or hard areas on the prostate, the physician will probably order a procedure called a *biopsy.* In a biopsy, a doctor removes a sample of tissue and examines the cells under a microscope to determine whether cancer is present.

In the most common biopsy procedure, a hollow needle is inserted along the rectum into contact with the prostate, where the needle cuts out a core of tissue. Most physicians perform the procedure on an outpatient basis. The patient receives an antibiotic to prevent infection by bacteria from the nearby rectum. The extremely thin biopsy needles now used cause so little discomfort that most patients do not need a painkilling drug.

If a biopsy reveals the presence of cancer cells, the next step is usually a battery of tests to determine if the cancer has spread to other parts of the body. The tests include *cystoscopy* (examination of the bladder using a viewing device called a *cystoscope*) and a *radionuclear bone scan* (images of the bones obtained by injecting a radioactive chemical that concentrates in areas of bone damage).

If a bone scan indicates that the cancer might have invaded the patient's bones, the doctor may order bone X rays. The doctor may also use advanced imaging techniques such as *computerized tomography* or *magnetic resonance imaging* to evaluate how much the disease has spread to other tissues. A surgeon will remove some of the lymph nodes near the prostate to see if cancer has spread there before doing surgery to remove a prostate tumor.

There are two blood tests that not only help determine the extent of the cancer but also later help evaluate the patient's response to treatment. The two tests are the PSA test and a similar test that measures a substance called *prostatic acid phosphatase* (PAP) in the blood. Only prostate cells—normal as well as cancerous—make both PSA and PAP. Cancerous prostate cells that have moved elsewhere in the body continue to make both substances.

Two to four weeks after a surgeon removes a man's prostate because of cancer, the patient's PSA level should drop to zero and his PAP level should fall significantly. If later tests show PSA or high amounts of PAP in the patient's blood, the surgery may have failed to remove all the malignant cells from the patient's body.

"Grading" and "staging" the cancer

The best treatment to combat prostate cancer depends on the aggressiveness of the cancer and the extent to which it has spread. Physicians can choose the most appropriate treatment and also predict the patient's chances of recovery based on two assessments called the *grade* and the *stage*.

The grade is a numerical rating of how abnormal and how aggressive the cancer cells look under a microscope. In about half of all cases, more than one type of malignant cell makes up the cancer. Examining biopsied tissue, a pathologist identifies the most common type of cancer cell in the sample and assigns it a number between 1 and 5. Cells most like normal tissue and slowest growing get a 1. Those most abnormal in appearance and most likely to spread rapidly receive a 5. The pathologist does the same for the second most common type of cancer cell found in the tissue, then adds the scores of the two most numerous cell types together for a tumor grade—called the *Gleason score*. The numbers range from 2 to 10. The higher the Gleason score, the more aggressive the cancer cells seem. Pathologist Donald F. Gleason originally developed the grading system, which is now standard practice.

Based on the patient's test results, doctors also determine the stage of the disease, using a letter score from A to D to indicate how much the cancer has spread before it was detected.

- **Stage A cancer,** which comprises 10 to 15 per cent of prostate cancer, is confined within the prostate and not detected by a rectal exam. This stage of cancer is detected only when a patient has surgery to remove overgrown prostate tissue, which is then examined for cancer cells.
- **Stage B cancer** is still limited to the prostate, but a physician can feel nodules or other abnormalities in a rectal exam. Between 20 and 30 per cent of prostate cancers are stage B.
- **Stage C cancer** has spread through most of the prostate and has broken through the prostate capsule, the fibrous shell around the gland. This stage accounts for about 25 to 30 per cent of prostate cancers. Many patients have begun to experience trouble urinating after they have reached stage C.
- **Stage D cancer** has spread to the lymph nodes surrounding the prostate and sometimes to the bones and lungs. The remaining 35 to 45 per cent of prostate cancers comprise stage D.

Survival depends on the stage and on the success of the treatment chosen by the physician and patient. Generally, the overall five-year survival rates are 78 per cent for patients with stage A prostate cancer; 68 per cent for stage B; 58 per cent for stage C; and 23 per cent for stage D. Since 1970, the survival rate for all stages combined rose from 48 per cent to 70 per cent, reflecting the fact that more prostate cancers are being discovered in earlier, more curable stages.

Treatment options for contained cancer

Treatments for prostate cancer vary widely, especially for early stages of the disease. If the patient has stage A cancer, with only a few areas of extremely slow-growing tumor cells, a physician may decide to do nothing to treat the disease, depending on the patient's age and the grade of the tumor. Many prostate cancers grow slowly. In older men, fewer cases of prostate cancer prove fatal, partly because most elderly men die of other causes first. Rather than subject an older patient to the risks of prostate surgery, the doctor may opt merely to keep a watchful eye on his condition, scheduling blood tests and rectal exams every six months or so. If an otherwise healthy man under age 60 has stage A disease, however, most doctors will try to rid the patient's body of cancer and achieve a complete cure, either with radiation or surgery.

In stage B, in which a localized tumor occurs in the prostate, surgeons often perform a procedure called a *radical prostatectomy*. This procedure involves surgical removal of the entire prostate gland, along with part of the urethra and *seminal vesicles* (small glands near the prostate where semen is stored). The bladder neck is attached to the remaining end of the urethra. The surgeon also removes nearby lymph nodes to check for metastasis.

A radical prostatectomy may take up to four hours to perform, because the gland is difficult to reach. The surgical team may approach the gland from behind the pubic bone with an abdominal incision, or through the *perineum* (the region between the scrotum and rectum). Radical prostatectomy often results in *impotence* (the inability to have or maintain an erection) because key nerves that carry nerve impulses to the pelvis may be cut. *Urinary incontinence* (inability to hold back urine) occurs in 10 to 20 per cent of cases.

Physicians often prescribe radiation therapy instead of surgery in treating stage A and B prostate cancer. The most frequently used method is *external beam radiation*, performed in the outpatient X-ray department of a hospital. In this procedure, an X-ray machine directs radiation at the cancerous area to destroy malignant cells. The patient receives treatment five days a week for seven weeks. Radiation therapy avoids the physical pain of surgery, as well as some of the emotional stress and complications. It does, however, cause side effects, including diarrhea, nausea, and loss of appetite. Impotence occurs in up to 50 per cent of cases treated with radiation therapy.

A more recent version of radiation therapy uses a long needle to implant radioactive "seeds," or irradiated metal pellets, into the prostate. The pellets deliver high doses of cancer-killing radiation to specific locations within the gland, thus minimizing the damage to nearby healthy tissue. The technique can be done on an outpatient basis. It seems to be most effective in destroying small prostate tumors that have not spread.

Treatment for advanced cases

In advanced stages—stages C and D—cancer has spread well beyond the prostate and cannot be cured. But treatment can relieve symptoms, slow the spread of the disease, and extend life. These less aggressive treatments take advantage of the fact that nearly 9 out of 10 prostate cancers cannot grow and spread without *testosterone*, the male sex hormone produced in the testicles. Therefore, doctors can remove the testicles to significantly slow the progress of prostate cancer. This procedure, known as a *bilateral orchiectomy*, is a safe operation that can be done on an outpatient basis. But it may result in the loss of a man's sex drive. Urologists have observed that most men—even those

Classification of prostate cancer

Physicians classify prostate cancer by *grade* and *stage*. On the Gleason grading system, a score from 1 to 5 indicates how abnormal and fast-growing the cancer cells seem. The grades for the two most numerous types of cells are added together to form a score from 2 to 10. The stage is a letter rating from A to D indicating how much the cancer has spread.

Grading: How abnormal the cells appear

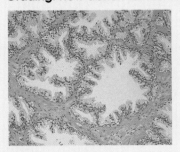 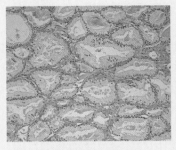 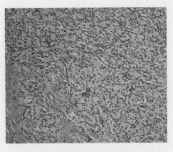

Normal prostate tissue, viewed under the microscope, shows pale, irregular islands of glandular tissue surrounded by smaller, dark pink muscle cells.

A Gleason grade 1 tumor shows the glandular areas becoming crowded and disorganized and the muscle cells beginning to break down.

A sample of prostate tissue containing a Gleason grade 5 tumor consists of densely crowded cancerous cells. Almost no glandular tissue remains.

Staging: How far the cancer has spread

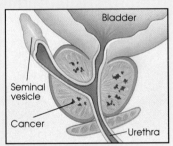 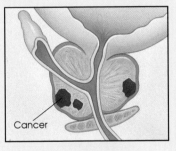 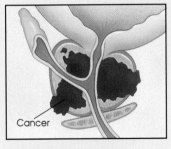

Stage A cancer is confined within the prostate and cannot be detected by a rectal exam. It is found only by microscopic examination of tissue.

Stage B cancer is still limited to the prostate, but a physician can feel bumps or other abnormalities in a rectal examination.

Stage C cancer has spread throughout most of the prostate and has broken through the *capsule*, the fibrous shell around the gland.

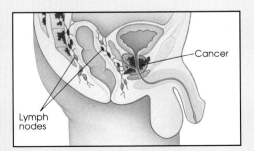

Stage D cancer has spread to the lymph nodes, and perhaps to the bones, lungs, and other organs.

Benign enlarged prostate:
A common disorder

Surgeons perform nearly half a million operations each year in the United States to remove noncancerous tissue from enlarged prostates. Four out of five of these procedures involve men over age 65, making prostate surgery one of the most common types of major surgery in that age group.

Enlargement of the prostate gland, known as *benign prostatic hyperplasia* or *benign prostatic hypertrophy*, both abbreviated *BPH*, is a condition that affects more than half of men over age 50 and about three-fourths of men over age 70. In only one-fourth of these men does BPH trigger symptoms severe enough to warrant surgery.

The cause of BPH is unknown, but scientists believe the condition is related to the action of male hormones. The prostate begins to enlarge slowly in most men while they are in their 30's, and it can produce problems for some by age 40. As BPH tissue grows, it pushes on and obstructs the urethra, the tube that carries urine down from the bladder and out through the penis. The bladder muscle then has to work harder to push urine through the system.

Eventually, the pressure on the urethra may make it impossible to empty the bladder with each urination, causing a condition called *urinary retention*. If untreated, the condition can eventually cause urine to back up into the kidneys. This can lead to kidney damage and even

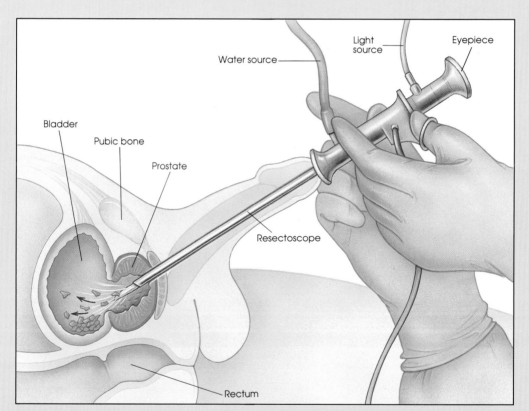

TURP surgery

The most common surgery for an enlarged prostate is called *transurethral resection of the prostate* (TURP). In this procedure, the surgeon runs an instrument called a *resectoscope* through the urethra to the area where excess prostate tissue has grown. The resectoscope cuts or burns off pieces of overgrown tissue, which are flushed out through the instrument with water.

kidney failure in advanced cases of the disorder.

The early symptoms of BPH resemble the symptoms of prostate cancer. These symptoms include the following:

- difficulty in starting urination;
- a weak or interrupted flow of urine;
- dribbling after finishing urinating;
- a feeling of incomplete emptying of the bladder; and
- the need to urinate frequently, including at night.

If these symptoms are mild and there is no evidence of cancer, physicians usually take a wait-and-see approach. Treatment is generally required when symptoms are severe. For men with moderate symptoms, the best plan of action is less clear cut. In mid-1991, the U.S. Agency for Health Care Policy and Research was in the process of drafting new guidelines to help physicians and patients decide when and how best to treat most cases of BPH.

Surgery to remove BPH tissue is relatively safe, but it does entail risks, including possible blood loss, infection, and complications from general anesthesia. The risks are greater in aging men. If surgery is warranted, the surgeon will most likely use a procedure called *transurethral resection of the prostate* (TURP), which literally means cutting the prostate by going through the urethra. A major advantage of this procedure is that it requires no incision, unlike procedures that involve cutting through the abdomen or the *perineum* (the area between the scrotum and the rectum) to reach the prostate.

In the TURP procedure, the patient is first placed under general anesthesia. Then, the surgeon runs an instrument called a *resectoscope* through the urethra to the prostate. The tip of the resectoscope is either very sharp or has an electric current running through it. It cuts or burns off pieces of the gland outwardly from the middle, much like slicing out the core of an apple. The pieces of tissue are washed out through the instrument.

An experimental procedure developed in Europe and now being tested in the United States employs microwave radiation to shrink the enlarged tissues. A thin tube carrying a microwave antenna is inserted into the prostate through the urethra. When the microwave is turned on, it heats the prostate cells to nearly 140 °F (60 °C), killing excess tissue. The microwave procedure requires only local rather than general anesthesia and can be done on an outpatient basis.

As an alternative to surgery, doctors treat some BPH patients with drugs called *alpha blockers*, which relax the muscles that cause urinary obstruction. Other patients undergo a procedure called *prostatic balloon dilation*. The doctor threads a thin, flexible tube into the portion of the patient's urethra that is constricted by excess prostate tissue. A balloon inside the tube is then inflated briefly, enlarging the urethral opening.

Still other patients may be given hormones that interfere with the prostate-stimulating effects of naturally produced male hormones. This helps shrink the prostate.

Researchers with Merck Sharp & Dohme Incorporated—a pharmaceutical company headquartered in Rahway, N.J.—reported in June 1991 that an experimental drug called Proscar may become another alternative to surgery. The drug reportedly shrinks enlarged prostates by blocking the production of a male hormone known as *dihydrotestosterone* within the prostate while hormone levels elsewhere in the body remain normal.
[W.H.A.]

Living with an enlarged prostate

Men with an enlarged prostate whose doctor advises against surgery may find the following advice helpful in living more comfortably with the condition:

- Limit fluids after 8 p.m. to cut down on nighttime trips to the bathroom.
- Limit consumption of alcoholic beverages and coffee.
- Urinate at three- to four-hour intervals.
- Get a checkup, including a digital rectal exam, every six months to monitor the condition of the bladder and the prostate and to check for signs of cancer.
- Notify your doctor if sudden changes of symptoms occur, such as a burning sensation during urination, bloody urine, an increased frequency of urination, fever, chills, or unusual fatigue.

who no longer consider sexual intercourse important—dread such a loss. For this reason, many men refuse the operation despite its proven effectiveness in slowing the cancer.

Instead, the doctor may try various forms of hormonal therapy to suppress testosterone production. One such hormone is *estrogen*, a female hormone. But many men find that estrogen treatment swells their breasts, decreases their sex drive, and inhibits the ability to have an erection. It can also cause fluid retention, aggravate underlying heart or artery disease, and cause potentially dangerous blood clots.

Newer hormone therapies produce fewer side effects. The most effective such therapy seems to be a combination of a substance that tricks the pituitary gland in the brain into shutting off production of testosterone in the testicles and an agent that interferes with the action of testosterone.

On a more experimental basis, some cancer specialists have used *chemotherapy* (treatment with cancer-killing drugs) without hormones to combat advanced prostate cancer. Recent studies have shown that anticancer drugs reduce pain, slow tumor growth, and increase survival time. But patients given these chemicals may suffer nausea, hair loss, and increased vulnerability to infections and blood clots.

Searching for causes

Although the growth of prostate cancer is stimulated by testosterone, the original cause of the disease remains unknown. Some researchers have suggested that dietary factors or exposure to certain chemicals in the workplace may play a role in the development of prostate cancer, but the evidence is not conclusive for any one cause.

Researchers are hunting for links between prostate cancer and various possible risk factors. A 1990 study of family connections showed that a susceptibility to prostate cancer may be inherited. Urologist Gary D. Steinberg of the Brady Urological Institute at Johns Hopkins Hospital in Baltimore headed the study. The research, which traced the disease among brothers, fathers, and sons, showed that a man with one blood relative with prostate cancer may have twice the normal risk of getting the disease. Other studies have indicated that the incidence rate is one and a half times greater in black men than in white men.

Researchers have also found that people in some parts of the world, such as eastern Asia, are less likely than people in North America to develop prostate cancer. If Asian men move to North America, they retain their low risk, but their sons end up having just as much chance of getting prostate cancer as other North Americans. That shift has led some scientists to conclude that a combination of genetic and environmental factors triggers the disease.

Research on colon cancer and other kinds of tumors has shown that human cells contain "cancer-suppressor genes," genetic instructions that appear to play a major role in keeping the cells growing normally. If a part of the suppressor gene is missing, the cells can become malignant and multiply rapidly. Scientists believe a malfunction in this gene may also be behind prostate cancer. If the process can be clarified, it may one day help medical scientists detect susceptible men and devise new treatments.

Until that day comes, the single best method to avoid the tragic consequences of prostate cancer is a routine annual rectal exam. Doctors now know that every man and his doctor must use constant vigilance to detect this widespread and deadly affliction, and that effective countermeasures must be launched quickly once it is discovered.

For further reading:

The Prostate. Ed. by John M. Fitzpatrick and Robert J. Kane. Churchill Livingstone, 1989.

Rous, Stephen N. *The Prostate Book: Sound Advice on Symptoms and Treatment.* Norton, 1988.

Siegel, Mary-Ellen. *Dr. Greenberger's What Every Man Should Know About His Prostate.* Walker, 1988.

For more information:

American Cancer Society
1599 Clifton Road
Atlanta, GA 30329

Office of Cancer Communications
Building 31, Room 10A-24
National Institutes of Health
Bethesda, MD 20892

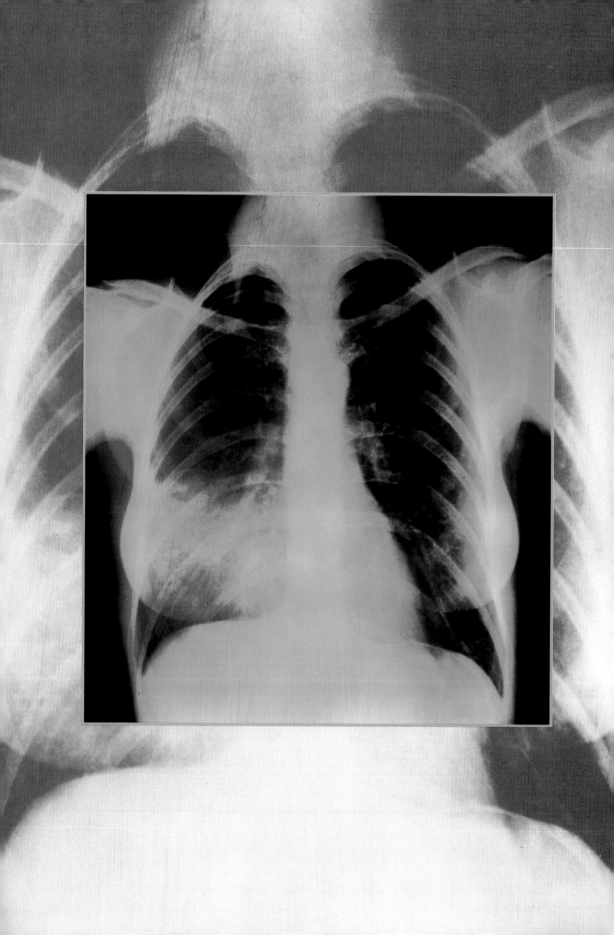

Most people no longer think of
pneumonia as a life-threatening illness.
But the ailment, which strikes about
2 million Americans each year, ranks
as the sixth leading cause of death.

Pneumonia
Still Can Be
A Killer

By Beverly Merz

When Jim Henson, creator of the Muppets, died suddenly in
the summer of 1990, the world was not only saddened, it was
shocked. Although people had become accustomed to reading
obituaries of celebrities who had died of cancer, heart attack, or
stroke, they found it hard to believe that Henson had suc-
cumbed to pneumonia—a disease not usually fatal to healthy,
middle-aged men. Henson's death left many people questioning
whether they, too, could be done in by pneumonia.

The answer is probably not. Jim Henson's pneumonia was an
uncommon and particularly deadly type caused by *Group A
streptococcus*, the bacterium that produces strep throat. This
type of pneumonia sometimes evades even the best medical
treatment. Henson's pneumonia began with deceptively mild
symptoms resembling influenza. But it worsened rapidly. When
Henson realized that he had more than the usual case of flu, he
headed for the emergency room of one of New York City's finest
hospitals. Despite the best efforts of a team of skilled physicians, Henson died only 20 hours after he had checked in.

Fortunately for the rest of us, Jim Henson's pneumonia was as
rare as his talent. Group A streptococcus produces fatal pneu-

monia in fewer than 1 in 1 million people. Most cases of pneumonia are traced to other causes and are routinely cured. In fact, with proper treatment 95 per cent of all people in the United States who contract pneumonia make full recoveries.

Although people should not be unduly afraid of pneumonia, they should take it seriously. The National Center for Health Statistics in Hyattsville, Md., estimates that in the United States in 1989 almost 74,000 people died of pneumonia, making it the nation's sixth leading cause of death.

Causes of pneumonia

The term *pneumonia* refers to any inflammation of the lung. The disease is caused by various microscopic organisms, including viruses, bacteria, fungi, and protozoa, as well as radiation, chemicals, or other irritants. Pneumonia develops when one of these substances enters the lung and begins a process that clogs up tiny microscopic air sacs called *alveoli.* This congestion prevents the alveoli from performing their job of adding oxygen to the blood and filtering carbon dioxide out of the blood when we breathe. If not reversed, pneumonia is dangerous because it can deprive the entire body of oxygen—in effect "suffocating" its victim.

The peak season for pneumonia, just as for colds and flu, is from late fall to early spring. However, contrary to folklore, soaking rains, icy gusts, and bone-chilling cold do not bring on pneumonia. Most cases are caused by a bacterium or virus that is inhaled from the air when someone carrying such a microbe coughs or sneezes. People tend to pass these microbes more frequently during cold weather months when they are likely to gather indoors and be in closer contact with each other.

Pneumonia may also occur if a person inhales or *aspirates* solids, liquids, or irritating vapors by accident (as when food, drink, or saliva goes "down the wrong pipe"). But the body usually quickly expels such matter by coughing or using other built-in defenses. Occasionally, though, a substance reaches the lungs and *aspiration pneumonia* results. This most often occurs in someone who has vomited while asleep or unconscious. If food or some other solid object is aspirated, a doctor usually extracts it using a *bronchoscope,* a long, thin tube placed down the throat and into the lungs.

The body's defenses against pneumonia

The severity of pneumonia depends on the agent causing it and the body's ability to fight off disease. Healthy people have several defenses against airborne microbes, particles, and chemicals. The very structure of the respiratory system presents several obstacles to invading organisms.

The author:

Beverly Merz is national editor, science and technology, for *American Medical News.*

Leading causes of U.S. deaths

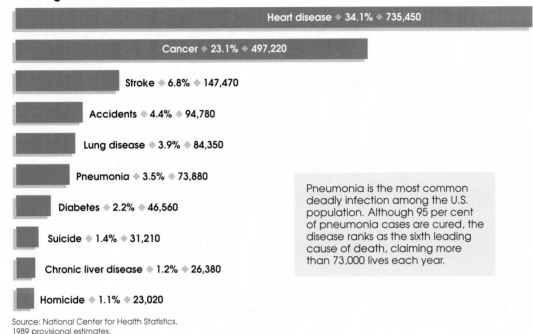

Heart disease ◆ 34.1% ◆ 735,450

Cancer ◆ 23.1% ◆ 497,220

Stroke ◆ 6.8% ◆ 147,470

Accidents ◆ 4.4% ◆ 94,780

Lung disease ◆ 3.9% ◆ 84,350

Pneumonia ◆ 3.5% ◆ 73,880

Diabetes ◆ 2.2% ◆ 46,560

Suicide ◆ 1.4% ◆ 31,210

Chronic liver disease ◆ 1.2% ◆ 26,380

Homicide ◆ 1.1% ◆ 23,020

Pneumonia is the most common deadly infection among the U.S. population. Although 95 per cent of pneumonia cases are cured, the disease ranks as the sixth leading cause of death, claiming more than 73,000 lives each year.

Source: National Center for Health Statistics, 1989 provisional estimates.

To get to the lungs, foreign substances must enter through the nose or mouth. Hairs lining the inside of the nose provide the first line of defense by trapping invading particles. While the hairs hold on to the particles, mucus engulfs the particles and prevents them from reaching the *trachea* or windpipe. Substances in the mouth are denied entry to the trachea by the *epiglottis*, a lidlike structure at the back of the throat that closes over the vocal cords and trachea when we swallow.

Particles that sneak past these checkpoints usually have free passage down the trachea, but find rough going in the *bronchi*, two tubes that branch from either side of the trachea into the lungs. The bronchi drench the invaders with more mucus and try to sweep them back into the throat with *cilia*, tiny hairlike projections that line the bronchi and move particles with a waving motion. The bronchi continue to branch into smaller and smaller *bronchioles*, which lead into the 300 million alveoli that fill with air every time we breathe. Another defense, coughing, assists the bronchi in expelling unwanted microbes and particles. Coughing brings up mucus—and the microbes in it—from the lungs and trachea.

The body's most sophisticated defense is called an *immune response*, which produces disease-fighting cells and *antibodies* (proteins specifically designed to neutralize invading microbes). Disease-fighting cells that are types of white blood cells patrol the entire respiratory system, ready to overpower any intruders.

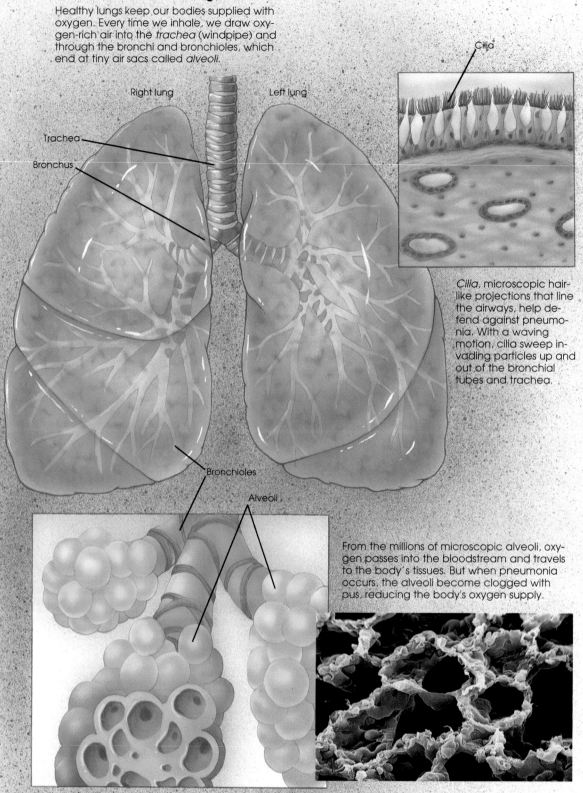

An inside view of the lungs

Healthy lungs keep our bodies supplied with oxygen. Every time we inhale, we draw oxygen-rich air into the *trachea* (windpipe) and through the bronchi and bronchioles, which end at tiny air sacs called *alveoli*.

Cilia

Right lung

Left lung

Trachea

Bronchus

Cilia, microscopic hair-like projections that line the airways, help defend against pneumonia. With a waving motion, cilia sweep invading particles up and out of the bronchial tubes and trachea.

Bronchioles

Alveoli

From the millions of microscopic alveoli, oxygen passes into the bloodstream and travels to the body's tissues. But when pneumonia occurs, the alveoli become clogged with pus, reducing the body's oxygen supply.

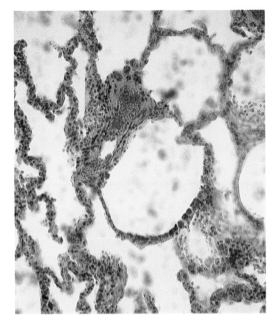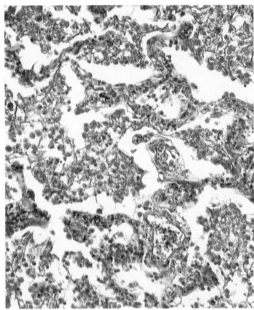

Healthy alveoli, *above left*, fill with oxygen when we inhale. But when the body's immune system attacks microbes infecting the lungs, the process reduces air space by filling the alveoli with fluid and dead or damaged cells, *above right*.

If the body's defenses are weakened, foreign particles may invade the lungs and cause pneumonia. Even so, most otherwise healthy people who receive proper medical attention recover in a week or two. However, if a person's immune system is depleted from other infections or damaged by a disease such as AIDS, a pneumonia may develop that is likely to be prolonged and is often fatal. Infants, whose immune systems are not fully developed, and elderly people, who have slower immune responses, also are likely to have more severe cases of pneumonia.

Smoking, drinking heavily, or taking sleeping pills also increase the risk of pneumonia. These practices keep the immune system, the bronchial cilia, and even the epiglottis, from functioning normally. People who have chronic lung diseases, such as emphysema, also are particularly susceptible to pneumonia. Unconscious or semiconscious patients who cannot cough, and bedridden patients whose cough reflex is weakened by illness, are at increased risk for the disease as well. Surgical patients may develop pneumonia if they breathe in irritating vapors or mucus while they are under general anesthesia. Because of this risk, patients are encouraged to cough and perform deep breathing exercises after surgery to help clear their lungs.

How pneumonia develops

Most cases of pneumonia proceed along the same course, regardless of the cause. When bacteria, viruses, or other irritants damage the lung, white blood cells enter the alveoli to rout out the irritants and repair the destruction. As the cells work, the alveoli fill with fluid, damaged cells, and dead microbes. This debris, or pus, clogs the alveoli and reduces the space for oxygen and carbon dioxide.

The infected person soon begins to feel the effects of the battle raging in the lungs. Breathing becomes difficult, and chest pains may accompany every breath. Attempts to clear the lungs result in violent coughing. The body's temperature increases as the immune system struggles to overcome the invader and repair the damage.

How pneumonia is diagnosed

People with these symptoms—shortness of breath, chest pain, cough, and fever—should suspect that they have pneumonia and call the doctor. Physicians can do several things to determine the type and severity of a pneumonia infection. They usually begin by noting a patient's symptoms and taking his or her temperature. Certain symptoms, such as a high fever with a cough producing large amounts of yellow-green or rust-colored *sputum* or *phlegm* (coughed-up mucus and saliva), signal pneumonia.

Doctors also listen to a patient's lungs with a stethoscope. With this instrument, the doctor is able to hear the crackling or rattling sounds that indicate fluid-filled lungs. By moving the instrument over the patient's chest, the doctor is able to determine which areas of the lungs are inflamed. An X ray of the chest often reveals more precisely the location and extent of the inflammation.

With this information in hand, the physician may use one of several terms to describe the patient's infection. An inflammation involving one or more of the three *lobes* (segments) of the right lung or the two lobes of the left lung is called *lobar pneumonia. Double pneumonia* refers to any infection in both lungs. *Bronchial pneumonia* or *bronchopneumonia* describes a smaller area of infection surrounding the bronchioles.

To treat pneumonia properly, physicians need to know what microbes are causing the disease. To find out, they ask patients to cough up some sputum into a small container. If physicians cannot obtain a good sample in this manner, they may use a bronchoscope to see inside the lungs and extract a sample of sputum to send to the laboratory. Technicians in the lab perform a variety of tests to identify the microbes in the sputum. Some tests take only a few minutes, while others may require one or two days.

Even before the laboratory results are available, physicians usually prescribe bed rest. Some patients may need to check into the hospital, but most people with pneumonia usually recover at home.

Major kinds of pneumonia

TYPE	CAUSE	SYMPTOMS	TREATMENT	TRANSMISSION
VIRAL	Variety of viruses, including those causing influenza, measles, and chicken pox.	Resemble an upper respiratory infection, or "cold." Headache, muscle aches, fever, cough that produces sputum (saliva mixed with mucus).	Bed rest, lots of fluids, pain reliever.	Usually person-to-person (breathing droplets in the air or touching recently soiled objects, such as tissues).
BACTERIAL	*Streptococcus pneumoniae* (pneumococcus). Causes about 90 per cent of bacterial pneumonias and often follows a cold.	Sudden, severe chill. Cough that produces sputum, often tinged with blood. Chest pain, fever, rapid pulse, and difficulty breathing.	Antibiotics: penicillin, erythromycin, or cephalosporins.	Person-to-person.
	Chlamydia trachomatis.	Cough.	Antibiotics: erythromycin.	Cervical infection transferred from mother to newborn at birth.
	Legionella pneumophila.	Headache, muscle pain, nausea. Fever, chills, and dry cough develop later.	Antibiotics: erythromycin or rifampin.	Air conditioners, humidifiers, and other water reservoirs, including lakes and streams.
	Mycoplasma pneumoniae.	Develops slowly. Fever, fatigue, sore throat, headache, cough that produces thick mucus.	Antibiotics: erythromycin or tetracycline.	Person-to-person.
	TWAR agent.	Cough, fever, sore throat, hoarseness. Chest pain and rattling sound in lungs.	Antibiotics: tetracycline or erythromycin.	Possibly person-to-person.
PROTOZOAN	*Pneumocystis carinii (PCP).*	Dry, hacking cough. Shallow, rapid breathing. Chest pain and sometimes a fever.	Pentamidine or trimethoprim-sulfamethoxazole.	Possibly person-to-person. Usually only strikes persons with a suppressed immune system.

Klebsiella pneumoniae bacteria

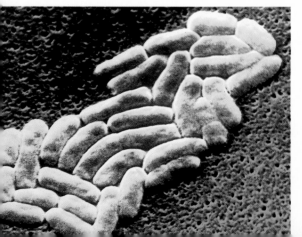

Influenza viruses

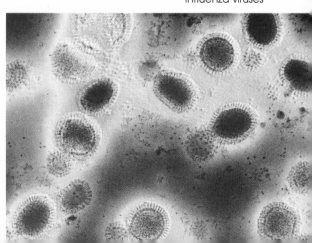

Viral pneumonia

About half of all pneumonias, and usually the mildest cases, are caused by viruses. Viruses are extremely primitive creatures—bits of genetic material shrouded in a protein coat—that cannot survive long outside a cell. The viruses that cause pneumonia are sometimes the same viruses that cause influenza. But to bring on pneumonia, they have managed to advance beyond the nose and throat into the lungs. Because viral pneumonia usually resembles a bad, lingering cold, its symptoms may not be severe enough to send people to bed or to the doctor. This is why it often is referred to as "walking pneumonia."

Once viruses get inside a cell, they act like an unruly punk rock band in a luxury hotel: They use all the amenities and then wreck the place. Viruses use a cell's reproductive machinery to make viral parts and assemble them into new viruses. As these new viruses break through the cell wall, the cell's contents spill out. This cell destruction places a burden on the immune system. The white blood cells of the immune system must come in to clean up the cellular debris. While they work, they release proteins that trigger a fever.

Although no effective drugs exist to combat most viral pneumonias, the body's immune system usually overcomes viruses within a week or two. Therefore, physicians usually treat patients with viral pneumonia the same way they treat patients with a cold. They recommend bed rest, lots of fluids, and, perhaps, a cough syrup.

Bacterial pneumonia

Unlike viruses, bacteria are complete cells that act like tourists in trailer caravans. They move in wherever they can find a campsite and then compete with the neighbors (the body's cells) for resources such as food and water.

When bacterial colonies move into the lung's alveoli, they gobble up nutrients from the bloodstream and crowd out the cells that exchange oxygen for carbon dioxide. They also pollute the region with poisonous wastes, called toxins, that further damage surrounding cells.

Once the immune system is alerted to a bacterial invasion, it moves in much the same way it does to rid the body of viruses. However, routing bacteria from the lungs usually takes longer than exterminating viruses, so people with bacterial pneumonia usually feel worse than those with viral infections. They are seized with chills and stabbing chest pains, and they may cough up blood-tinged sputum. People with bacterial pneumonia usually realize they have something worse than a cold or flu and seek medical attention.

Attending to bacterial pneumonia quickly is a good idea, because this infection is nothing to trifle with. Before antibiotics became available in the 1940's, people often died of this form of pneumonia. Because each antibiotic works somewhat differently, doctors want to know the exact type of bacterium they are dealing with. About 90 per cent of all bacterial pneumonias are caused by *Streptococcus pneumoniae*, commonly called pneumococcus. Seen under a microscope, the pneumococcus bacterium looks something like a short chain of beads.

Penicillin usually gets rid of pneumococci in a few days. Patients who are allergic to penicillin may receive *erythromycin*, a different antibiotic. Some pneumococci have become resistant to or unaffected by these medications and must be treated by a newer antibiotic called *vancomycin*.

Although antibiotics have reduced the number of deaths, about 40,000 people die every year from bacterial pneumonia caused by pneumococci, according to the Centers for Disease Control (CDC) in Atlanta, Ga. Infants, the elderly, and those who are already sick from other illnesses face the greatest risk of dying from this infection.

Rarer forms of pneumonia

A less common bacterium that causes pneumonia is *Mycoplasma pneumoniae*. Mycoplasmal pneumonia occurs most often among children and young adults, especially those in communal living situations, such as day-care centers, military barracks, and college dormitories. This pneumonia is rarely fatal and generally less severe than that caused by pneumococcus. In fact, some cases are so mild that they may last only a few days and be mistaken for a cold.

Mycoplasmal pneumonia begins slowly, with a fever, headache, and cough. Within a few days, the infected person may have chest pains and cough up thick mucus. Although penicillin is useless against mycoplasmal infections, erythromycin and another antibiotic, *tetracycline*, usually work.

Another type of pneumonia is caused by a bacterium known as *Legionella pneumophila*, so named because it was responsible for an outbreak of pneumonia among veterans attending an American Legion convention in Philadelphia in 1976. Legionella thrive in air conditioners, humidifiers, and virtually any type of water-storage facility. Because legionella are transmitted when water from these reservoirs evaporates or sprays into the air, Legionnaires' disease can usually be prevented by regularly cleaning and disinfecting water-storage systems.

Legionnaires' disease usually begins like the flu, with a headache, muscle aches, and loss of appetite. As it progresses, the infected person may develop a high fever, chills, and a dry cough. This pneumonia can be treated with erythromycin and some other antibiotics.

Like some other forms of pneumonia, Legionnaires' disease is

Diagnosing pneumonia

Doctors sometimes use X rays or a procedure called bronchoscopy to diagnose pneumonia. A chest X ray, *right*, reveals a cloudy area (designated by arrow) that indicates the presence of pneumonia in a patient's lower right lung.

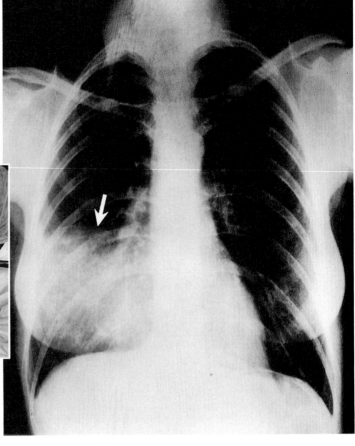

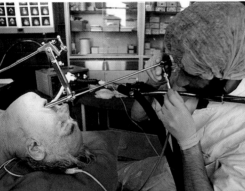

A doctor uses a long, thin tube called a *bronchoscope* to examine a patient's *bronchioles,* a network of airways in the lungs where pneumonia can develop.

more severe in people weakened by chronic illnesses, such as kidney disease or diabetes. It rarely strikes people younger than 20 years old, and the most severe cases occur in people who are older than 50.

Bacteria called *chlamydia* also can cause pneumonia. A fetus whose mother is infected with *Chlamydia trachomatis,* an organism that may dwell in the female genital tract, can pick up the microbe during birth and develop pneumonia after delivery. The infection, which is mild in most infants, generally improves without treatment, although doctors will prescribe erythromycin in some cases.

Another type of chlamydia called the *TWAR agent* also causes a mild pneumonia. Like mycoplasmal pneumonia, it most often affects young people living in groups, is rarely fatal, and can be cured with tetracycline or erythromycin.

Tetracycline is also used to treat *psittacosis,* another form of pneumonia caused by a species of chlamydia. The infection is commonly known as parrot fever because the disease occurs in such birds as parrots, parakeets, lovebirds, pigeons, poultry, and

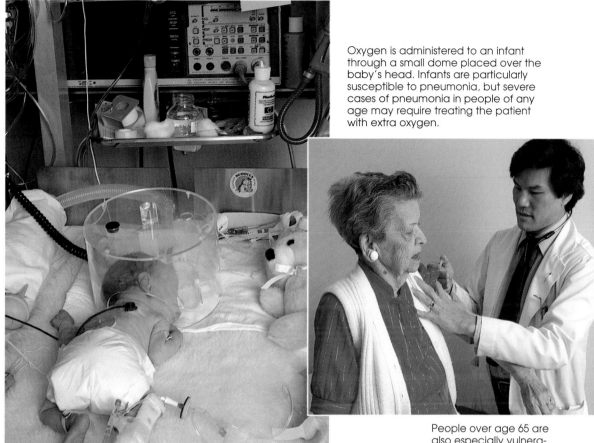

Oxygen is administered to an infant through a small dome placed over the baby's head. Infants are particularly susceptible to pneumonia, but severe cases of pneumonia in people of any age may require treating the patient with extra oxygen.

People over age 65 are also especially vulnerable to pneumonia. For them, doctors advise vaccinations that protect against some forms of pneumonia, such as that caused by the influenza virus.

canaries. Human beings become infected by inhaling contaminated dust from the feathers or from droppings of these birds.

Malnourished and sickly infants, as well as people with AIDS and other conditions that cripple the immune system, are susceptible to a pneumonia caused by *Pneumocystis carinii*, a type of *protozoan* (single-celled parasite). In the absence of a healthy immune system, which would easily sweep the protozoa out of the respiratory system, the microbes sneak into the spaces between the cells. As they multiply, the lungs become heavy and lose their elasticity, making breathing difficult. Although *Pneumocystis carinii* pneumonia (PCP) rarely occurs in well people, it strikes 60 per cent of those with AIDS.

People who are susceptible to PCP can undergo preventive treatments with a drug called *pentamidine*, which they breathe in from a device called a *nebulizer*. To fight PCP that is already established in the lungs, doctors may give pentamidine or other drugs intravenously (directly into the bloodstream).

Many rare forms of pneumonia are caused by microbes associated with other diseases, such as the viruses responsible for measles and chicken pox. In other cases, bacteria that normally stay in the nose, mouth, throat, or digestive system, including *Klebsiella pneumoniae*, *Streptococcus pyogenes*, and *Staphylococcus aureus*, may invade the lungs to cause pneumonia—especially if a person is already suffering from influenza.

Determining which of several types of antibiotics will be effective against these rarer pneumonias depends on identifying the bacterium involved. Because it takes time for laboratory technicians to rule out common microbes, identification of the more unusual types of pneumonia may take awhile. Unfortunately, by the time health care workers pinpoint the bacterium, the infection may be too well established to treat with the usual methods.

For example, oral antibiotics may not be effective in advanced cases of pneumonia because high concentrations in the bloodstream are required to combat the infection. Taken orally, antibiotics may not reach great enough concentrations to control the rapidly multiplying bacteria. Thus, patients with severe infections may need high doses of antibiotics delivered intravenously through narrow tubes inserted into the veins. Intravenous treatments are usually given in the hospital.

Some patients may also need treatment with oxygen. For adults, this is usually supplied through a small tube attached to the nose. Children who might not tolerate a tube can be placed inside a see-through oxygen tent.

Extremely ill patients who have accumulated large amounts of fluid in their lungs might need more intensive oxygen treatment with a *ventilator*, a machine that pumps a mixture of oxygen and nitrogen directly into the lungs. To prepare a patient for ventilation, the physician places a tube into the patient's trachea through the mouth or through an incision in the throat. The tube is then attached to the ventilator. Patients on ventilators cannot speak because the tube blocks the air supply to the vocal cords. However, as the infection subsides and the lungs begin to function normally, the physician removes the tube.

Occasionally, any type of pneumonia may rage out of control and spread its microbes through the bloodstream to other organs, such as the heart and kidneys. When this occurs the damage is no longer limited to the lungs, and the infection can become fatal. This is what happened to Jim Henson.

Vaccines against pneumonia

One of the best strategies against pneumonia is prevention, and vaccination is one of the most successful preventive measures. Vaccines are preparations that contain killed or weakened viruses or bacteria of a particular type. Sometimes they contain only certain parts of these microbes. Except in rare cases, vaccines cannot cause disease. But when they are injected or swallowed, they stimulate the body's immune system to produce antibodies that easily overpower the harmless microbes in the vaccine. The "primed" immune system then can produce these antibodies in abundance if any potent microbes of the same type invade the body in the future.

A few vaccines offer protection against pneumonia. One works against the influenza virus, which is responsible for many cases of viral pneumonia. Because the flu virus changes slightly from year to year, a new version of the vaccine is created annually. The CDC recommends that people over age 65, and others who are at high risk for acquiring pneumonia, receive flu vaccinations every autumn. This vaccine is prepared in hens' eggs and should not be given to people who are allergic to eggs.

A different vaccine is designed to combat the pneumococcus bacterium. This vaccine works against the types of pneumococcus responsible for 87 per cent of all pneumococcal pneumonia cases, and patients need to receive it only once. As with the flu vaccine, the CDC recommends this vaccination for all people over age 65, and for those with weakened immune systems or chronic illnesses. But many physicians recommend the vaccine for people over age 55, because the risks associated with pneumonia begin to increase sharply after this age.

The measles (rubeola) vaccine, recommended for all children aged 15 months or more, usually offers lifetime protection against pneumonia caused by the measles virus. But health experts caution that pregnant women or people whose immune systems are not functioning normally should not receive this vaccine.

Protection through good health habits

Other simple measures also reduce the chances of getting pneumonia. To keep the immune system working at peak efficiency, doctors advise that people should eat a well-balanced diet, get sufficient exercise and rest, and develop good methods for handling stress. The best way for smokers and heavy drinkers to prevent pneumonia is to give up these habits. Although both smoking and drinking can damage the respiratory system's cells, many of the cells recover rapidly when these practices are stopped.

Pneumonia still can be a devastating and fatal disease. But knowing that many effective methods can prevent it and treat it should help us all breathe a little easier.

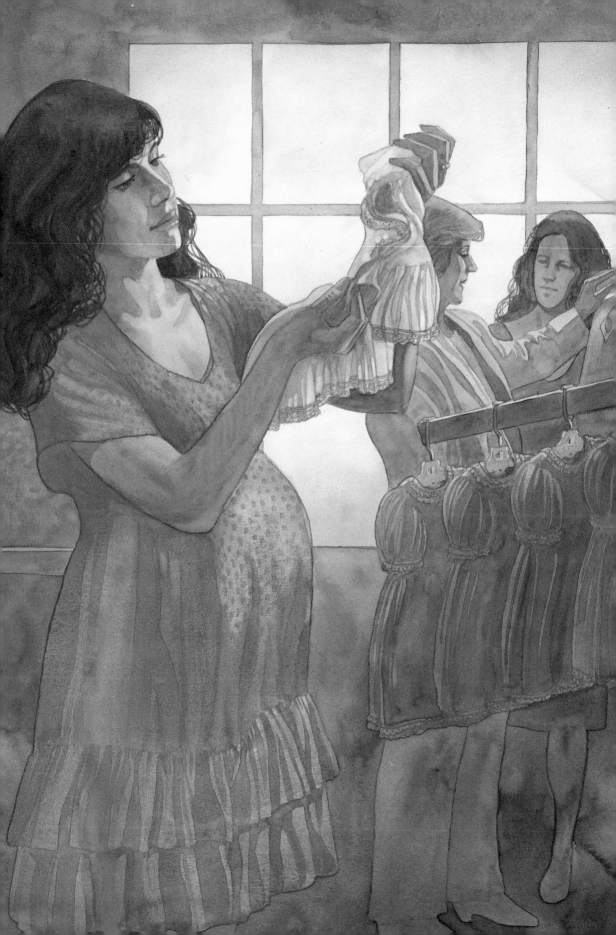

By taking care of their own health and seeking prenatal care, women today have far greater opportunities than ever before to have a healthy baby.

Healthy Mothers, Healthy Babies

By Cristine Russell

Forty-year-old Jocelyn was living the hectic existence of a municipal bond trader on New York City's Wall Street when she added a new challenge to her busy life. In addition to rising at 5 a.m., commuting from Connecticut, working madly until the market closed, and returning home to care for her two children, she had to manage morning sickness. Jocelyn and her husband had decided to have another baby.

Although the nausea seemed the same as it did during her last pregnancy 10 years earlier, Jocelyn found that she now had much more control and many more options along the way to creating a new member of the family. Advances in medicine and technology allow today's prospective parents—even those in their 40's—to plan a pregnancy, monitor its progress, avoid known hazards to the unborn infant, and choose the style and setting for childbirth that best meets their personal needs. While the choices available today promote potentially healthier offspring, there is no magic formula for success for Jocelyn or the more than 4 million American women who give birth each year.

Doctors today consider the months before *conception* (when the egg is fertilized by the sperm) as an important time to pre-

The author:

Cristine Russell is special health correspondent for *The Washington Post* and a free-lance science writer.

pare for a healthy baby. Preconceptual planning allows a woman and her health-care provider to identify and treat any medical conditions or health habits that might decrease the chances of conceiving and carrying a normal, healthy child.

Prepregnancy planning also includes determining what type of health-care professional will supervise the pregnancy, labor, and delivery. Most women use an obstetrician, but many family physicians also provide obstetrical care. Some women are choosing midwives, once the standard maternity caregivers. Certified nurse-midwives, who have formal training in obstetrical care, can provide an alternative to physician care in low-risk pregnancies. Nurse-midwives typically emphasize *natural childbirth* (childbirth with little or no medical intervention) but are usually affiliated with obstetricians who can intervene if a woman needs more medical attention. Before a woman becomes pregnant, she can talk with various doctors or nurse-midwives to learn about their qualifications and understand their approach to pregnancy and childbirth.

Health care before and during pregnancy

After a woman has selected a health-care provider, she should schedule a prepregnancy appointment. According to a recent U.S. Public Health Service report, a healthy pregnancy depends greatly on a woman's general health before pregnancy. "The [prepregnancy] visit may be the single most important health-care visit when viewed in the context of its effect on pregnancy," the report noted.

This visit could address such topics as nutrition, potential hazards in the workplace, stress, family history, life style, and treatment for other medical conditions. For example, high blood pressure or diabetes should be controlled before a pregnancy starts. If a woman has never been exposed to *rubella* (German measles), her doctor may suggest that she receive a rubella vaccination at least three months before becoming pregnant. Testing for exposure to rubella is important, because if a woman is exposed to the virus or the vaccine during pregnancy, it can seriously harm the fetus.

The prepregnancy visit may also include genetic counseling to obtain information about diseases that can be inherited. A couple who previously had a child with certain genetic or developmental defects—or who have relatives with those conditions—may have a heightened chance of producing offspring with the same characteristics. In this case, the couple may have the option of a screening test to determine their risk of passing a particular disorder on to the baby.

When a woman suspects that she is pregnant, she should confirm her condition as soon as possible. Laboratory blood tests can verify pregnancy as soon as 6 or 7 days after conception. A

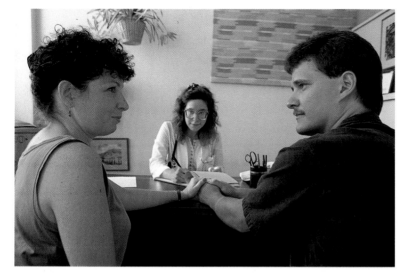

A visit to a doctor before pregnancy helps a couple plan for a healthy baby. A physician can provide guidelines for prenatal care and identify and treat medical conditions that might cause problems during pregnancy. In addition, genetic counseling benefits couples whose age or family history puts them at risk of passing on genetic defects.

urine test, which is only slightly less accurate than a blood test, may detect pregnancy as early as 10 days after conception. Some women perform a urine test using a home pregnancy test kit. These kits are quite accurate, but still should have medical confirmation. The blood test and urine test both measure the level of a hormone called *human chorionic gonadotropin.*

Women should plan a doctor's visit early in pregnancy. A woman's health during those first weeks is crucial to normal fetal development. By the end of the first eight weeks, the fetus is already forming its brain and many other body structures that can be affected by the mother's health and habits.

Many doctors schedule prenatal visits monthly for the first 28 weeks of pregnancy, every 2 weeks from 28 to 36 weeks, and weekly during the last month, following the guidelines of the American College of Obstetricians and Gynecologists (ACOG). A controversial 1989 U.S. Public Health Service report questioned the need for such frequent visits among healthy pregnant women, particularly those who have previously given birth. For low-risk pregnancies, the report recommended more visits early in pregnancy and fewer in the later stages. The ACOG suggests that the traditional schedule can serve as a guideline, which a doctor may deviate from according to a woman's individual medical needs.

An initial pregnancy visit usually includes a medical history, blood and urine tests, a Pap test, and a physical examination. A urine test screens for protein and sugar, which could indicate diabetes. Blood tests check for *anemia* (a decrease in the number of red blood cells), *Hepatitis B* (a liver disease), and *syphilis* (a sexually transmitted disease that can harm the fetus). They also reveal immunity to rubella and the *Rh blood factor* (a substance in the red blood cells of most people).

If a woman who is Rh negative (lacks the Rh factor) has a baby with a man who is Rh positive (has the factor), her body can form antibodies that will attack the fetus's red blood cells. Although the first baby of such parents normally is not harmed, subsequent babies are at risk. Physicians can usually prevent this hazard by giving an Rh-negative woman an injection of a blood product called *Rh immunoglobin* during and after pregnancy. This prevents antibodies from forming.

During prenatal visits the doctor routinely checks weight and blood pressure. He or she may also repeat the urine test to check for diabetes. The doctor listens to the fetus's heartbeat and measures the mother's abdomen to determine the fetus's growth and position. A doctor estimates the date of delivery based on the date of the woman's last menstrual period and the size of her uterus. Delivery is calculated to occur 280 days, or 40 weeks, from the first day of the last menstrual period.

Testing for fetal disorders

Doctor visits may also include tests to detect possible problems with the fetus. One of the most common problems is *Down syndrome*, a genetic flaw that causes mental retardation and some physical abnormalities. Although any pregnant woman, no matter what her age, may have a child with Down syndrome, the risk of having a baby with this disorder increases with a woman's age. A pregnant woman at age 40, for example, faces a 1 in 106 chance of delivering a Down syndrome baby; at age 41, the chances of this outcome increase to 1 in 82. However, results of a large Canadian study published in March 1991 showed that women over age 35 are at no increased risk of bearing children with certain other birth defects.

The *alphafetoprotein test* is usually offered to all pregnant women. This blood test is performed between 15 and 18 weeks of pregnancy to screen for Down syndrome and brain and spinal cord malformations known as *neural tube defects*. If the test results are abnormal, the doctor may repeat the test or order a dif-

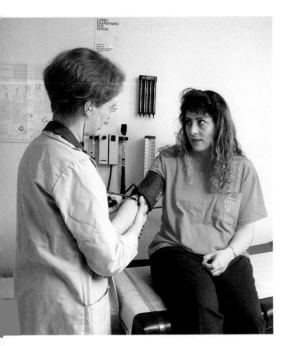

A doctor checks the blood pressure of a pregnant woman during a routine visit. During pregnancy, a woman should keep regular appointments with a health-care provider, who will monitor the woman's health and look for problems that require special care.

ferent type of procedure to determine if any problem actually exists.

An *ultrasound* exam uses sound waves, inaudible to the human ear, to create pictures of the fetus, its heartbeat, or the pattern of blood flow through the umbilical vessels. Ultrasound can help confirm the number of babies the mother is carrying, the position and growth of the fetus, and the delivery date. Studies in 1990 showed that ultrasound could also detect certain birth defects, such as neural tube defects and Down syndrome.

When ultrasound reveals a potential problem, a woman may undergo the test again to confirm the condition or monitor its progress. No studies have found that ultrasound—in use for more than 20 years—poses any threat to the mother or fetus.

Other tests also can reveal genetic defects and a baby's sex. In *amniocentesis*, a doctor inserts a thin needle through the mother's abdomen and into the uterus to withdraw a small amount of amniotic fluid from the sac surrounding the fetus. The fluid contains cells shed by the fetus and can be tested for genetic

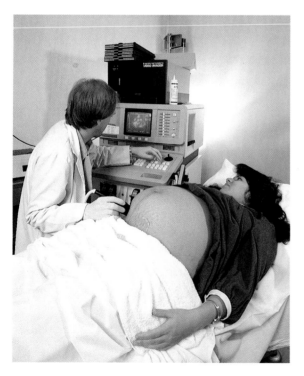

Ultrasound "sees" the fetus

In an ultrasound procedure, *left*, a doctor positions a sensor that sends harmless sound waves into a pregnant woman's abdomen. The pattern of waves reflected by the fetus forms images on a monitor. The pictures may reveal the size, sex, and position of the fetus, as well as the presence of some abnormalities or multiple fetuses. Twins, for example, are detectable in an ultrasound image showing the curved outlines of two heads, *below*.

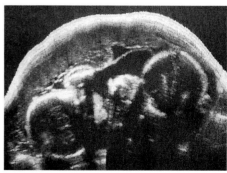

disorders, such as Down syndrome and neural tube defects.

Amniocentesis is a relatively safe procedure. Mild complications—such as cramping or bleeding—or more serious ones, such as damage to the fetus—are rare. Amniocentesis increases the risk of miscarriage by less than 1 per cent. If a doctor recommends this test, it is usually performed in the hospital or the office between the 14th and 18th weeks of pregnancy, and the doctor can report the findings in 3 or 4 weeks.

A woman may undergo an earlier alternative to amniocentesis from 9 to 12 weeks into her pregnancy. In this procedure, called *chorionic villus sampling* (CVS), an obstetrician places a needle through the abdomen, or inserts a thin, flexible tube through the vagina, to reach the uterus and take a sample of the *chorionic villi*, feathery projections of placental tissue. Lab technicians analyze the tissue sample for genetic abnormalities. Studies have shown that CVS is slightly more likely than amniocentesis to cause miscarriage.

Information on probable birth defects can help couples to plan for the future care of the baby or to end the pregnancy. However, according to the ACOG, only 2 to 3 per cent of babies born in the United States have serious birth defects. In any case, a woman can do many things to promote the health of her baby.

Nutrition and weight gain

Eating well is a basic but crucial habit for an expectant mother to develop, obstetricians say. Pregnant women need to eat the right foods and eat enough of them. Women who do not eat enough to gain sufficient weight may deliver a baby with a low birth weight (less than 5.5 pounds or 2.5 kilograms). Such babies are at increased risk of dying during the first year of life, primarily because their less-developed organs have more difficulty adjusting to life outside the womb. They cannot, for example, handle infections as well as bigger, more robust babies.

Since the 1960's, most doctors have advised women to gain 20 to 25 pounds (about 9 to 11 kilograms) during pregnancy. But a 1990 report from the National Academy of Science's Institute of Medicine recommended figuring appropriate weight gain based on the woman's size before pregnancy. Most women of normal weight for their height should gain 25 to 35 pounds (about 11 to 16 kilograms) during pregnancy, according to the report. Thinner women should aim for 28 to 40 pounds (about 13 to 18 kilograms), while overweight women should gain only 15 to 25 pounds (about 7 to 11 kilograms).

To maintain a healthy diet during pregnancy, a woman of average weight will need to add only about 300 more well-balanced calories a day to her diet, according to the ACOG. A good overall diet includes a variety of vitamin-rich fruits and vegetables, complex carbohydrates, such as whole-grain breads and

Daily dietary needs for pregnant women

Type of food	Fruits and vegetables	Whole-grain or enriched bread and cereal products	Milk and milk products	Meat, poultry, fish, eggs, nuts, and beans
Important functions	Helps fight infections; promotes healthy skin and good eyesight.	Supplies energy; provides fiber to prevent constipation.	Builds bones and teeth; aids growth of new tissue and repair of body cells.	Helps build new body tissue; prevents anemia.
Nutrients	Minerals Vitamins	Carbohydrates Minerals Vitamins Protein	Calcium Phosphorus Protein Vitamins	Protein Iron Vitamins
Daily servings	4 or more	4 or more	4 or more	3 or more
Sample food choices	Select at least one serving rich in vitamin A (dark yellow or green, leafy vegetables, such as broccoli, spinach, carrots, or winter squash) and one serving rich in vitamin C (grapefruit, oranges, tomatoes, cantaloupe, or strawberries).	Select from a variety of foods in this category: bread, rolls, muffins, crackers, rice, cold and hot cereals, pancakes, pasta, and tortillas.	Choices include milk or other dairy products, such as yogurt, cheese, custard, cottage cheese, or ice cream.	Meat, poultry, and fish can be alternated with other protein sources to provide comparable nutritional benefits. Eggs, peanut butter, nuts, tofu, and legumes (such as peas, pinto beans, soybeans, or kidney beans) are good choices.
Examples of serving size	■ 1 cup raw, dark green, leafy vegetables ■ ½ cup cooked vegetables or fruit ■ ½ grapefruit or 1 medium-sized fruit, such as an apple, orange, or banana ■ ½ cup fruit juice	■ 1 slice bread, biscuit, or roll ■ 1 oz. (¾ cup) cold cereal ■ ½ cup cooked rice, pasta, or cereal such as oatmeal or grits ■ 2 graham crackers	■ 1 8-oz. glass milk ■ 1⅓ cups cottage cheese ■ 1½ slices cheese ■ 1½ cups ice cream	■ 2 or 3 oz. meat, fish, or poultry ■ 1 cup cooked legumes ■ 4 tbs. peanut butter ■ 2 eggs

Recommended dietary allowances for pregnant women

Nutrient	Amount	Nutrient	Amount
Protein (g)	60	Vitamin E (mg)	10.0
Calcium (mg)	1,200	Vitamin C (mg)	70.0
Phosphorus (mg)	1,200	Thiamin (mg)	1.5
Magnesium (mg)	300	Riboflavin (mg)	1.6
Iron (mg)	30	Niacin (mg)	17.0
Zinc (mg)	15	Vitamin B_6 (mg)	2.2
Vitamin A (μg)	800	Folate (μg)	400.0
Vitamin D (μg)	10	Vitamin B_{12} (μg)	2.2

Recommendations are for nutrients derived from food sources.
Any need for vitamin supplements should be determined by a physician.
g = gram; mg = milligram ($^{1}/_{1,000}$ gram); μg = microgram ($^{1}/_{1,000}$ milligram)

Sources: American College of Obstetricians and Gynecologists; National Academy of Sciences.

cereals, calcium-rich milk and dairy products, and high-protein foods such as meat, poultry, fish, eggs, nuts, and beans. An expectant mother also needs to drink six to eight glasses of liquid—such as water, milk, and fruit or vegetable juices—per day. "Junk food," such as potato chips, sweets, and soda pop, quickly increase caloric intake while offering little nutrition.

Contrary to popular belief, pregnant women should not decrease the amount of sodium in their diet. The body actually needs more sodium during pregnancy to meet the needs of the fetus and to regulate fluids in the mother. Women with high blood pressure can be an exception, however, and should consult their doctor about salt intake.

According to the Institute of Medicine report, a well-rounded diet usually provides pregnant women with a sufficient amount of vitamins and nutrients, with two possible exceptions: iron and folate. "Iron is the only known nutrient for which requirements cannot be met reasonably by diet alone," the report said. Therefore, it recommended daily low-dose supplements (30 mg) of ferrous iron during the second and third *trimesters* (the three-month periods into which pregnancy is roughly divided). The report also noted that some studies have shown that increased folate intake before pregnancy may help prevent neural tube defects. The ACOG also recommends only supplements of iron and folate during pregnancy and suggests that a woman discuss with her doctor the possible need for other supplements.

Benefits of moderate exercise

In addition to new standards for weight gain and nutrition, recent studies have indicated that appropriate exercise during pregnancy does not harm the fetus and can help the mother feel better. As with all people, exercise can improve appearance and posture, heighten feelings of well-being, and reduce backache and fatigue. However, a pregnant woman needs to observe some cautions in her physical activities to guard both her health and her baby's.

An ACOG guidebook states: "This is not a good time to take up a new, strenuous sport, but if you were active before your pregnancy, you should be able to continue, within reason." For those who had not been active before pregnancy, walking is a good exercise. Recreational swimmers, joggers, tennis players, and golfers can continue their sports in moderation. Snow skiing, water skiing, and surfing are risky because of the increased chance of taking a hard fall and injuring the fetus.

Regular, moderate exercise is more beneficial than sudden spurts of strenuous activity followed by periods of inactivity. The ACOG advises pregnant woman to avoid jerky, bouncy, high-impact activities as well as deep knee bends, full sit-ups, double leg raises, and straight-leg toe touches. These can strain leg and back muscles that already are handling more than their normal load.

Certain exercises help strengthen abdominal muscles and relieve backache, a common pregnancy complaint. In one such exercise, the "pelvic tilt," a woman stands or kneels with her hands on the floor. By pulling in the abdomen and tightening the buttocks, she tilts her pelvis upward and takes pressure off the lower back. The position is held for 10 seconds and repeated several times. Some women find that getting on their hands and knees and arching the back also helps relieve backache.

What to avoid

A healthy pregnancy also requires shunning potentially harmful substances and activities. Health experts say pregnant women should avoid the following hazards:

Cigarettes. Cigarette smoke contains harmful chemicals, such as carbon monoxide and nicotine, which reduce oxygen to the fetus. Smoking can slow fetal growth, reduce birth weight, and raise the risk of miscarriage, premature delivery, and bleeding in the mother. A 1990 report from the U.S. surgeon general said that women who stop smoking before becoming pregnant deliver babies of the same birth weight as those born to women who have never smoked. Quitting completely in the first three or four months of pregnancy may decrease the chances of having a low-birth-weight baby.

Alcohol. Simply put, the less a pregnant woman drinks, the better. Evidence has shown that heavy drinking during pregnancy can lead to *fetal alcohol syndrome*, which causes a variety of physical deformities and mental problems in the infant. Since doctors suspect but do not know for sure whether moderate or light drinking causes birth defects or other conditions unfavorable to a fetus, they believe the safest course is to not drink any alcoholic beverages during pregnancy.

Illegal drugs. Babies of women who smoke marijuana or use cocaine are likely to be born prematurely and be small for their age. Infants born to addicts of drugs such as heroin, methadone, or PCP (angel dust) may be addicted

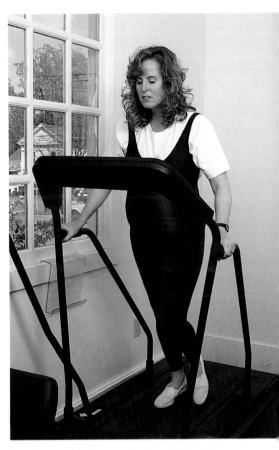

Regular, moderate exercise can improve a pregnant woman's fitness and reduce some of the discomforts of pregnancy. Physicians advise against beginning a new, strenuous sport during pregnancy but say that most women can safely continue the level of activity they maintained before pregnancy.

105

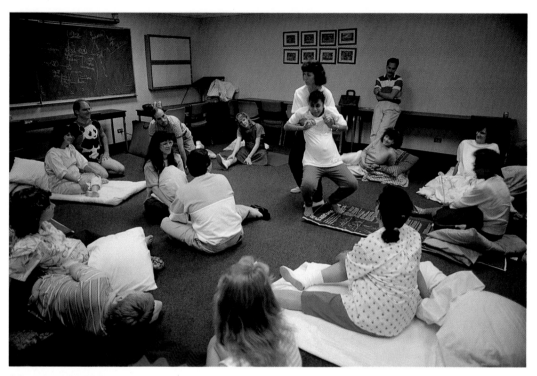

A Lamaze childbirth class helps mothers and their partners prepare for labor and delivery. Such classes provide a realistic preview of the birthing process and teach natural pain-control techniques for use during childbirth.

themselves and undergo withdrawal after birth. Crack, a form of cocaine that is smoked, can kill an adult and is particularly dangerous to a fetus. A baby that survives crack exposure may have birth defects or breathing and neurological problems.

Nonprescribed medication. Pregnant women should avoid prescription and over-the-counter medications unless a doctor advises otherwise. Even common, seemingly harmless remedies can pose potential dangers. For example, aspirin taken late in pregnancy may complicate delivery by causing excessive bleeding. A drug prescribed for acne, isotretinoin (also known as Accutane), can cause miscarriages and birth defects. Tetracycline, a common antibiotic, can affect the fetus and prevent proper tooth development later on. Women with health problems requiring medication should discuss their situation with a doctor, ideally before becoming pregnant.

X rays. An X-ray examination of a pregnant woman's teeth, arms, or legs usually poses no threat to the fetus, particularly if standard precautions are taken and the abdominal area is shielded. But an X ray of the abdomen, hip, or back can place the fetus in direct line with radiation that could cause genetic defects leading to retarded growth and intellectual development.

Infectious and toxic agents. *Toxoplasmosis*, a disease transmitted by a parasite in raw or undercooked meat and in cat feces can cause death or severe neurological problems in a fetus. Thorough hand washing after handling raw meat helps prevent transmission of the toxoplasmosis parasite. Cats can pick up the parasite by eating mice. Pregnant women who own a cat should try to keep the animal indoors and have another family member change the litter box.

Chemicals in the home, workplace, or environment may also present a risk to a developing infant. Pregnant women should read and heed warnings on paint, glue, cleaning agents, and other such household products.

Hot tubs and saunas. The body's effort to keep cool in the heat generated by whirlpools and saunas can result in blood— and therefore oxygen—being drawn away from the uterus.

A man's habits may also affect offspring. Studies have indicated that alcohol, radiation, lead, and some chemicals, may alter sperm and lead to birth defects.Therefore, a man might be wise to avoid toxic chemicals and limit or suspend alcohol consumption several weeks before he attempts to father a child.

Coping with the discomforts of pregnancy

For nine months, a woman's body makes tremendous accommodations to the growing baby inside. A certain amount of discomfort is inevitable, particularly in the first and last trimesters, but some common symptoms can be minimized.

Many women experience nausea or vomiting during the first three months of pregnancy. A woman can reduce nausea by not letting her stomach become completely empty. Eating crackers or dry toast first thing in the morning, and small meals or snacks throughout the day, helps ward off that queasy feeling.

Heartburn—a burning feeling in the chest, just below the breastbone—is a common complaint during pregnancy, especially in the later months. Eating several small meals rather than a few large ones lessens the load on the digestive system and helps prevent heartburn. Antacids should not be used during pregnancy unless a doctor recommends them.

Constipation is another typical problem women encounter most often in the late stages of pregnancy. Plenty of water and a diet that includes fresh fruits, vegetables, and other high-fiber foods will help remedy this problem.

During the last months of pregnancy, a woman may have trouble finding a comfortable position in which to sleep. When lying on her side, a pillow under the abdomen and another between the knees offers extra support.

A pregnant woman can reduce discomfort from varicose veins (twisted, widened veins in the legs, common in pregnancy) by not sitting or standing in one place for a long time, by putting her feet up whenever possible, and by wearing support hosiery. She should avoid wearing stockings with tight bands.

More serious discomforts or complications require careful medical monitoring. *Preeclampsia*, a condition characterized by

Infant mortality in the United States

In April 1991, the United States National Center for Health Statistics offered welcome news on U.S. *infant mortality*, deaths of babies who are less than 1 year old. The number of infant deaths decreased 6 per cent in one year, from 9.7 deaths per 1,000 live births in 1989 to 9.1 deaths per 1,000 births in 1990, the most significant annual drop in these rates since 1980. However, despite this decline, more than 20 other industrialized nations have a lower infant mortality rate than that of the United States.

Government health experts attributed much of the decrease in the death rate to new drugs that successfully treat lung problems in premature babies. Unfortunately, many of the conditions that lead to infant deaths are not easily treated, and each year nearly 40,000 U.S. babies die before their first birthday. Black infants are twice as likely to die as whites, and mortality is also high among babies of native American and Puerto Rican mothers.

The causes of infant mortality are complex. Inadequate prenatal care, teen-age pregnancy, drug and alcohol abuse, untreated medical conditions, and AIDS (contracted from infected mothers) are major contributors. A lack of early prenatal care may lead to prematurity and low birth weight and is a serious problem among some minorities.

The latest figures from the National Center for Health Statistics show that in 1988 only about 60 per cent of black, American Indian, Puerto Rican, and Mexican women living in the United States received prenatal care during the first three months of pregnancy. In contrast, nearly 80 per cent of white, Cuban, and Asian women started their care early in pregnancy.

In March 1991, President George Bush announced that he had proposed $171 million in grants for a "Healthy Start" program that would help provide prenatal care and help prevent infant mortality. The Bush Administration said $25 million would be distributed in 1991 to 10 communities with the highest infant mortality rates. Government officials expected substantial increases for 1992.

Washington, D.C., had the highest infant mortality rate based on the average number of deaths per 1,000 live births in 1988. Detroit, Philadelphia, Cleveland, and Memphis exhibited the next four highest rates for that year.

While federal, state, and local governments are grappling with the infant mortality problem, some privately funded efforts are pioneering new, inexpensive approaches for improving the health of babies. In New Haven, for example, the Hospital of St. Raphael began "Project MotherCare," a cooperative effort with Yale University, the local health department, and other medical facilities. The project sends a mobile clinic into seven of the city's poorest neighborhoods and offers free prenatal and primary medical care to needy pregnant women.

The project is the brainchild of Wilfred Reguero, a Puerto Rican physician who heads the department of obstetrics and gynecology at St. Raphael's. "It is quite clear from medical literature that the best way to reduce the infant death rate is by giving prenatal care—the earlier, the better," says Reguero.

Programs such as these may help not only to reduce infant mortality, but they also can provide care that decreases the incidence of birth defects and health problems in both mothers and their newborns. [C. R.]

very high blood pressure and swelling in the ankles and feet during the last few months of pregnancy, demands medical attention. Uncontrolled, this condition may progress to *eclampsia*, which is a serious disorder characterized by coma or seizures.

Women with diabetes should have the condition well managed before becoming pregnant—and carefully monitored by a physician during pregnancy. Uncontrolled diabetes may lead to premature delivery, miscarriage, birth defects, or a large baby that is difficult to deliver. Some women develop a type of diabetes called gestational, or Type III diabetes, during pregnancy. Those who are seriously overweight, who have previously had a baby weighing more than $9\frac{1}{2}$ pounds, or who have a family history of diabetes, are at increased risk for developing the disease. Gestational diabetes usually disappears after childbirth, but some women may develop another form of diabetes later in life.

Vaginal bleeding may not indicate a serious problem, but a woman should always report any such bleeding to her health-care provider. Early in pregnancy, bleeding is common but it may signal a possible miscarriage. Late in pregnancy, it may signal premature labor or a placenta that has pulled away from the uterine wall, a situation that calls for urgent medical care.

Preparing for childbirth

Apart from attending to her body's physical needs during pregnancy, a woman can help herself and her baby by preparing for labor and delivery. Childbirth classes provide information on various pain-control techniques, such as breathing and relaxation. These natural methods can reduce or eliminate the need for pain medication, which may slow the baby's reflexes and breathing as well as the overall birthing process.

Childbirth education also offers a realistic look at what to expect during labor and delivery, including the possibility of a *Caesarean section* (surgical removal of the baby through an incision in the abdomen and uterus). Caesareans are the most common surgery in the United States, accounting for about 25 per cent of all births. Although a vaginal birth is normally the desired goal of pregnancy, a woman should prepare for the possibility that a Caesarean delivery may be medically necessary.

The presence of a *doula*, a woman who provides emotional support during labor and delivery, can also be helpful. A medical report published in 1991 said that women who had a doula with them during labor were at significantly decreased risk for having a Caesarean section. They also needed less medical intervention, had shorter labors, and delivered babies with fewer health problems.

Care during pregnancy has come a long way since the early 1900's. Before then, women risked their lives giving birth and often lost their babies. As Jocelyn and many other women have learned, a healthy life style, combined with the medical community's growing skill, knowledge, and technology, now paves the way for nurturing new life.

For further reading:
ACOG Guide to Planning for Pregnancy, Birth, and Beyond. The American College of Obstetricians and Gynecologists, 1990. (For information about ordering, call: 1-800-762-2264.)

Hotchner, Tracy. *Pregnancy and Childbirth,* Avon Books, 1990.

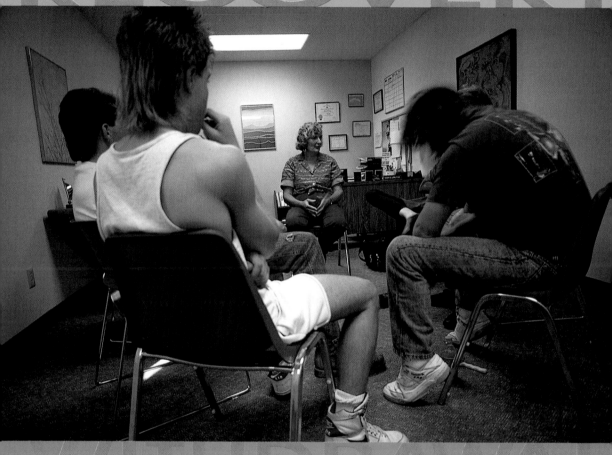

GROUP
THERAPY
REHABILITATION
RECOVERY

WITHDRAWAL
DETOX
COCAINE
ANONYMOUS

Breaking the devastating habit of drug abuse can be a daunting—and sometimes deadly—challenge. But for many people, the right drug treatment program can make the difference.

Defeating Drug Dependency

By Dianne Hales

A suburban high school student. A professional athlete. A young stockbroker. An inner-city teen-ager. A rock musician. For these individuals, the war on drugs is not simply a national priority or a newspaper headline, but a deeply personal and wrenching reality. Along with millions of other Americans, they are waging a physical, psychological, and spiritual battle to overcome the grip of drug addiction. Their struggle to recover is a long and hard one, but advances in understanding and treating addiction are providing new hope for all who are trying to break free of drugs.

On both an individual and a national level, the war on drugs is far from over. According to a 1990 study of drug use among American adults conducted by the National Institute on Drug Abuse (NIDA) in Rockville, Md., the number of illegal drug users has dropped from approximately 23 million in 1985 to 13 million in 1990. Yet the National Academy of Science's Institute of Medicine in Washington, D.C., estimates more than 5.5 million Americans are addicted to drugs—that is, they abuse drugs to the point of suffering physical and psychological distress if they stop drug use. According to a September 1990 report by the institute, 3.3 million of these people are between the ages of 18 and 34; and 1 in 5 is in trouble with the law.

In addition, cocaine addiction may be on the rise. In 1991, the Office of National Drug Control Policy in Washington, D.C., estimated that there are 1.7 million cocaine addicts in the United States. Whether due to undercounting or an actual increase in addicts, this is triple the estimated number in 1990.

Therapists today view addiction—once damned as a shameful failure of will or virtue—as a chronic but treatable disease that affects both body and mind. Most drug users are ordinary people who try drugs out of curiosity, boredom, or a desire simply to go along with their pals. At highest risk are the young and the poor, especially those who live in communities where drugs are widely used or where there are few economic opportunities. But celebrities such as champion boxer Sugar Ray Leonard, former first lady Betty Ford, and New York Mets pitcher Dwight Gooden have shown the world that even famous and successful people can develop a drug problem.

Yet no one—rich or poor, young or old—ever sets out to become an addict. Users invariably believe they're too smart, too strong, or too lucky to lose control. Addiction isn't a matter of intelligence, willpower, or luck, however, but a complex mixture of physical and psychological dependence.

Such dependence arises from the pleasurable feelings or calming effects drug users experience when taking drugs. It also results from the extreme physical and psychological distress—symptoms of *withdrawal*—that they feel when they try to quit or cut back. According to most drug addiction experts, drug addicts commonly develop both physical and psychological dependence, the mix depending on which drugs they abuse.

Drug addicts with a physical dependence suffer physical symptoms when they try to quit. This is due to a process called *tolerance*. With regular use, the body's response to a drug diminishes. As a result, individuals take larger and larger amounts of the drug to feel the drug's pleasurable effects. The body then becomes dependent upon, or addicted to, the drug. If an addicted person stops taking the drug, he or she experiences withdrawal symptoms that, depending on the drug, can last from a few days to several months.

Symptoms of withdrawal are often painful and can even be deadly. They range from chills, sweats, cramps, and body aches associated with heroin withdrawal to insomnia, convulsions, and delirium associated with withdrawal from severe addiction to *barbiturates* (drugs that give rise to a sense of calm or induce sleep). Drug users with a physical addiction usually continue taking drugs to avoid withdrawal.

About 90 per cent of drug addicts have a physical dependence

The author:

Dianne Hales, a free-lance writer from California, has written several books and numerous articles covering the subjects of drugs and drug abuse treatment.

on drugs, according to Richard Frances, professor of clinical psychiatry at the New Jersey Medical School in Newark. This physical dependence is usually coupled with some degree of psychological dependence.

Only about 10 per cent of addicts become psychologically addicted without becoming physically dependent on drugs, according to Frances, who is also founding president of the American Academy of Psychiatrists in Alcoholism and Addictions in Greenbelt, Md. Drug users with a psychological addiction take drugs to feel good or to relieve stress and anxiety. Even in cases where quitting drugs would cause only minor withdrawal symptoms, these addicts feel they cannot cope without drugs and continue to use them even when it interferes with work or family obligations. Some drug addicts become hooked on different combinations of drugs that produce a mixture of physical and psychological dependence.

Drugs that present a particularly high risk of physical addic-

Drug abuse in the United States

The federal budget for drug prevention and treatment has steadily increased since 1985, though enforcement efforts command most of the funds targeted for preventing illegal drug use, *below left*. A survey of people who admitted using illicit drugs at least once shows that in 1990, marijuana and cocaine were the most commonly used potentially addictive drugs, *below*.

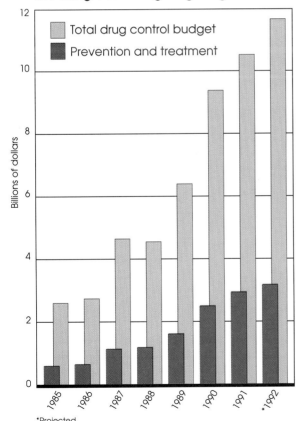

The rising costs of fighting drug abuse

- Total drug control budget
- Prevention and treatment

Billions of dollars

*Projected.
Source: Office of Management and Budget.

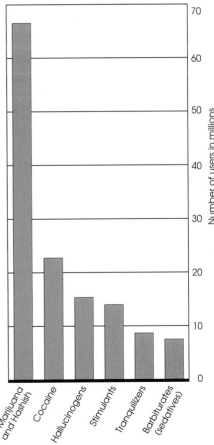

Nonmedical drug use, 1990

Number of users in millions

Marijuana and Hashish · Cocaine · Hallucinogens · Stimulants · Tranquilizers · Barbiturates (sedatives)

Source: National Institute on Drug Abuse.

Some commonly abused drugs

	Name	What they do	Immediate health effects	Long-term health effects	Withdrawal symptoms
STIMULANTS	**Amphetamines** (Dexedrine, Benzedrine)	Speed up physical and mental processes, lessen fatigue, boost energy, create sense of excitement.	Loss of appetite, blurred vision, headache, dizziness, sweating, sleeplessness, trembling, anxiety, hallucinations.	Malnutrition, depression, brain damage, stroke, heart failure.	Irritability, depression, disorientation, long periods of sleep, apathy.
	Cocaine and crack	Speed up physical and mental processes, create sense of heightened energy and confidence.	Headaches, exhaustion, blurred vision, nausea, seizures, loss of appetite, loss of sexual desire, impaired judgment, extreme suspiciousness, violence.	Damage to nasal lining, heart attack, stroke, hepatitis or AIDS (if injected). If used in pregnancy, danger of miscarriage, mild mental impairment, flat moods, emotional poverty for fetus.	Restlessness, cravings, irritability, depression, long periods of sleep, apathy.
DEPRESSANTS	**Barbiturates** (Nembutal, Seconal)	Produce mild intoxication, drowsiness and lethargy, decrease alertness.	Drowsiness, poor coordination, slurred speech, slowed breathing, weak and rapid heartbeat, impaired judgment, confusion, irritability.	Disrupted sleep, dangerously impaired vision. Risk of fatal overdose. If used in pregnancy, can cause birth defects.	Extreme anxiety, insomnia, delirium, and convulsions. Risk of death if withdrawal is abrupt.
	Tranquilizers (Valium, Xanax, Librium)	Slow down the central nervous system and relax muscles. Decrease alertness.	Slurred speech, drowsiness, stupor. Impaired judgment.	Physical and psychological dependence, fatal overdose.	Anxiety, insomnia, tremors, delirium, convulsions, coma, risk of death if withdrawal is abrupt.
CANNABIS	**Marijuana and hashish**	Relax the mind and body, heighten perceptions, alter mood.	Faster heartbeat and pulse, impaired perception and reactions, nausea, possible hallucinations, panic attacks, decreased motivation.	Impaired memory and coordination, increased heart rate and blood pressure. If used in pregnancy, babies are more likely to have lower birth weight and slower growth rate.	Occasional insomnia, hyperactivity, decreased appetite, mental confusion.
OPIATES	**Heroin, morphine, opium, codeine, and synthetic narcotics**	Relax central nervous system, relieve pain, produce sense of well-being.	Restlessness, nausea, vomiting, slowed breathing, weight loss, lethargy, mood swings, slurred speech, sweating.	Physical dependence; malnutrition; lower immunity; infections of the heart lining and valves; skin abscesses; congested lungs; tetanus; liver disease; hepatitis or AIDS (from contaminated needles); and fatal overdoses.	Watery eyes, runny nose, yawning, loss of appetite, irritability, tremors, panic, chills, sweating, cramps, nausea, diarrhea.
HALLUCINOGENS	**LSD and PCP**	Alter perceptions and produce hallucinations, which may be frightening or pleasurable.	Increased heart rate, nausea, sweating and trembling on LSD. PCP can produce delusions of great strength and invulnerability.	LSD may trigger disturbing flashbacks. Effects on fetus not known. PCP can cause stupor, increased heart rate, coma, convulsions, heart and lung failure, brain damage.	These drugs are not known to cause physical withdrawal symptoms.

tion include the *opiates*, such as heroin, morphine, and codeine. Drugs whose danger is chiefly psychological include marijuana and hallucinogens such as PCP and LSD. Drugs that present a risk of both physical and psychological addiction include cocaine and crack (which is derived from cocaine), amphetamines, barbiturates, and the class of drugs called *benzodiazepines*. This group of drugs includes alprazolam (Xanax), diazepam (Valium), and similar agents used for anxiety, panic attacks, or sleep problems. Ultimately, however, whether the dependence is physical, psychological, or both, the need for a drug can become so overpowering that nothing matters except getting more.

The most difficult step in breaking their habit is for drug users to acknowledge that they have a problem. Denial is one of the chief psychological symptoms of addiction. Refusing to admit even to themselves that they've lost control, users convince themselves that they're not hooked—and keep on using drugs.

Sometimes a crisis, such as an overdose or a medical emergency, forces users to recognize what drugs are doing to their lives. More often, family, friends, or co-workers must confront drug users and insist that they do something about their problem. Such intervention can be a turning point for addicts and their loved ones.

But even when drug users want to quit, finding help can be difficult. Although federal funding for treating drug abuse increased from $459 million in 1985 to $1.5 billion in 1991, the National Association of State Alcohol and Drug Abuse Directors in Washington, D.C., estimates that more than 66,000 addicts are on waiting lists for publicly supported treatment programs, including clinics for treating heroin addicts with *methadone*, a substitute drug that helps ease withdrawal from heroin and decreases addicts' craving for the drug. In some areas, the wait may be as long as five months.

Those who have private insurance or can afford the costs have more options available, including about 9,000 private residential treatment programs in the United States. These facilities are housed in hospitals or in separate centers that combine a campuslike atmosphere with that of a health-care organization. The average stay is 28 days and is often limited by the type of insurance the patient has. Fees range from $5,000 to $20,000 for a four-week stay, but about 80 per cent of these facilities also offer outpatient programs at much lower rates. Most residential treatment centers also provide one or two years of follow-up care—usually counseling designed to relieve the stress of withdrawal and to prevent relapses.

Treatment programs generally follow the same pattern, starting with *detoxification* (gradual, supervised withdrawal) and, if necessary, medications to help overcome physical dependence.

These measures are usually followed by intensive counseling, education, group support, psychotherapy, and self-help programs made up of former drug users, all in an attempt to break psychological dependence.

A combination of several approaches is most likely to be effective. "The challenge is finding the right combination for the right patient," explains addiction specialist Frances. "One of the reasons I feel more and more hopeful about drug therapy is that we are getting much better at matching the right patients with the right treatment approach."

For example, in the past, treatment often focused exclusively on drug use—even though, as researchers at the National Institute of Mental Health in Rockville, Md., reported in November 1990, half of all people with substance abuse problems also have a mental illness such as depression or anxiety. "These patients need treatment for drug dependence and for their psychiatric problem," says Frances. "One won't work without the other. Now they're much more likely to get both."

For many drug users, the first stage in the recovery process—withdrawal—remains the hardest. Individuals suffering from medical or psychiatric conditions or who are at high risk of fatal side effects from physically addictive drugs may require hospitalization. But most drug users do not have to be hospitalized as long as they receive careful monitoring and strong emotional support. However, a qualified psychiatrist should decide whether a person needs to enter a hospital for withdrawal.

Although withdrawal is commonly associated with physical symptoms and pain, the attempt to quit some drugs produces what many drug addiction specialists regard as psychological symptoms. These can be more difficult to treat than physical symptoms, according to experts. The most troublesome drugs in this category are the stimulants, including amphetamines and cocaine. Withdrawal from cocaine, which produces anxiety, irritability, and intense cravings, is especially hard to treat, health experts note.

Once heavy users of cocaine or crack cut down or stop using the drug, they "crash" for one to three days. They feel irritable, anxious, tired, and restless. They may sleep for long stretches or not be able to sleep at all. Some become severely depressed, extremely suspicious, even suicidal; their cravings become an all-consuming hunger. Although the cravings diminish after a few days, depression, anxiety, and irritability may persist for a week or more. During this time, former cocaine users describe themselves as feeling empty and incapable of enjoyment.

According to drug addiction experts, there is currently no medication universally recognized as an effective treatment for the craving cocaine addicts suffer during withdrawal. Because a major symptom of cocaine withdrawal is depression, some psychiatrists prescribe drugs from a class of medications called *tricyclic antidepressants* to ease that symptom.

For those addicted to heroin and other opiates, substitute-drug therapy with methadone is standard practice for withdrawal. Methadone, a synthetic opiate that reduces cravings for its stronger chemical relatives, eases the irritability, restlessness, depression, and flulike symptoms that accompany heroin withdrawal. Physicians gradually lower the dose of methadone, but do not necessarily eliminate it entirely. Methadone, unlike heroin, can be taken orally, and a dose can last as long as two or three days versus six to eight hours for heroin.

Because it blunts the euphoric effects of stronger opiates, methadone helps addicts resist the temptation to use heroin. When taken in the proper doses, it also produces a more balanced effect on users—unlike the dazed condition resulting from heroin use. This may allow some recovering drug abusers to lead relatively normal lives while still taking methadone.

Methadone has drawbacks, however. Because it is also an opiate, discontinuing the drug after prolonged use can cause symptoms that mimic those of heroin withdrawal, including shaking, chills, and cramps. Methadone withdrawal symptoms also last longer—up to two weeks—compared to five or six days for heroin withdrawal. For this reason, many methadone patients are never able to come off the drug.

Cocaine or heroin detoxification, though difficult, is rarely life-threatening. But withdrawal from other drugs can be. The greatest risk may come from benzodiazepines, the most commonly prescribed drugs in the United States. These drugs are classified as *depressants* because they depress, or slow down, body functions. They are legally prescribed as tranquilizers and sleeping pills. About 11 per cent of Americans take a benzodiazepine at least once in a 12-month period, reports Carl Salzman, an associate professor of psychiatry at Harvard Medical School in Boston. Salzman says that while 80 per cent of these people take them for less than 60 days and rarely develop a problem, some patients can end up taking too high a dose for too long a time. If they try to quit abruptly, they run the risk of seizures, coma, and death.

The key to safe detoxification from benzodiazepines is a very gradual, supervised reduction in dose over a period of weeks or months. During the initial stage of withdrawal, individuals may develop nausea, vomiting, malaise, weakness, anxiety or irritability, dizziness on standing, twitching of the tongue and eyelids, and severe insomnia. Yet even those who have been dependent on benzodiazepines for years do not crave the drug during withdrawal, as cocaine or heroin addicts do.

"Detox" from drugs—whether in a hospital or other drug treatment facility—is only the beginning of recovery. After their bodies are drug-free, most former users enroll in further treatment programs designed to help them through the initial period of abstinence. The most common are residential and outpatient programs.

Residential programs generally follow what is known as the "Minnesota model," a treatment approach developed in the 1950's at the Hazelden Rehabilitation Center, a recovery center in Center City, Minn. It offers a multidisciplinary approach that addresses the physical, emotional, spiritual, family, and social concerns of patients; offers a supportive community; and has a goal of abstinence and health.

Residential treatment usually includes individual *psychotherapy* (treatment for mental and emotional problems), *group therapy* (psychotherapy conducted with a group of patients), as well as *family therapy* (a form of group therapy conducted with members of a family). Individual psychotherapy aims to uncover and resolve some of the conflicts that may have led to a patient's drug abuse. Group therapy has a similar aim and allows patients to benefit from other patients' experiences. Family therapy stresses more open communication among a patient's family members to help resolve conflicts that may have led to the drug abuse.

Residential programs may also use relaxation techniques designed to help patients learn to reduce some of the stress that may lead to the desire to take drugs. Psychiatrists may also administer drugs to ease withdrawal.

Good residential programs usually provide follow-up care, or "aftercare," which begins after a patient leaves the facility. Aftercare usually includes weekly counseling sessions, as well as regular attendance at group support meetings held by organizations such as Narcotics Anonymous. These meetings are attended by people working together to overcome their addiction.

Long-time addicts may need more time away from the environment that helped produce their drug habit. To achieve this, some former addicts spend up to two years in publicly funded "therapeutic communities," which are run with a rigorous, almost military discipline. According to Dr. George De Leon, director of research and training for Therapeutic Communities of America in New York City, an organization for the advancement of therapeutic communities, most patients at these facilities are former cocaine addicts. But other recovering drug abusers can also benefit from them, he says. Many patients dislike the strict discipline in therapeutic communities, but others can find security and stability, as well as individual and group therapy, drug counseling, and job training at these facilities.

Cocaine babies

Their tiny faces contort. Their pencil-thin limbs quiver. Their mouths open in a cry, but they are so weak that they barely make a sound. Often born months too early and struggling to stay alive, these "crack babies"—whose mothers used crack or other forms of cocaine while pregnant—are the most poignant and innocent victims of drug addiction.

According to the President's 1990 National Drug Control Strategy Report, approximately 100,000 babies exposed to cocaine are born each year. All forms of cocaine affect an unborn child directly and indirectly. "Cocaine crosses the placenta (the organ by which a fetus is attached to the wall of the uterus) and causes fetal blood vessels to constrict, which can result in birth defects, strokes, and heart attacks," explains Ira Chasnoff, director of the National Association for Perinatal Addiction Research in Chicago. "Cocaine also can cause acute hypertension, constriction of blood vessels, and rapid heartbeat in the mother, all of which can impair blood flow to the fetus," he says.

As a result of prenatal drug effects, babies of crack-using mothers are at high risk of being stillborn, born prematurely, having low birth weight (less than 5.5 pounds, or 2.5 kilograms), birth defects, or breathing and neurological problems; and dying of *sudden infant death syndrome* (the medical term for the sudden, unexplained death of an apparently healthy baby).

About 18 per cent require weeks or months of intensive care after they're born. According to a 1989 study by the United States Department of Health and Human Services' Office of the Inspector General, costs for these babies during their first five years, including special education and hospital and foster care, average $166,000 per child. And treatment for emotionally disturbed children older than 5 years can cost even more—between $25,000 and $47,500 a year, according to the study.

No one knows what the future may hold as crack babies grow older, but experts caution that the widespread notion that such infants are permanently damaged has not been supported by good studies. "A lot depends on whether they get early intervention: speech therapy, physical therapy, neurological therapy, early education," observes Chasnoff, who has been studying crack babies from birth to age 5. "In general, development is normal, but they have some behavioral problems—short attention spans, difficulty following a sequence—that indicate they're at risk for learning disabilities and other problems," he says.

Ultimately, the best hope is prevention by providing drug treatment for pregnant women. "Therapy does work," emphasizes Chasnoff. "We've found that if pregnant women enter treatment and become drug-free by the sixth month, their babies avoid most medical complications. It's really best if the mother becomes drug-free by the fourth month. We provide parenting classes, home visits, and training in lifestyle skills, so that the mothers can learn how to take care of their babies and how to function in the world without turning to drugs."   [D. H.]

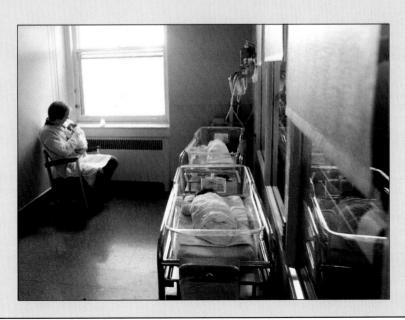

A volunteer "baby holder" at a New York City hospital cradles a "crack baby," *right*, an infant whose mother took crack cocaine during pregnancy. Exposure to crack and other forms of cocaine before birth may result in mental and physical impairment in newborns.

An experimental program at Lincoln Hospital in New York City uses acupuncture to treat cocaine addiction. Needles inserted in addicts' ears, *right*, seem to calm patients and help ease withdrawal from the drug.

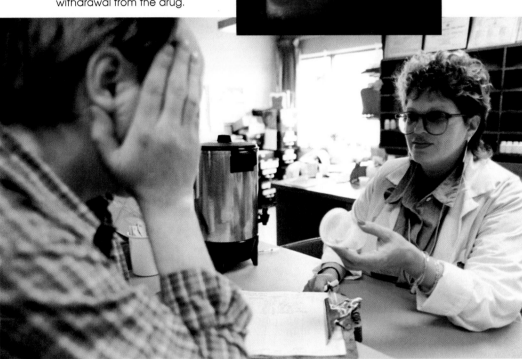

A counselor at a drug clinic dispenses methadone, a drug that reduces the craving for heroin and other opiates. Although methadone itself can cause addiction, experts agree that, if taken properly, its effects are less severe than those of heroin.

Many drug users prefer outpatient (nonresidential) programs, which permit them to go on with their daily lives as they undergo treatment. Outpatient programs usually resemble those at residential centers, with self-help groups, individual therapy, family therapy, and education programs. Most include regular urine testing to ensure that participants aren't using drugs. Some people in outpatient programs attend drug abuse treatment sessions four or five nights a week for six weeks at a treatment center; others participate in seven to eight days of eight-hour sessions followed by weekly group therapy. Drug abuse experts have found that outpatient programs are best suited for patients who can rely on supportive family members and friends, and who have not failed a previous attempt at outpatient treatment.

Experts disagree on the value of individual psychotherapy in treating drug abuse. Some maintain that psychotherapy can help people understand problems that contribute to the desire to

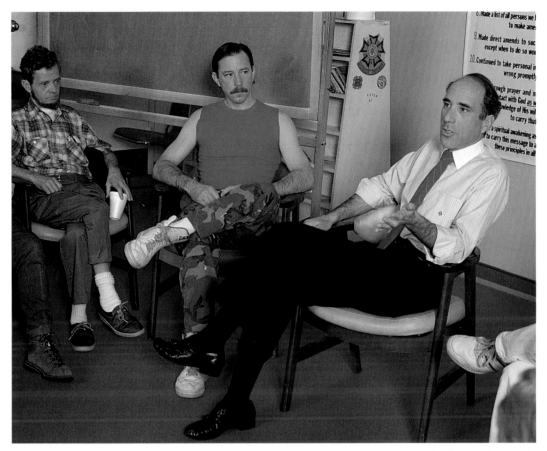

Under the guidance of a counselor, addicts in a therapy group share experiences and discuss their feelings about their addictions. Most treatment programs for substance abuse include such therapy to help members resolve problems that may have led to addictive behavior.

take drugs, and for those with a "dual diagnosis"—addiction plus a mental disorder—psychotherapy can be an essential part of recovery. Psychotherapy often centers on either *behavioral* or *cognitive* therapy.

Behavioral therapy focuses on correcting the way a person responds. Behavioral therapists believe that drug addicts can learn to refrain from drugs when faced with undesirable consequences as a result of continued drug use. One type of behavioral therapy is *contingency contracting* between a drug user and a therapist. With this method, the user signs a contract promising to stop taking drugs. The contract also states that the patient will give up something valuable, such as a car or a large sum of money, if he or she begins using drugs again. The patient then submits to urine tests to ensure compliance.

Cognitive therapy focuses on the way a person thinks and works to help a patient replace unrealistic thoughts with more realistic ones. For drug abusers, cognitive approaches emphasize education, such as identifying situations and feelings that lead to use or relapse and then learning how to avoid these situations or conquer the disturbing feelings. Many programs also teach social skills, such as assertiveness training, to be able to with-stand peer pressure to use drugs.

Group therapy brings together individuals with similar experiences to share their problems with honesty and empathy. As former users, members can spot attempts to lie or make excuses and can confront participants who aren't being honest. Some small groups use role-playing, in which individuals pretend to play other people's roles (such as that of a long-suffering spouse) to reveal hidden conflicts and emotions. A professional therapist guides the sessions.

Family therapy brings together drug users and their families so that addicts can better understand the damage their drug habit has done to their relationships. This process may be especially useful for the children of drug users, who may otherwise grow up trapped in unhealthy behavioral patterns caused by living with an addicted parent.

Self-help programs, many modeled after Alcoholics Anonymous (AA), also play a role in treating drug abusers. Founded in 1935, AA is the oldest, largest, and most successful self-help program in the world. As many as 200 other programs, including Narcotics Anonymous and Cocaine Anonymous, are based on the spiritual 12-step program of AA.

The basis of all 12-step programs is the idea that members are powerless when it comes to their drug-using behavior and that only a "higher power" can help them stop taking drugs. Members are free to define their "higher power" as they wish, but the desire to stop must come from the drug user. People generally attend meetings every day when they first begin recovery; most programs recommend 90 meetings in 90 days. Many people taper off to one or two meetings a week as their recovery progresses.

What are the odds that someone hooked on drugs will break the habit for good? The Comprehensive Assessment of Treatment Outcome Research (CATOR) in St. Paul, Minn., a research organization that tracks the effectiveness of drug treatment programs, estimates that about half of those who complete a treatment program of any sort remain drug- and alcohol-free a year later. Ten to 20 per cent of people in this group return to drugs during the next two to five years. But the most important factors in drug treatment, according to CATOR Executive Director Norman Hoffmann, is time. The longer drug abusers remain free of drugs in a treatment program or self-help support group, says Hoffmann, the better their chances of staying off drugs.

CATOR tracked 1,900 drug patients released from 21- and 28-day residential treatment facilities in 1987 and 1988 and found that 76 per cent of those who attended weekly meetings of support groups such as Narcotics Anonymous were still drug-free one year later. This compares with 52 per cent for those who attended no such meetings, reports Hoffmann.

Some therapists believe that addicts are never truly cured, but as with diabetics or arthritics, they can learn to live fulfilling lives in spite of their illness. Doing so demands self-esteem, confidence, and motivation. "Drug addiction is a highly treatable disease when patients are motivated and have something to lose if they go back to drugs," says Frances. "Addicts have to feel there's something better than drugs."

But the sober reality is that even the best treatment may never help all drug abusers. According to the Institute of Medicine's 1990 report, drug abuse and dependence are chronic, relapsing disorders. "As with medical therapies for cancer and other diseases," the report notes, "the best interventions work only partially—some of the time and for some of the people."

After two, three, or more attempts at quitting, many drug users do find a method that helps them quit drugs and rebuild their lives. Often the toughest programs yield the greatest success. At Phoenix House, a therapeutic community in New York City, the rules and regulations are so strict that as many as 40 per cent of the residents leave within the first 90 days. Among those who hang in and complete the program, however, 75 per cent remain drug-free, crime-free, and employed five years after graduation from the program. For them—as for all the others who overcome a drug habit—treatment proves to be both an end and a beginning: the end of a past haunted by drugs and the beginning of a future brightened by hope.

For more information:
Groups and organizations that offer help and advice concerning drug abuse treatment include:

The American Council for Drug Education
204 Monroe St., Suite 110
Rockville, MD 20850
(301-294-0600).

Narcotics Anonymous
P.O. Box 9999
Van Nuys, CA 91409
(818-780-3951).

National Council on Alcoholism and Drug Dependence
12 W. 21st St.
New York, NY 10010
(212-206-6770).

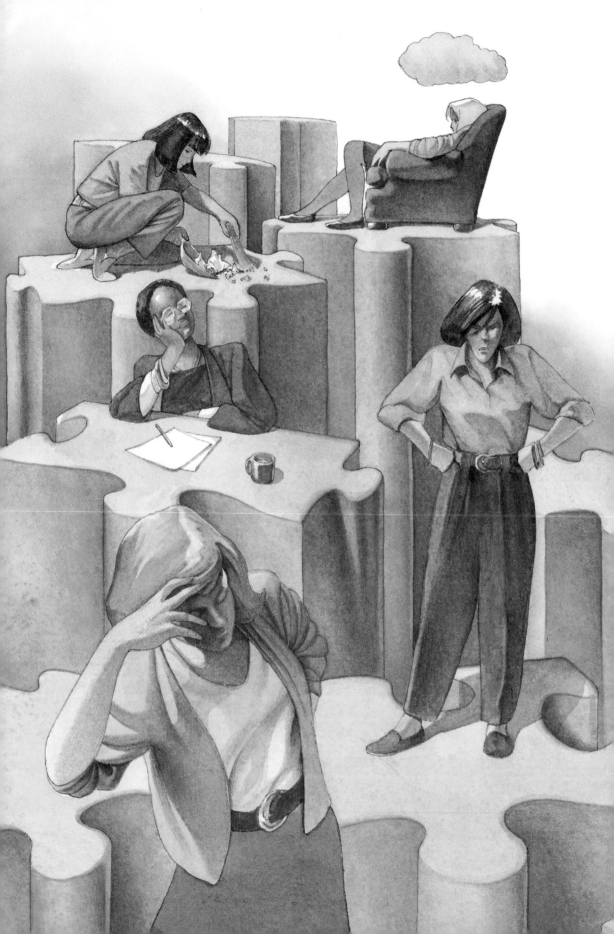

The Puzzle of PMS

By Sally Squires

Although researchers have not yet
identified the cause of premenstrual
syndrome—nor a cure—many women
have found effective ways to cope
with this frustrating condition.

Florence, a busy and successful physician, noticed a disturbing
pattern in her behavior. Like many women, Florence was accustomed to irritability, feelings of sadness, and breast tenderness
for a few days before her menstrual period began. But recently,
her symptoms had become worse.

Now, in the week before her period was to start, Florence felt
profoundly depressed. Her breasts became painfully sore, and
she often developed throbbing headaches that left her nauseous
and unable to tolerate light. Even more troubling to Florence—
as well as to her husband and two young daughters—were her
swift mood changes. Normally a calm and organized person, she
found that routine family matters could suddenly overwhelm
her. But within about a day after her menstrual period began,
she felt better.

Florence's problem? Premenstrual syndrome (PMS)—a group
of physical and psychological symptoms that fewer than 10 per
cent of women experience in the 7 to 10 days before the start of
their menstrual period. Despite 50 years of study, PMS remains
both vexing and controversial. Researchers still have not identified the cause of PMS—or even determined whether there is one

Glossary

Biobehavioral problem: A condition with both physical and emotional effects.

Estrogen: One of a group of female hormones that have many effects on female sexual development and reproduction.

Follicular phase: The first phase of the menstrual cycle, which begins on the first day of menstrual bleeding.

Luteal phase: The final phase of the menstrual cycle, which begins after ovulation.

Menstrual cycle: The repeating cycle of changes that prepare a woman's body for pregnancy.

Ovulation: The process by which a mature egg is released from an ovary.

Progesterone: A female hormone that prepares the *uterus* (womb) so a fertilized egg may implant in it.

The author:

Sally Squires is a health and medical writer for *The Washington Post.*

cause or many. Nor do researchers know why some women develop PMS and others do not.

In part, the lack of answers stems from a historic failure of many doctors to take women's complaints about menstrual problems seriously, as well as from a lack of funding for studies of health issues affecting women, including PMS. Another factor contributing to our poor understanding of PMS is the poor quality of some earlier studies of premenstrual problems. For example, some researchers failed to rule out whether the women in their study suffered from other medical problems that may produce symptoms similar to those linked to PMS. As a result, these studies produced erroneous or misleading conclusions.

The confusing nature of the syndrome itself has made it difficult for scientists to find answers. Nearly 150 symptoms have been associated with PMS by various researchers. Some women experience only two or three symptoms. Other women experience more. The symptoms may vary in number and intensity from month to month in the same woman.

Some researchers have even questioned whether PMS actually exists as a medical condition. Others have debated whether it is a medical or psychological condition. Some observers, while agreeing that PMS exists, have argued against classifying PMS as an illness at all because of fears that such a categorization would be used to justify job discrimination against women.

B y the mid-1980's, however, many women's health experts had come to classify PMS as a *biobehavioral problem*—that is, a condition with both physical and emotional effects. Common physical changes include breast tenderness, food cravings and binge eating, headaches, fatigue, constipation, acne, hot flashes, and abdominal swelling and water retention that can cause bloating and temporary weight gain. Among the most commonly reported behavioral changes are irritability, anxiety, tension, depression, mood swings, inability to concentrate, sleep disturbances, and a change in sex drive.

PMS and ordinary "premenstrual tension"—the temporary changes that are a normal part of the week or so before a menstrual period—share many symptoms. The difference between the two is a matter of degree. In women with PMS, the symptoms are severe enough to interfere with everyday activities and to disrupt relationships with others to some extent. But just as the overwhelming majority of women with premenstrual tension manage to tend to their families, jobs, and other daily responsibilities, so too, most women with PMS manage their lives without becoming derailed by their condition. Women with PMS may feel more vulnerable to stress, however, and may need to make an extra effort on some days.

Symptoms of PMS can appear at any time during a woman's

childbearing years, but once they occur, they usually continue monthly until a woman stops menstruating. A number of studies have shown that, for unknown reasons, the risk of PMS increases with age; most sufferers are in their 30's or 40's. Studies also show that the more children a woman has, the greater is the likelihood that she will experience some PMS symptoms—though the reason is unclear.

Women who have a history of *postpartum depression* (depression after childbirth) or a psychological disorder such as depression are more likely than other women to suffer from PMS, several studies have found. Women who have a close relative with depression are also more likely to develop the condition. Scientists have found that the syndrome is more common among divorced or separated women than among single and married women. Again, researchers are not sure why.

The idea that the days preceding menstruation could pose physical and psychological problems for some women is not new. The ancient Greek physician Hippocrates (460?-377? B.C.), who is considered the father of Western medicine, linked menstruation with delusions, mania, and suicidal thoughts. Other references to the menstrual cycle's effects on women's behavior can be found in ancient religious works. Generally, however, these comments were not attempts to explore a health issue affecting women. Instead, they often served as justification for the view that women are weaker and more emotional than men.

In the 1900's, however, premenstrual symptoms began to generate serious interest among researchers. In 1931, two American physicians, endocrinologist Robert T. Frank and psychiatrist Karen Horney, separately described versions of what is now called PMS. British physi-

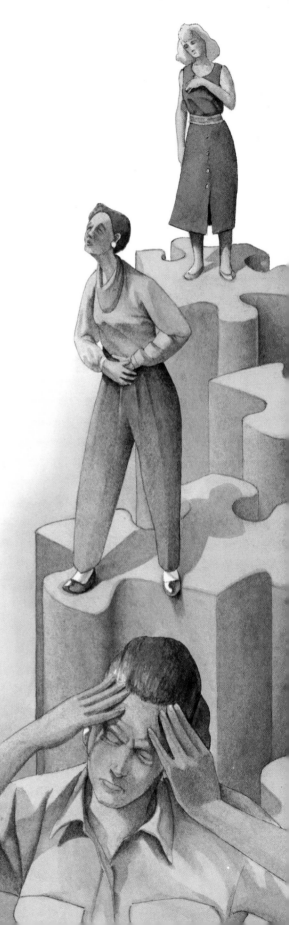

Physical symptoms

Women with PMS may suffer a variety of physical symptoms. These include headaches, breast soreness, constipation, back pain, fatigue, and water retention that can cause abdominal swelling and temporary weight gain.

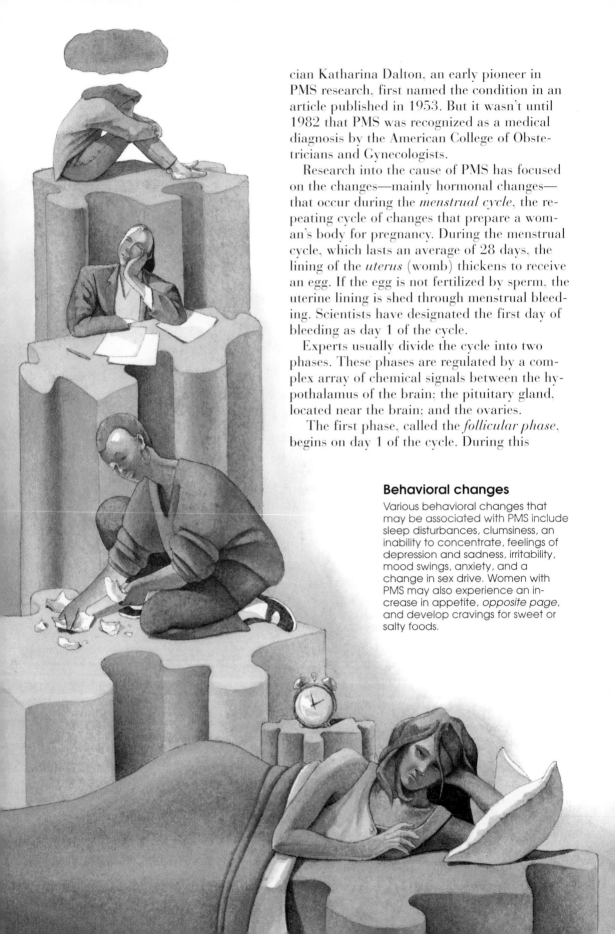

cian Katharina Dalton, an early pioneer in PMS research, first named the condition in an article published in 1953. But it wasn't until 1982 that PMS was recognized as a medical diagnosis by the American College of Obstetricians and Gynecologists.

Research into the cause of PMS has focused on the changes—mainly hormonal changes—that occur during the *menstrual cycle*, the repeating cycle of changes that prepare a woman's body for pregnancy. During the menstrual cycle, which lasts an average of 28 days, the lining of the *uterus* (womb) thickens to receive an egg. If the egg is not fertilized by sperm, the uterine lining is shed through menstrual bleeding. Scientists have designated the first day of bleeding as day 1 of the cycle.

Experts usually divide the cycle into two phases. These phases are regulated by a complex array of chemical signals between the hypothalamus of the brain; the pituitary gland, located near the brain; and the ovaries.

The first phase, called the *follicular phase*, begins on day 1 of the cycle. During this

Behavioral changes

Various behavioral changes that may be associated with PMS include sleep disturbances, clumsiness, an inability to concentrate, feelings of depression and sadness, irritability, mood swings, anxiety, and a change in sex drive. Women with PMS may also experience an increase in appetite, *opposite page*, and develop cravings for sweet or salty foods.

phase, an egg matures in one of two ovaries. At the same time, cells in the ovary increase their production of the hormone *estrogen*. Menstrual bleeding stops as estrogen levels rise, and on about day 5 of the cycle, the lining of the uterus begins to thicken again to receive a fertilized egg.

The egg is released from the ovary on about day 14 of the cycle, a process called *ovulation*. After ovulation, the second part of the menstrual cycle, the *luteal phase*, begins. During this phase, the production of the hormone *progesterone* rises as the egg is released from the ovary. This causes an increase in blood supply to the uterus, along with other changes that help prepare the body for pregnancy. Meanwhile, the egg leaves the ovary and travels down a Fallopian tube to the uterus.

If the egg is fertilized by a sperm, it may implant in the wall of the uterus and develop into a fetus. If the egg is not fertilized, estrogen and progesterone levels fall, and the lining of the uterus—and the unfertilized egg—are shed.

Although researchers have discovered what appear to be links between PMS and excesses or deficiencies of certain body chemicals, the cause of the syndrome remains frustratingly unclear. Many researchers have theorized that PMS may be caused by either inadequate or excessive levels of progesterone because symptoms appear during the luteal phase of the menstrual cycle—when progesterone levels rise—and disappear around the onset of menstrual bleeding—when levels of the two hormones fall. But studies of progesterone levels in women with PMS have failed to demonstrate that the women have either inadequate or excessive levels of the hormone.

Similarly, most women with PMS who have been given either drugs to reduce progesterone levels or progesterone supplements in research studies have not obtained relief from their symptoms. For example, researchers at the National Institute of Mental Health (NIMH) and the National Institute of Child Health and Human Development, both in Bethesda, Md., reported in 1989 that about half of the women

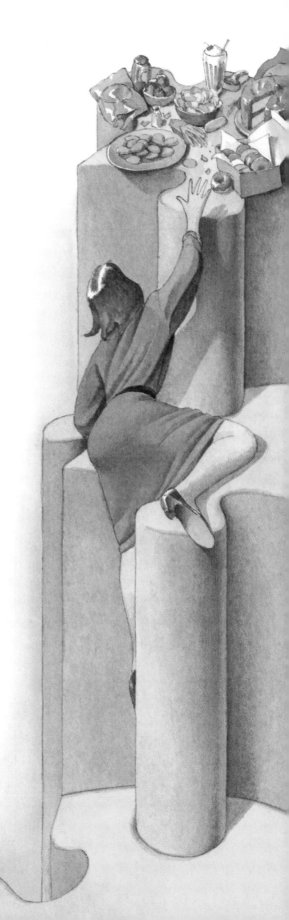

in their study who were given a drug to block the production of progesterone still experienced PMS symptoms. Moreover, six of seven small studies conducted between 1975 and 1986 failed to confirm that progesterone supplements were any more effective than a *placebo* (an inactive substance) in treating PMS. The seventh study, which involved 23 women, found that progesterone helped reduce swelling, hot flashes, and water retention.

Although all but one of these studies failed to demonstrate the effectiveness of progesterone therapy for women with PMS, some researchers and physicians continued to promote the use of the hormone. They argued that the studies of the therapeutic value of the hormone were flawed because of their small size and the low doses of progesterone given to the women.

But a more recent study of progesterone therapy—the first large-scale evaluation of the hormone as a PMS treatment—also found no benefit. Researchers from the University of Pennsylvania in Philadelphia reported in July 1990 that they had divided 168 women with PMS into two groups. The first group used progesterone daily on days 16 through 28 of two menstrual cycles. The second group of women used a placebo. The researchers reported that the progesterone was no more effective than the placebo in easing PMS symptoms.

Another line of research into the cause of PMS has focused on *prolactin*. This hormone, produced by the pituitary gland, is essential for the development of the breasts during pregnancy and for the production of breast milk after childbirth. Some researchers suggested that prolactin might play a role in causing the water retention, bloating, and breast tenderness associated with PMS. But studies failed to show that women with PMS have higher levels of prolactin than do women without the syndrome. On the other hand, some studies have found that the drug *bromocriptine*, which reduces prolactin levels, can ease breast swelling and tenderness. Bromocriptine can also produce such unpleasant side effects as nausea, dizziness, and nasal congestion, however.

Researchers have also explored whether vitamin deficiencies can trigger hormonal changes that may, in turn, cause the symptoms of PMS. Supplements of vitamins E and B_6, for example, have often been touted as a remedy. A 1986 study by researchers at North Charles Hospital in Baltimore found that women who took vitamin E for three months reported that they experienced a 27 to 42 per cent reduction in the severity of their symptoms. But there has been little other research on vitamin E's effect on PMS.

Studies of the effectiveness of vitamin B_6 have been more extensive, but the results have been inconclusive. A 1972 British study and a 1985 Scandinavian study both found that women

The menstrual cycle

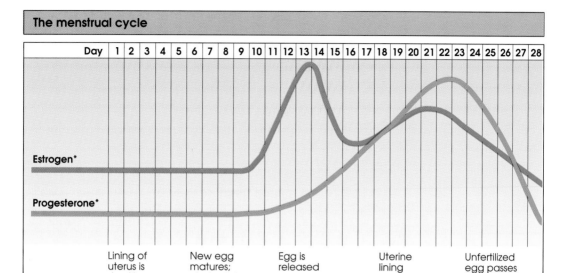

Day	1	2	3	4	5	6	7	8	9	10	11	12	13	14	15	16	17	18	19	20	21	22	23	24	25	26	27	28

Estrogen*

Progesterone*

Lining of uterus is shed by menstrual bleeding

New egg matures; uterine lining thickens

Egg is released

Uterine lining thickens further

Unfertilized egg passes through uterus

*Shows relative changes in hormones over time, not actual amounts.

with PMS who took vitamin B_6 supplements obtained no more relief from their symptoms than did women who took a placebo.

One chemical that continues to intrigue PMS researchers, however, is *serotonin*, a *neurotransmitter* that helps regulate mood and appetite. (Neurotransmitters are chemicals that permit messages to be carried from one nerve cell to another.) Scientists have found that people who are depressed may not be able to break down serotonin as efficiently as people who are not depressed.

In 1987, obstetrician Andrea J. Rapkin of the University of California at Los Angeles reported that blood levels of serotonin in a group of 14 women with PMS dropped in the few days before menstrual bleeding began. In contrast, serotonin levels remained constant in the women in a control group. Rapkin's study suggests that an imbalance in serotonin may be linked to the feelings of depression and the severe mood swings associated with PMS. Future studies with larger numbers of women may clarify what role, if any, serotonin plays in PMS.

Some researchers suggest that serotonin, which suppresses the desire for carbohydrates, may also be linked to the food cravings and binge eating sometimes associated with PMS. Studies have shown that drugs that increase serotonin levels—including a drug called *d-fenfluramine*—can suppress the appetite for carbohydrates. This drug, which is permitted only for experimental use in the United States, is used in some other countries for the treatment of a condition called *carbohydrate-craving obesity*.

A team of researchers headed by neuroscientist Richard

The menstrual cycle
This approximately monthly cycle prepares a woman's body for pregnancy. Its phases are regulated mainly by changing levels of the hormones estrogen and progesterone. Scientists believe that subtle abnormalities in the levels of such hormones during the second half of the menstrual cycle may be linked to the symptoms of PMS, though studies have thus far failed to support this hypothesis.

Wurtman of the Massachusetts Institute of Technology in Cambridge, Mass., administered d-fenfluramine to 17 women with PMS over the course of three menstrual cycles. All the women had been suffering from carbohydrate cravings and depressed moods. The women also received placebos for another three menstrual cycles. The researchers found that d-fenfluramine significantly reduced the feelings of depression and carbohydrate cravings in the women. But because this drug eases only some PMS symptoms, it is not considered a cure for PMS.

Some PMS researchers have focused their attention on *beta-endorphin*, one of the *opioids*, chemicals produced by the brain that help relieve pain and promote feelings of well-being. Obstetrician C. James Chuong of the Baylor College of Medicine in Houston in the 1980's showed that blood levels of beta-endorphin dropped sharply in many women with PMS during the luteal phase of their menstrual cycle. In contrast, the levels of the chemical in women without PMS symptoms remained high.

In a 1989 study, Chuong also found that when women with PMS took *naloxone*, a drug that prevents the breakdown of beta-endorphin and other opioids in the body, blood levels of beta-endorphin stayed high in about 70 per cent of the women studied. At the same time, the women reported that the severity of their PMS symptoms dropped sharply. The findings suggest that beta-endorphins play some role in causing PMS. But even if this is the case, the chemicals cannot be the sole cause, because not all the women in the study benefited from naloxone.

Diagnosing PMS
Women suspected of having PMS are urged to track their symptoms daily for several months to determine if a pattern exists, *opposite page*. Tracking increases awareness of what symptoms exist and when they may appear; most women with PMS experience symptoms only during the second half of the menstrual cycle. Women may also record which coping strategies they follow and how effectively these steps relieve their symptoms.

Although most researchers continue to argue for a direct connection between PMS and the menstrual cycle, a study published in April 1991 suggested that such a linkage is far from clear-cut. Researchers at NIMH and the National Institute of Child Health and Human Development administered a drug called *mifepristone* to women with PMS in the middle of their luteal phase. The drug triggered the onset of menstrual bleeding within 72 hours, thus shortening the luteal phase. The researchers found, however, that the women continued to experience the PMS symptoms they normally experienced—though their symptoms usually disappeared with the onset of bleeding.

The researchers suggested two explanations for their findings. They theorized that the hormonal changes responsible for PMS symptoms may occur early in the luteal cycle. Or, they speculated, PMS may be a cyclic mood disorder that is synchronized with—but not caused by—the menstrual cycle.

Researchers also remain puzzled over the cause of *late luteal phase dysphoric disorder* (LLPD), believed to be a severe form of PMS that affects less than 5 per cent of women with the syndrome. Several studies have linked LLPD with *bipolar disorder* (also known as *manic-depressive disorder*), a form of depression

Tracking Symptoms of PMS

Tracking and scoring symptoms

Symptoms commonly associated with PMS are listed on the left side of the chart. There are also blank spaces for inserting additional symptoms. Each day, women should note which symptoms, if any, they experience and rate their severity.

A rating of 1 indicates mild discomfort; 2, moderate discomfort that does not interfere with normal activities; 3, serious discomfort that interferes with normal activities; 4, disabling symptoms. Day 1 is the first day of menstrual bleeding. Circle the remaining menstrual period days.

	Day	1	2	3	4	5	6	7	8	9	10	11	12	13	14	15	16	17	18	19	20	21	22	23	24	25	26	27	28	29	30	31	32	33	34	35	36
Symptoms	Anxiety and tension																																				
	Binge eating and food cravings																																				
	Bloating																																				
	Breast Soreness																																				
	Feelings of depression																																				
	Headache																																				
	Inability to concentrate																																				
	Irritability																																				
	Sleep disturbances																																				

Coping strategies

Steps often taken to ease the symptoms of PMS are listed on the left side of the chart. Also included are blank spaces for inserting additional steps. Each day, women should note which steps, if any, they took and rate how helpful the steps were. A rating of 1 indicates not helpful; 2, moderately helpful; 3, very helpful.

	Day	1	2	3	4	5	6	7	8	9	10	11	12	13	14	15	16	17	18	19	20	21	22	23	24	25	26	27	28	29	30	31	32	33	34	35	36
Coping strategies	Exercised																																				
	Relaxed																																				
	Received support from others																																				
	Avoided caffeine																																				
	Reduced salt and sugar intake																																				
	Ate regular, well-balanced meals																																				
	Pampered self																																				
	Got enough sleep																																				

Critically reviewed by Jean Endicott, Ph.D., New York State Psychiatric Institute.

that affects both men and women. These patients alternate between deep depression and feelings of euphoria. As a result, some researchers have theorized that there may be a biological or genetic factor that makes women vulnerable to both bipolar depression and LLPD.

In a 1985 study of 35 women with PMS, clinical psychologist Jean Endicott and her colleagues at the New York State Psychiatric Institute in New York City found that women with bipolar depression were much more prone to severe mood changes prior to their menstrual periods than were women who had not been diagnosed as being depressed. They also found that women in the study who experienced moderate to severe mood changes prior to monthly bleeding were much more likely to have had an episode of major depression.

As research continues into PMS, many scientists are concluding that the syndrome probably describes a set of symptoms caused by a wide range of problems. PMS could reflect imbalances and irregularities in the ratios of a variety of hormones and other chemicals in the body. These, in turn, could work independently or together to trigger changes in the brain and elsewhere that could produce symptoms. As the ability to measure and identify substances involved in the menstrual cycle improves, researchers believe that they will be better able to pinpoint the cause—or various causes—of PMS.

But for now, the lack of a specific biological abnormality detectable by a medical test makes diagnosing PMS somewhat difficult. Generally, doctors first rule out other medical conditions that could cause symptoms similar to those of PMS. One of the

Easing symptoms

Although there is no cure for PMS, certain changes in daily habits can help ease symptoms and improve a woman's ability to cope with the syndrome. These life-style changes include getting enough sleep, practicing relaxation techniques, exercising regularly, and eating well-balanced meals. Watching salt and sugar intake can also reduce water retention and help prevent weight gain.

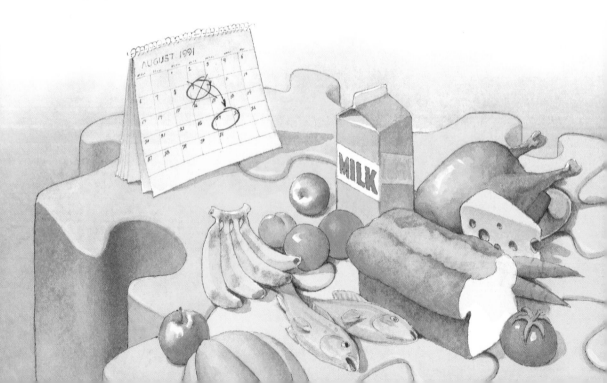

most common of these conditions is *fibrocystic breast changes*, a condition in which noncancerous lumps of tissue in the breast swell and cause pain. Another condition that may cause PMS-like symptoms is *endometriosis*, in which tissue similar to that found in the lining of the uterus grows in the ovaries, Fallopian tubes, and other areas of the abdominal cavity. During menstrual bleeding, this tissue bleeds lightly, irritating nearby tissue and causing pain. *Dysmenorrhea*, painful menstrual cramps, is also sometimes confused with PMS. Other health problems that may produce PMS-like symptoms include allergies, thyroid problems, diabetes, depression, and stress.

The key to diagnosing PMS is finding a pattern. The best way for a woman who suspects she has PMS to do this is to keep a diary and record her daily symptoms for two or three cycles. This involves tracking what symptoms she has, when they occur, and how severe they are. Some women also jot down their feelings in a daily log. They note days when they feel angry or upset or have emotional outbursts.

If a woman's symptoms last throughout the month, PMS can

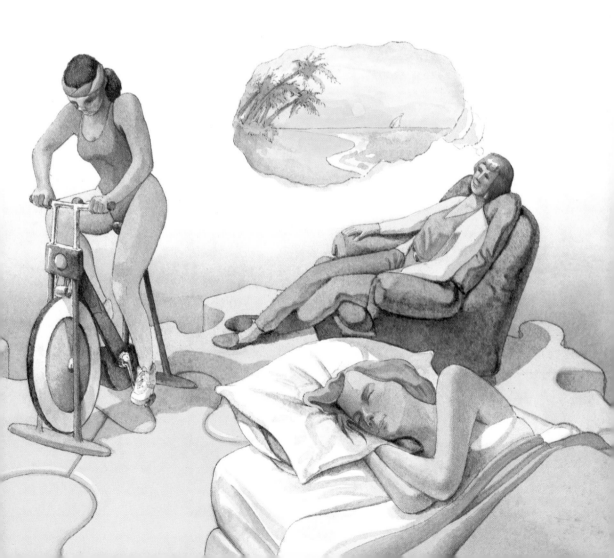

usually be ruled out. The overwhelming majority of women with PMS experience at least two symptom-free weeks during each menstrual cycle. In addition, symptoms cluster during the second half of the menstrual cycle. Relief also follows a pattern; symptoms almost always subside either the day before, the day of, or the day following the start of menstrual bleeding.

Once PMS has been diagnosed, a doctor will attempt to help the woman find a way to relieve her symptoms. Although there is no proven treatment for PMS, most women with the syndrome benefit from a combination of three therapies: life-style changes, medication, and counseling and support.

Physicians advise that life-style changes, such as getting enough sleep, can not only ease the symptoms of PMS but also help reduce the stress associated with the syndrome. Exercising regularly can reduce stress and muscle tension, help control appetite, and create a sense of well-being. Progressive relaxation, a technique that involves deep breathing exercises and gradual relaxation of muscles, can also help alleviate stress and sometimes reduce symptoms.

Dietary changes may also benefit some women with PMS. For example, eating five or six small, well-balanced meals during the day may help prevent the hunger that may lead to binge-eating. Some doctors also recommend that women with PMS reduce the amount of caffeine and salt in their diet. Too much caffeine may aggravate such PMS symptoms as anxiety, insom-

Emotional support

Women who are troubled by PMS symptoms may find participating in a support group helpful. Such groups provide an opportunity for women with PMS to share their feelings about their symptoms and to learn new coping strategies.

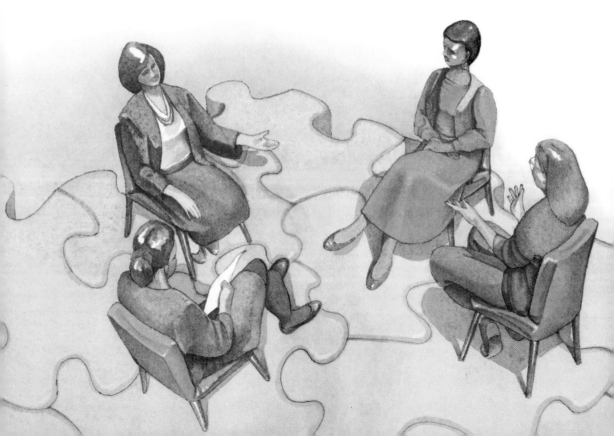

nia, nervousness, and irritability. Caffeine can also worsen headaches or even lead to rebound headaches, which appear about 12 to 24 hours after the last dose of caffeine is consumed.

By reducing salt intake, some women find that they can reduce some of the bloating and water retention associated with PMS. Nutritionists recommend eating fresh food rather than processed foods, which generally contain higher amounts of salt.

Doctors also caution against drinking too much alcohol, which can be relaxing in small amounts but in larger quantities may lead to hangovers and increased irritability. Candy, cookies, and other sweets should be avoided or eaten in moderation. These foods may temporarily lift spirits, but once the sugar "high" wears off, they can leave PMS sufferers feeling worse than ever.

Many women also find over-the-counter painkillers, such as *ibuprofen*, helpful in alleviating the headaches and muscle and joint pain that may accompany PMS. If taken in large amounts or for long periods, however, these drugs can produce such serious side effects as stomach ulcers and kidney damage.

Other options include prescription drugs. *Diuretics*, which stimulate urine output, can help reduce bloating. But some women find that bloating increases again for several days after they have stopped taking these drugs. *Antidepressants* (drugs that alleviate the symptoms of depression) and *tranquilizers* (drugs that produce a calming effect) may help control some of the mood swings and depression associated with PMS. The antidepressant medication *Prozac* is one of the most commonly prescribed drugs for women with PMS. However, people taking this drug should be carefully monitored by their doctor for possible side effects. In addition, tranquilizers may be addictive.

One of the most helpful coping strategies for women with PMS may be the simplest: support groups. These groups help women realize that they are not alone in their problem and enable them to share their feelings about their experience. Some women also turn to psychotherapy to help them deal with their mood swings and depression.

Sometimes simply planning ahead can help. Knowing that symptoms are likely to occur on certain days can help women with PMS work around their problem. They can, for example, be sure to get enough sleep and postpone major decisions. Knowing that there is a time limit on their symptoms also helps many women with PMS feel more in control of their discomfort.

For further reading:

"Premenstrual Syndrome." The American College of Obstetricians and Gynecologists, 409 12th Street SW, Washington, DC 20024-2188

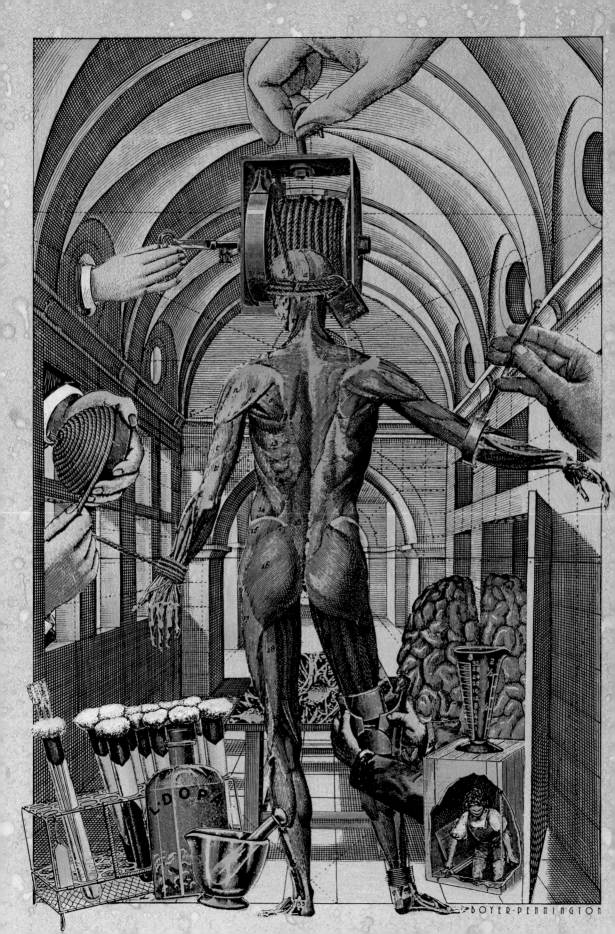

Scientists believe they are close to
finding the cause—or causes—of
Parkinson's disease, a brain disorder
that results in a gradual loss of
muscle control.

Closing in on Parkinson's Disease

By Michael Woods

Deep within the brain, something goes wrong. Slowly, imperceptibly, cells producing an important brain chemical deteriorate and die. As the damage progresses, muscle movements, orchestrated by the brain, become increasingly erratic, and the patient experiences a growing feeling of helplessness. Once the ruler of his or her body, the person may now feel more like a puppet manipulated by unseen strings.

This is *Parkinson's disease*, one of the most common of all nervous system disorders. Some 500,000 people in the United States, most of them over age 50, suffer from this disorder, which afflicts men and women equally. Although Parkinson's disease is rarely fatal, it can so weaken patients that they may die from infections or other complications.

For many years, Parkinson's disease remained a mystery; researchers could find no reason why the chemical-producing cells died, and doctors could offer patients no hope for recovery. Sufferers took drugs that temporarily improved their symptoms and learned as best they could to cope with the disease when the symptoms grew worse—as they inevitably did.

Today, Parkinson's disease is still a mystery, but scientists

Glossary

Basal ganglia: A group of structures in the center of the brain that are involved in coordinating movement.

Dopamine: A neurotransmitter that is in short supply in the brains of Parkinson's disease patients.

L-dopa: A drug that is converted to dopamine in the brain and used to treat many Parkinson's disease patients.

Neuron: A nerve cell in the brain or in another part of the nervous system.

Neurotoxin: A substance that harms or kills neurons.

Neurotransmitter: A chemical "messenger" that transmits nerve impulses from one neuron to another.

Substantia nigra: A dopamine-producing group of cells in the basal ganglia.

The author:

Michael Woods is science editor of the *Toledo Blade* and the author of many articles on scientific and medical topics.

think they are well on the way to solving it. Evidence compiled since the early 1980's lends increasing support to the theory that many cases of the disorder are caused by *toxins* (poisons) in the environment that may slowly kill certain brain cells. While investigators continue to pursue this line of research, other scientists are developing new surgical and drug treatments for Parkinson's disease. For the first time, there may be hope that this devastating condition might be prevented or cured.

Symptoms of the disease

Parkinson's disease is named for James Parkinson, a British physician who first described the disorder. In his "Essay on the Shaking Palsy," published in 1817, Parkinson wrote of patients afflicted by "involuntary tremulous motion, with lessened muscular power."

Symptoms are usually mild at first and progress slowly. In hindsight, many patients cannot pinpoint the time when their symptoms began. The first signs may include neck and shoulder pain, fatigue, and a feeling of exhaustion after mild exercise. Patients may have difficulty fastening buttons, brushing their teeth, or performing other tasks requiring dexterity.

Many patients have such symptoms for months before being diagnosed with Parkinson's disease. The physician may attribute a patient's vague complaints to overwork, depression, or other disorders. There is no X-ray scan or other test to diagnose the disorder; such tests are useful only to rule out the possibility of other conditions that can be confused with the early stages of Parkinson's disease. In most cases, the patient is not diagnosed until one or more of the three hallmarks of Parkinson's disease—*tremor, rigidity,* and a general slowness of movement called *bradykinesia*—finally appears.

Tremor, a trembling of the limbs, usually begins in one hand or foot. Hand tremors are often a more complex back-and-forth movement of the thumb and fingers, as if the patient were rolling a marble between the thumb and forefinger. Physicians of the 1800's, who used the same motion to prepare medicines by hand, described the tremor as "pill rolling," a term still applied today. Tremors tend to occur when a limb is at rest and diminish when it is in motion. They disappear during sleep or when the patient is at ease and become more severe during stress.

Rigidity is a specific type of muscle stiffness that afflicts Parkinson's disease patients, preventing smooth, even movements of the limbs. Physicians describe it as "cogwheel rigidity." When, for instance, the doctor rotates the patient's hand in an arc, the hand resists and moves with a succession of jerks, as though the cogs of a gear were catching in the wrist joint. Muscles look and feel stiff because they are flexed even when at rest.

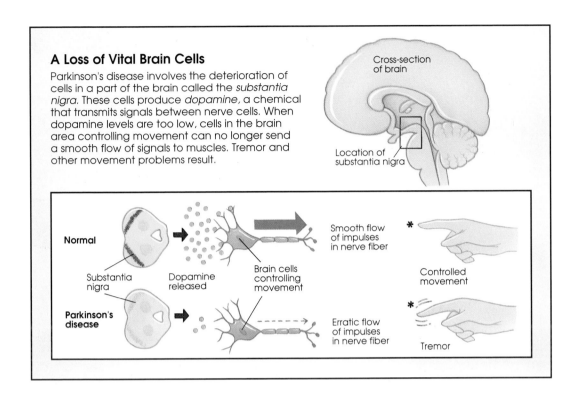

A Loss of Vital Brain Cells

Parkinson's disease involves the deterioration of cells in a part of the brain called the *substantia nigra*. These cells produce *dopamine*, a chemical that transmits signals between nerve cells. When dopamine levels are too low, cells in the brain area controlling movement can no longer send a smooth flow of signals to muscles. Tremor and other movement problems result.

Cross-section of brain

Location of substantia nigra

Normal

Substantia nigra

Dopamine released

Brain cells controlling movement

Smooth flow of impulses in nerve fiber

Controlled movement

Parkinson's disease

Erratic flow of impulses in nerve fiber

Tremor

Patients may suffer from headaches and backaches resulting from the chronic contraction of the muscles of the head, neck, and spine.

Bradykinesia is a term derived from the Greek words *brady* (slow) and *kinesis* (movement). Patients with bradykinesia have trouble starting and performing body movements. They are likely to experience difficulty moving their arms and legs and may have to think out every muscle movement needed to turn over in bed or rise from a chair. Walking also becomes an effort. Patients walk with a shuffling, short-stepped gait, as if trying to avoid falling forward, and, as the disease progresses, they may sometimes "freeze" while walking.

A variety of other symptoms also occur. For example, automatic movements such as blinking, swallowing, and smiling or frowning are likely to diminish. Patients thus may develop dry and irritated eyes, drool, and have an expressionless, masklike face. Patients also tend to speak in a low monotone, and their handwriting becomes small and difficult to read.

The symptoms of Parkinson's disease are not all physical. Some patients experience memory loss and other kinds of intellectual decline, and most undergo personality changes. People who formerly took a keen interest in world events or were avid readers may sit for hours staring into space or at the television set. They are also apt to be depressed, fearful, and more passive and to have difficulty making decisions.

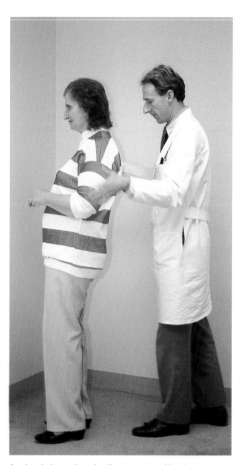

A physician checks the sense of balance of a woman with Parkinson's disease to evaluate the status of her condition. The symptoms of the disease include difficulties in walking normally or standing in an erect position without tilting or wobbling. Because there is no definitive laboratory test for Parkinson's, doctors look for such symptoms to diagnose the disorder.

The physical manifestations of the disease result from the malfunction of *neurons* (nerve cells) in the *basal ganglia*, a group of structures in the center of the brain that help control muscle movements. The basal ganglia act as a sort of switchboard, coordinating signals to and from the spinal cord and the *cerebral cortex*. The cerebral cortex, which overlies the basal ganglia, is the folded outer layer of the brain where thinking—including decisions concerning body movements—takes place. When the basal ganglia can no longer carry out this coordinating and processing function, nerve signals to the muscles become erratic, and as a consequence muscle control is lost.

Loss of an essential brain chemical

Researchers have found that the problem begins in the cells of a small, heavily pigmented segment of the basal ganglia called the *substantia nigra* (Latin for "black substance"). The pigmentation comes from cells rich in melanin—the substance that gives skin cells their color—that produce and store *dopamine*. Dopamine is a *neurotransmitter*, a chemical messenger that carries impulses from one nerve cell to another. In Parkinson's disease, the substantia nigra's cells deteriorate and die. As the damage progresses, the substantia nigra—which at autopsy may appear to be bleached almost white—can no longer supply an adequate amount of dopamine to other areas of the brain, including the neighboring parts of the basal ganglia. It is a deficiency of dopamine, scientists learned, that causes the cells of the basal ganglia to malfunction and leads to the symptoms of Parkinson's disease.

That much has been known about Parkinson's disease since the mid-1960's. With most cases of the disease, however, researchers have been at a loss to explain what factors cause the dopamine-producing cells of the substantia nigra to die.

Dopamine can become depleted in the brain for several reasons. Certain medications, for example, can affect the substantia nigra and produce symptoms resembling those of Parkinson's disease. Doctors know of several tranquilizers that cause this side effect, though dopamine levels return to normal after patients stop using the drug. In a more recent and more troubling drug finding, medical researchers at the University of Colorado in Denver reported in 1991 that three medications used to treat schizophrenia, a severe form of mental illness, may cause permanent damage to the substantia nigra. A permanent loss of dopamine-producing cells can also be caused by other conditions, notably brain tumors, strokes, carbon monoxide poisoning, and head injuries.

Searching for the cause of Parkinson's disease

These are all special circumstances, however, and do not explain why most people with Parkinson's disease developed their illness. For years, scientists sought in vain for a common thread among the great majority of Parkinson's cases. Many medical researchers think that Parkinson's disease may actually be a group of similar disorders, each caused by a different agent. Some investigators theorize that some cases of Parkinson's—as well as of several other degenerative brain disorders such as Alzheimer's disease—may result from infections by so-called *slow viruses.* Unlike the more common viruses that cause colds, influenza, and many other illnesses, slow viruses do their damage so gradually that years or decades pass after the initial infection before symptoms appear.

Some studies point in other directions. In 1990, for instance, Blaine Beaman, a microbiologist at the University of California at Davis, suggested that the cause of Parkinson's disease may be a common soil bacterium called *Nocardia.* Beaman found that at least 25 strains of *Nocardia* cause Parkinson's symptoms in laboratory mice. Examination of the animals' brains showed that the microorganism had infected their substantia nigra cells. Whether *Nocardia* bacteria can have—or do have—the same effect on the human brain is not known.

Scientists were intrigued by the *Nocardia* discovery, but it seems unlikely that the microorganism will turn out to be a major player in Parkinson's disease. Likewise, slow viruses, though yet to be counted out, are not in the forefront of Parkinson's research. Judy Rosner, executive director of the United Parkinson Foundation in Chicago, says many neuroscientists are now betting that further studies will show environmental toxins to be involved in most cases of the disease.

Researchers were steered onto that avenue of investigation by an unusual group of medical cases that occurred in California in the early 1980's. In the summer of 1982, a young drug user in northern California injected herself with a synthetic version of heroin manufactured in an "underground" laboratory. After taking the drug, she suffered from hallucinations and blurred vision, and her arms and legs jerked uncontrollably. The woman never used the synthetic heroin again, and for about a year thereafter she seemed to be in good health.

Then other strange symptoms began: Unaccountably, the woman was plagued by muscle aches, tremors, slowed speech, and stiffness in her arms and legs. Her posture became stooped, and sometimes she froze in midstride when walking. The symptoms were indistinguishable from those of Parkinson's disease.

As the year wore on, dozens of other young people in northern California who had used the same drug began to turn up with Parkinson's symptoms at hospitals and neurology clinics. Doctors were baffled; this strange syndrome was completely new to their experience.

An investigation soon revealed what had happened. The synthetic heroin taken by the drug users was tainted with a chemical called *MPTP*. Studies showed that MPTP, though not itself toxic, is converted in the brain to another compound, *MPP+*, that damages the same brain areas affected by Parkinson's disease. Tragic as it was for the victims, the MPTP incident led to some of the most dramatic advances in scientists' understanding of Parkinson's disease in more than 150 years.

Medical researchers quickly realized that they could use MPTP to produce the same damage in animal nerve cells that occurs in the brains of Parkinson's patients. With MPTP, they created a new and more realistic "animal model" for the testing of promising new drugs against Parkinson's disease.

Other studies with MPTP led investigators to new insights into the course of the disease and the damage it does to nerve cells. Perhaps most important, the discovery of MPTP's effects on the brain sharpened the focus of scientists' efforts to unmask the cause of most cases of Parkinson's disease.

Studies implicate environmental toxins

Mulling the experience of the unfortunate drug addicts, some researchers theorized that an environmental toxin—and most likely more than one—caused Parkinson's disease. Like MPTP, it would be a *neurotoxin*, an agent that damages nerve cells.

The neurotoxin theory gained increased acceptance in the late 1980's. One piece of supporting evidence came from studies of the native Chamorro people, who live on the remote islands of Guam and Rota in the western Pacific Ocean. During the first half of the 1900's, a mysterious nerve disorder occurred with great frequency among the Chamorro. The condition, named *ALS-PD*, had characteristics of Parkinson's disease, Alzheimer's disease, and another degenerative brain disease called *amyotrophic lateral sclerosis* (ALS, also known as Lou Gehrig's disease) that also greatly impairs movement. In 1987, scientists linked ALS-PD to a neurotoxin they identified in the seeds of large palmlike plants called cycads, which the Chamorro used

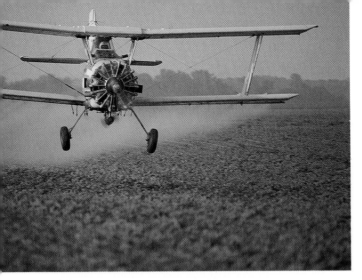

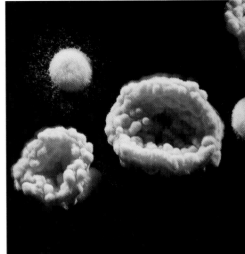

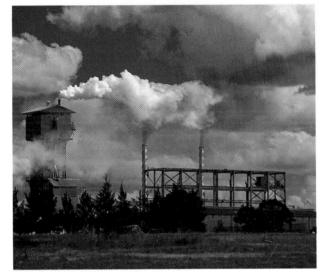

Studies indicate that environmental *toxins* (poisons) such as agricultural chemicals, *above left*, and industrial pollutants, *left*, may be involved in many cases of Parkinson's disease. Researchers speculate that the chemicals may cause the disorder in people with an inherited or acquired susceptibility to such toxins. Other research has shown that the soil bacterium *Nocardia*, *above*, causes Parkinson's symptoms in laboratory mice. No evidence, however, links the microorganism to the disease in human beings.

in native foods and traditional medicines. By the mid-1950's, as the Chamorro adopted a Western diet and modern medicines, the incidence of the devastating nerve disease had declined.

More than a dozen studies in the 1980's and 1990's have found a link between Parkinson's disease and exposure to various industrial chemicals, some of which may be neurotoxins. Several studies suggest, in particular, that farmers and rural residents who are exposed to pesticides and fertilizers in their jobs or by drinking contaminated well water have an increased risk of developing Parkinson's disease.

One such investigation was reported in 1990 by William Koller, a neurologist at the University of Kansas Medical Center in Kansas City. Koller studied 300 Kansans, half of whom had Parkinson's disease. He found that the Parkinson's patients were twice as likely as the individuals without the disease to have grown up in farming areas and to have drunk well water.

The possibility that poisons we encounter during the course of our lives can cause Parkinson's might explain why physicians did not report the disease until the early 1800's. The disorder may have been rare until the factories of the Industrial Revolution began discharging massive amounts of toxic wastes into the environment.

Even if researchers prove that certain toxins in the environment play a role in Parkinson's disease, scientists will be left with a great riddle: Many people are exposed to such substances, but relatively few develop Parkinson's disease. Scientists are thus working to identify factors that predispose people to the disease.

Some evidence suggests that the livers of Parkinson's victims may be unable to break down toxic chemicals into less harmful compounds. Other findings indicate that Parkinson's disease occurs in people who have abnormal *mitochondria* in their cells. Mitochondria are the cell's power plants, tiny structures that supply energy critical for a cell's maintenance and survival. Mitochondria already weakened by a defect might be more vulnerable to an environmental toxin. Animal research with MPTP supports this theory; scientists have determined that the chemical kills nerve cells by damaging their mitochondria.

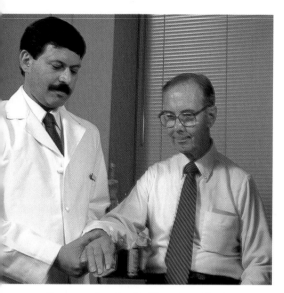

Doctors check a Parkinson's patient who has been taking the drug *deprenyl* to see if it has reduced tremors and rigidity in his upper limbs. Studies suggest that deprenyl protects nerve cells from destruction and thus might be able to prevent the onset of symptoms if prescribed soon enough—though such early treatment would require new and better diagnostic techniques.

Although medication for Parkinson's disease helps control symptoms for a while, the illness always progresses. Writing samples, *right,* show how a patient's manual dexterity deteriorated as his condition worsened.

earth. The octave of prayer must be fulfilled - as the strains of music project upward into the heavens, a golden light is ever present. To be able to just see the image, kill it forever on film so others may know of its spiritual meaning. Perhaps I should stop - never to ever take another photograph just to be a real voyeur - perhaps like the ever present sidewalk zombies, always watching, not doing anything; just

This is a sample of my handwriting now, one year later. It is typical of Parkinson script. The first letter always big then smaller as I go along. As I write the tremors are significant and my writing arm is tired.

May 1st, 1991

The evidence implicating defects of the liver and the mitochondria in Parkinson's disease raises still another question: Are these deficiencies somehow acquired after birth or are they genetically determined? If a genetic flaw underlies the disorder, and if the gene or genes involved can be located, a screening test might enable physicians to identify people who are at risk of developing Parkinson's disease. Those individuals could then be counseled to minimize their exposure to environmental toxins. Further in the future, it might be possible for scientists to correct the hereditary defect so the disease could not develop.

Drugs aid Parkinson's sufferers

Until the day arrives when Parkinson's disease can be prevented, better treatments are patients' best hope. Drugs have long been used to combat the disorder. Beginning in the late 1800's, doctors prescribed chemicals derived from plants to relieve the symptoms of many Parkinson's patients. The first modern drugs that proved effective against the disorder were developed in the 1940's. These synthetic *anticholinergic drugs* were similar to the plant compounds. Anticholinergic drugs counteract another neurotransmitter, *acetylcholine*, the influence of which increases in nerve cells that have been depleted of dopamine. Excessive acetylcholine activity contributes to muscle stiffness and tremor.

In the 1960's, drug researchers developed a new compound, *amantadine*, that became a standard medication for Parkinson's disease. Although amantadine was originally introduced as a drug to prevent one form of influenza, doctors soon learned that it also relieves Parkinson's symptoms in patients whose disease is still at an early stage. Administered by itself or in combination with anticholinergic drugs, amantadine works by stimulating the release of dopamine stored in nerve fibers in the brain. But amantadine loses its effectiveness as that limited supply of dopamine starts to run out.

Since the basic problem in Parkinson's disease is a lack of dopamine, why not just give

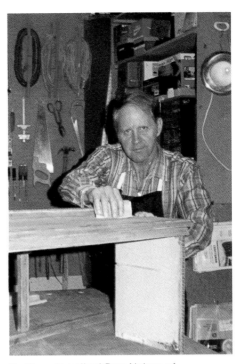

Parkinson's patient Don Nelson of Denver, *above*, pursues his hobby of woodworking. His trembling hands were unable to handle tools before he received a brain-tissue implant in 1988. He was the first person in the United States to undergo this still-experimental procedure in which dopamine-producing fetal brain cells are implanted deep in the brain. The implanted cells continued to produce dopamine, compensating for the deficiency caused by the disease.

How Parkinson's patients cope

Parkinson's patients learn a number of coping techniques that enable them to continue living a reasonably normal life. Walking difficulties, for instance, can be overcome with the aid of a wheeled cart that can also be used to carry various items, *right*.

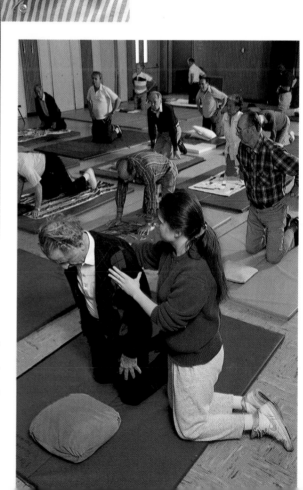

Eating utensils that many Parkinson's patients find helpful include large-handled spoons that provide a better grip, *above right*, and beverage glasses fitted with a lid and drinking spout that prevent trembling hands from causing spills, *above*.

A therapist assists a Parkinson's patient during a group exercise session, *right*. By maintaining muscle tone and strength, regular exercise helps patients remain mobile.

patients dopamine? In fact, scientists once thought that might be the answer. They quickly discovered, however, that dopamine is ineffective as an administered drug because it cannot cross the *blood-brain barrier*, a protective physical and biochemical blockade that prevents potentially harmful substances in the blood from entering brain tissues.

Researchers overcame that problem in the late 1960's with the development of a drug called *levodopa* (L-dopa), which is able to pass through the blood-brain barrier. Enzymes in the brain then convert L-dopa into dopamine. Doctors prescribe L-dopa for a patient as the disease progresses and anticholinergic drugs and amantadine cease to have an effect.

When it was introduced, L-dopa was hailed as a miracle drug, and indeed it revolutionized the treatment of Parkinson's disease. L-dopa reduced the Parkinson's death rate by about 50 per cent and greatly reduced patients' symptoms.

But L-dopa can also be converted to dopamine in other parts of the body. This presents a twofold problem: It reduces the amount of L-dopa available to the brain, and it exposes the entire body to a potent neurotransmitter. Dopamine circulating through the body can cause a variety of side effects, including nausea, vomiting, and *dyskinesia*, involuntary muscle movements that can be worse than the symptoms of the disease. Some patients who develop dyskinesia say they have felt as though their arms and legs were being pulled from their sockets. So Parkinson's patients usually take L-dopa in combination with a second drug, *carbidopa*. Carbidopa inhibits the chemical breakdown of L-dopa into dopamine outside of the brain.

Unfortunately, L-dopa tends to lose its effectiveness over time. For that reason, and because of the drug's potentially serious side effects, physicians usually delay prescribing the drug until patients' symptoms are fairly pronounced.

High hopes for a new drug: deprenyl

In 1989, the U.S. Food and Drug Administration approved a new drug, *deprenyl* (also called Eldepryl), for the treatment of Parkinson's disease. That same year, a federally funded study at 28 medical centers in the United States concluded that deprenyl may slow the progression of the disease. Researchers found that only 25 per cent of the patients taking deprenyl worsened to the point where they needed L-dopa within one year, compared with 44 per cent of those who did not receive the drug. The results suggest that deprenyl protects nerve cells from destruction and, if administered early enough, may actually be able to prevent Parkinson's disease. Another advantage of the drug is that, at proper dosages, it produces almost no side effects.

But as yet, there are insufficient data on deprenyl. Further studies will be required to confirm that the drug is really as effective as it seems to be and to learn how it works in the body.

The prospect of preventing Parkinson's disease with deprenyl or some other, as yet undiscovered, drug makes the search for a diagnostic test all the more urgent. Doctors believe that most Parkinson's patients have had the disease for years or decades before symptoms begin. By the time of diagnosis, the typical patient has already lost dopamine production in about 80 per cent of the substantia nigra cells. Early diagnosis and treatment could protect nerve cells when damage is still minor and thereby head off the appearance of symptoms.

Researchers have discovered a few clues about the disease on which a diagnostic test might be based. For instance, Parkinson's patients apparently have a defective enzyme in their blood *platelets*, disklike structures that help blood to clot. The enzyme could perhaps be useful as a telltale sign of the disease that could be detected in a blood test.

Brain-tissue implants show promise

While drug studies continue, some scientists are investigating the possibility of using transplants of dopamine-secreting nerve cells to restore dopamine production in the brains of Parkinson's patients. In the 1980's, doctors in Sweden and Mexico attempted to treat Parkinson's by extracting cells from patients' own adrenal glands and implanting them into the patients' brains. The adrenals, situated just above the kidneys, produce dopamine as well as adrenalin and other hormones. For a short time, the technique raised hopes, but the patients experienced many complications and showed only slight improvement.

In the late 1980's, the Swedish researchers developed a more promising implantation procedure using dopamine-secreting nerve cells taken from the brain tissues of aborted fetuses. The cells, mixed with a liquid similar to the fluid that bathes the brain, are injected through a slender tube into a section of the basal ganglia, where they grow and produce dopamine. Several patients in the United States with advanced Parkinson's disease have received fetal-cell implants. Their doctors report that the patients' symptoms have been greatly reduced, enabling the people to resume many of their former activities.

The technique is still experimental, however, and far from being widely accepted. Many experts say there are too many uncertainties about the long-term effectiveness of the procedure. Furthermore, the very fact that implants involve the use of tissue from aborted fetuses makes the operation controversial from an ethical standpoint. The U.S. government has banned the use of federal funds for research on fetal-cell implants, and some states forbid all such work, even if funded with private money.

The techniques of genetic engineering might offer a way to implant human cells without using fetal tissues. Researchers think it may be possible to insert a gene for the production of dopamine into cells that can be cultured in large quantities in the laboratory. This approach would have the added benefit of making larger amounts of tissue available for implantation.

Learning to live with Parkinson's

As they await new developments that could ease their suffering, Parkinson's patients can do much to make life with the disease more manageable. Health experts advise patients to remain physically active so as to maintain muscle strength and mobility. Other coping strategies include learning to adjust to the disease's symptoms. Walking, for example, may require a deliberate effort to place the heel down before the toe—a natural motion for most people but not for people with Parkinson's disease. Patients also learn to allot extra time to getting dressed and performing other everyday tasks.

Mechanical aids can simplify daily life for Parkinson's patients. These include Velcro patches rather than buttons or zippers for fastening clothing, handrails in the bathroom, and special knives and forks with large handles.

Naturally, people with Parkinson's disease don't want to cope, they want to be cured. How close researchers are to that objective is a question that no one can answer. But research into drug treatments and cell implants holds out hope that physicians will someday—and perhaps soon—be able to offer patients relief from many symptoms of the disease. The ultimate aim, of course, is to prevent the disease altogether. As more is learned about Parkinson's disease and its possible causes, that no longer seems like such an unrealistic goal.

For more information:

Godwin-Austen, Richard. *The Parkinson's Disease Handbook.* International Health, 1989.

The American Parkinson's Disease Foundation provides information on the disease as well as patient referrals to specialists and other services. The foundation is located at 116 John St., New York, NY 10038. The toll-free telephone number is 1-800-223-2732.

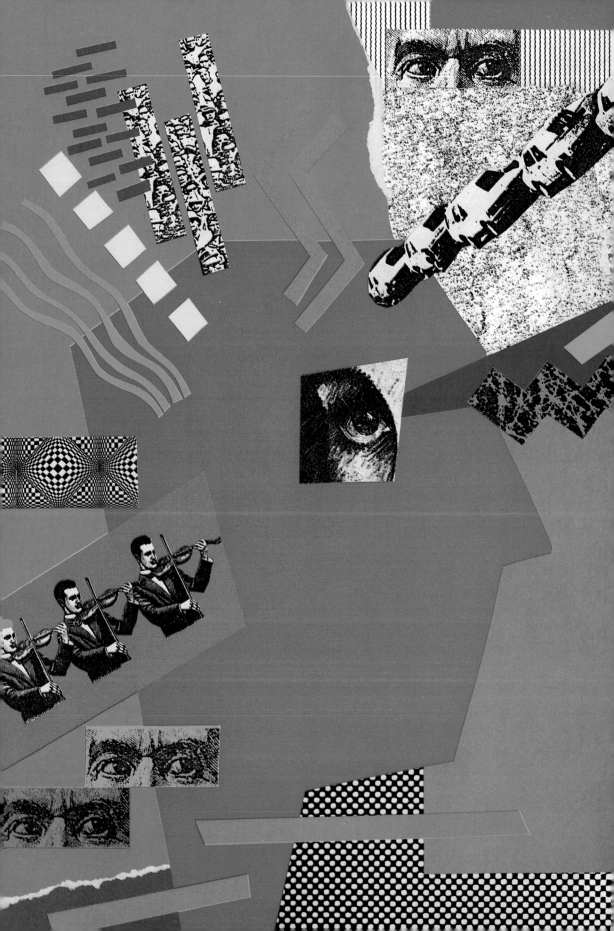

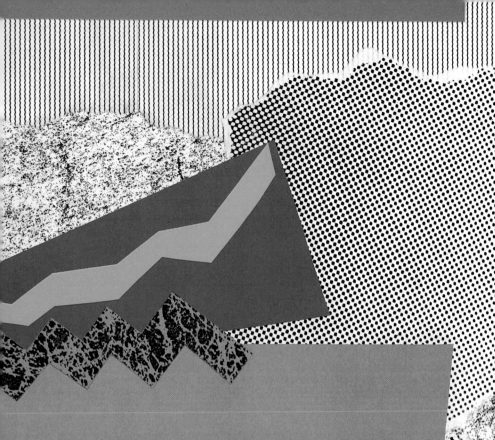

Schizophrenia's symptoms—
delusions, hallucinations,
and profoundly disorganized
thoughts—bring anguish to
patients and their families.
But there is hope for recovery.

Learning
to Treat
Schizophrenia

By Bruce Bower

The author:

Bruce Bower is the behavioral sciences editor for *Science News* magazine.

Every day, Ted stands on a city street corner, swathed in blankets, his belongings stuffed into a large plastic bag. Passers-by avoid the intense, unkempt man who talks to no one in particular, his incomprehensible banter reaching a fever pitch when voices only he can hear taunt and criticize him. Ted attended college in his early 20's, but his behavior began to deteriorate rapidly, and he shuttled in and out of a mental hospital for several years. Now in his 30's, he usually sleeps in a doorway or on a steam grate unless a frigid night forces him into a shelter for the homeless.

Shelly, on the other hand, lives in a supervised home. In 1984, she began to experience bizarre delusions (irrational beliefs not in accordance with reality) that took over her life for weeks at a time. At one time, Shelly became convinced that an evil spirit inhabited the home, and that to expel the imagined demon she must perform strange rituals and enlist the help of her neighbors. With medication, however, her delusions have become less frequent. At age 32, Shelly now performs occasional volunteer work and attends a community center where she learns tactics for successful behavior at work and with friends and family. A psychiatrist who monitors her progress expects her to be able to find a full-time job within the next year.

The lives of these two people, and those of more than a million other Americans, have been turned upside down by a devastating mental disorder that has long perplexed mental health professionals and scientists—schizophrenia. People with schizophrenia suffer great mental and emotional anguish. The lives of people with schizophrenia are usually disrupted for years as they try to learn how to live with and overcome the illness. Because of this, the lives of their families and friends are disrupted as well.

The Swiss psychiatrist Eugen Bleuler first coined the word *schizophrenia* in 1911. In Bleuler's definition, schizophrenia means split or fragmented mind, not a "split" or multiple personality in which a person acts as if he or she were two or more distinct individuals. Bleuler described schizophrenia as a mental disease that shatters the meaningful connection of thought, feeling, and behavior most people take for granted. While this definition is still helpful as a general description, mental health experts have narrowed the definition of the illness.

Today, most mental health officials agree schizophrenia is an illness marked by delusions, hallucinations, disturbed thinking and communication, and by inadequate social skills such as an inability to interact with others and a neglect of personal hygiene and appearance. According to a 1987 report by the National Institute of Mental Health (NIMH) in Bethesda, Md., schizophrenia is an illness that destroys "the inner unity of the mind" and weakens "the will and drive that constitute our essential character."

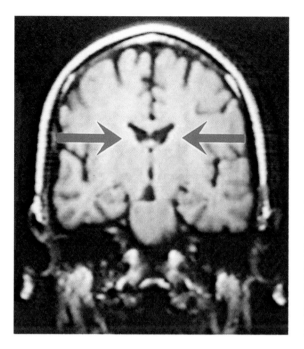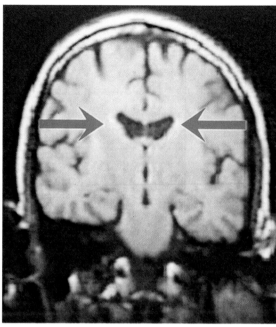

Many people with schizophrenia show a marked lack of emotion—or show emotions that are inappropriate in various situations—and are unable to carry out many normal tasks of day-to-day living. They might smile pleasantly while cursing, or announce calmly that electrical currents from outer space control the thoughts of everyone in the room. Someone suffering from schizophrenia may falsely perceive that he or she hears voices and stay up all night answering them.

Schizophrenia is both a personal tragedy and a serious public health problem. About 1 in 100 persons will develop schizophrenia sometime during their lives, and approximately 1.2 million Americans suffer from the disorder at any one time, according to psychiatrist E. Fuller Torrey of the NIMH. That's more than 4 times the number of people hospitalized each year from lung cancer and 1½ times the number hospitalized for heart attacks. More people are hospitalized for schizophrenia than for ailments such as pneumonia, for which 924,000 people are hospitalized each year, according to the National Center for Health Statistics in Hyattsville, Md.

Estimates of schizophrenia's cost to society vary, but all signs point to an enormous financial strain. Annual expenses for treatment and social services, as well as lost wages and job productivity, range from $20 billion, as calculated by the NIMH, to $48 billion, as calculated by the Institute of Medicine of the National Academy of Sciences.

Many theories exist about the cause of schizophrenia, but scientists are still unsure whether it has one cause or several. Although some regard schizophrenia as a single brain disorder, most researchers now believe it comprises a group of related mental illnesses. Most investigators also believe that psychological stress combined with a brain disorder—either inherited, or caused by environmental factors such as a childhood virus, or both—allows schizophrenia to develop.

The emphasis on a physical basis for the illness contrasts sharply with theories popular from the 1950's into the 1970's that blamed the development of schizophrenia nearly entirely on psychological factors such as a poor family environment or the state of society in general. In the 1960's, for instance, the late British psychiatrist R. D. Laing influenced many people with the notion that schizophrenia represents a "sane response to an insane world," and not a mental illness or brain disease. These theories, especially those that attribute the illness only to an improper upbringing, have been largely discredited. Although research suggests nonphysical environmental factors such as mental stress may contribute to the onset of the illness, most studies in the 1980's and 1990's have focused on physical causes.

Diagnosing schizophrenia

Three-quarters of schizophrenia sufferers first develop symptoms between the ages of 17 and 24. Many investigators think schizophrenia always occurs before age 45, although some evidence suggests a form of the disorder can appear after 50 years of age. Although the illness can strike before the age of 17, this is rare. Schizophrenia affects about as many men as women, but men tend to develop the illness sooner and display more chronic, severe symptoms.

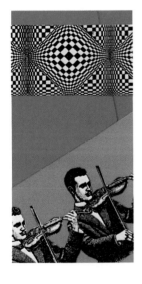

Because psychiatrists cannot identify schizophrenia with a physical test, they must base their diagnosis on emotional symptoms and behaviors. Opinions about who meets the criteria for schizophrenia still vary, but the most cited guidelines in the United States come from the American Psychiatric Association's (APA) latest manual of mental disorders, published in 1987.

The APA manual describes two main phases of schizophrenia—active and residual. In the *active phase*, which according to the guidelines must last for at least one week, a person displays symptoms of *psychosis*, a marked loss of contact with reality. These symptoms may include delusions that others control one's thoughts, for example, visual and auditory *hallucinations* ("seeing" and "hearing" imaginary sights and sounds), incoherent thoughts and speech, and inappropriate emotional reactions. A decrease in the ability to carry out normal daily tasks also generally accompanies these symptoms.

During the *residual phase*, the psychotic symptoms of the active phase ease, but other symptoms linger. Unlike active symptoms, these residual (remaining) symptoms often do not respond well to medication. Residual symptoms include social withdrawal, inability to function at work or school, talking continuously to oneself in public, apathy, or dulled feelings.

According to the APA manual, a patient's symptoms, active or residual, must be present for at least six months before doctors can make a definite diagnosis of schizophrenia. The aim of this diagnostic rule is to avoid misdiagnosing someone who may have signs of shorter-lived mental disorders that share some of the same symptoms.

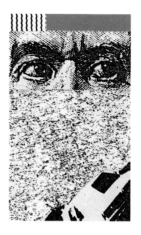

The psychiatric manual also cites four main types of schizophrenia. The *catatonic* type features an absence of physical movement, a rigid posture, and a lack of response to others. *Disorganized* schizophrenia includes incoherent thoughts, confused behavior, and an inability to behave in a generally accepted manner around people. The *paranoid* type revolves around a preoccupation with delusions of persecution or grandeur. *Undifferentiated* schizophrenia involves hallucinations, nonparanoid delusions, and confused behaviors.

Possible causes of schizophrenia

Scientists have yet to uncover clear, uncontested causes for this mysterious illness. Theories currently focus on a variety of factors that may contribute to the development of schizophrenia, including genetic factors, abnormalities in brain structure, and alterations in chemical communications among brain cells.

The possibility of an inherited vulnerability to schizophrenia has attracted special scrutiny since the mid-1980's. Interest in a possible genetic predisposition stems from several family studies showing that children of a parent with schizophrenia have a 1 in 10 chance of developing schizophrenia themselves, far greater than the 1 in 100 chance for the general population. And studies of identical twins, who possess exact copies of one another's genes, find that if one twin has schizophrenia, the other also develops schizophrenia 35 to 50 per cent of the time. Scientists note that the twin studies suggest that nongenetic factors also play a role in determining who develops the illness. If genes were the sole factor, they point out, schizophrenia would always afflict both members of a pair of identical twins.

A team of scientists led by psychiatrist Hugh Gurling of the University of London created a stir in 1988 when they claimed to have found a specific gene that makes its bearers more likely to develop most forms of the disorder. Gurling and his team studied five Icelandic and two English families with a high incidence of schizophrenia. They found evidence linking a tendency of certain family members to develop schizophrenia with the presence of a gene or genes on one of their chromosomes. Human beings have 23 pairs of chromosomes in their body cells. These chromosomes carry approximately 100,000 genes. The

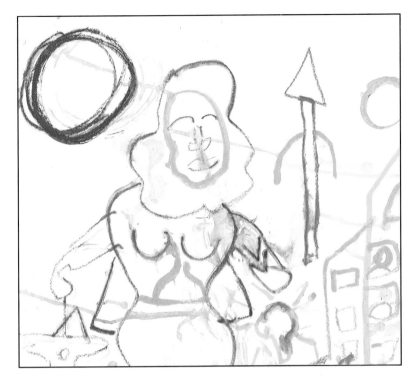

Drawings by a patient with schizophrenia, *right and opposite page*, reveal how the disease disrupts perceptions of people and situations, so that everyday life seems disorganized, distorted, frightening, or strange.

University of London researchers believed the genetic defect involved in schizophrenia was on chromosome 5.

But a 1988 study, led by psychiatrist Kenneth K. Kidd of Yale University in New Haven, Conn., found no connection between genes on chromosome 5 and schizophrenia in several generations of a large Swedish family. Two subsequent studies of schizophrenia-prone families, reported in 1989 by researchers at the University of Utah in Salt Lake City and the University of Edinburgh, Scotland, also failed to uncover a link with chromosome 5. Even if Gurling or others succeed in proving that a gene on chromosome 5 predisposes some families to develop schizophrenia, Kidd and other scientists believe that it is highly unlikely that a single gene is responsible for so complex and varied a disorder as schizophrenia. A number of genes may work together to set the stage for schizophrenia, Kidd maintains. Furthermore, precisely what these hypothetical genes do—whether they alter the development of the brain's anatomy or disrupt the brain's chemistry—is still a mystery.

Some researchers have found evidence that factors other than genes play a role in schizophrenia. In 1990, a team led by Daniel R. Weinberger of the NIMH presented results from brain scans of 15 sets of identical twins, eight male and seven female, with one schizophrenia sufferer per pair. Using a scanning technique called magnetic resonance imaging to take pictures of the twins' brains, the researchers found that all but one of the twins

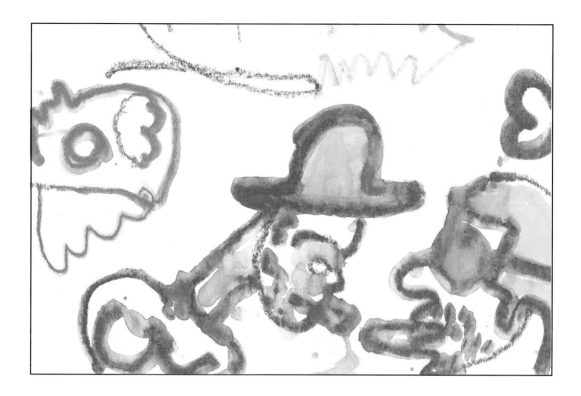

with schizophrenia had slightly larger *ventricles* (fluid-filled cavities in the center of the brain), compared with their healthy siblings. The twins with larger ventricles also showed less mass in several parts of the brain that are considered to be crucial in regulating emotion and motivation.

Weinberger proposes that early in brain development—either in the womb or shortly after birth—brain cells migrate to the wrong destinations, possibly due to a viral infection, a disorder in the body's immune system, injury at birth, or some other environmental factor. Then, he suggests, full-blown symptoms are triggered when an individual undergoes the physical changes of puberty. So far, however, the evidence doesn't completely support this theory. For instance, not all people with schizophrenia have large ventricles, while some people with other brain diseases, such as Alzheimer's disease, possess bloated ventricles similar to those seen in Weinberger's study.

Other scientists have uncovered different clues that hint that environmental factors play a role in schizophrenia. These include the observation that birth complications and childhood head injuries occur at an unusually high rate among people later hospitalized for schizophrenia. Researchers have also found that people with schizophrenia are more likely to have been born in the winter or early spring, when viral infections more frequently occur. But whether any of these factors lead to schizophrenia remains to be proved.

The area of schizophrenia research that has captured the most attention is the search for clues in the brain's chemistry—especially clues that pertain to chemicals that brain cells use to communicate with each other. Studies suggest that many people with schizophrenia may have a brain abnormality that makes them extra sensitive to *dopamine*, a brain chemical that carries certain messages among brain cells and helps control responses to stress. Dopamine conveys its messages by locking onto *receptors* (proteins on the brain cell surface that bind to specific molecules). In 1986, Johns Hopkins University scientists in Baltimore, aided by *positron emission tomography*, a technique that creates color-coded images of the brain at work, found an increased number of dopamine receptors on the brain cells of patients with schizophrenia. These extra receptors may make some individuals oversensitive to dopamine, scientists believe.

Drug treatment and supervised care

Theories that dopamine plays a role in schizophrenia date to the early 1950's, when French psychiatrists discovered that the drug chlorpromazine acted as a *neuroleptic*, a drug that reduces symptoms of psychosis. Chlorpromazine and most of the 19 other neuroleptics now in use block dopamine receptors in the brain. These drugs are structured like the dopamine molecule and are thus able to latch onto dopamine receptors. When the drug enters the brain, it apparently takes dopamine's place on many of the receptors—thus blunting dopamine's effect.

Most patients' hallucinations and delusions decrease in intensity after one or two weeks of neuroleptic treatment. But nearly one-third of schizophrenia sufferers do not improve when given conventional neuroleptics, and residual symptoms such as apathy usually remain for most patients.

Neuroleptics can also cause a variety of side effects, including tremors, muscle rigidity, restlessness, and a sensation of dulled emotions. They may also lead to a serious condition known as *tardive dyskinesia*, characterized by spasmodic movements of the mouth, tongue, and body. An estimated 20 per cent of patients who take neuroleptics develop tardive dyskinesia and, in rare instances, it can be disabling. About one in three patients taking neuroleptics stop taking the drugs, largely because of such side effects.

Scientists do not completely understand why some neuroleptics cause muscle rigidity and tremors, but a 1991 study provides a clue. Researchers from the University of Colorado in Denver found that three neuroleptics chemically resemble a toxic chemical that can cause Parkinson's disease. Parkinson's disease is a disorder of the brain that reduces muscle control. Its symptoms include trembling hands, rigid muscles, slow movement, and balance difficulties.

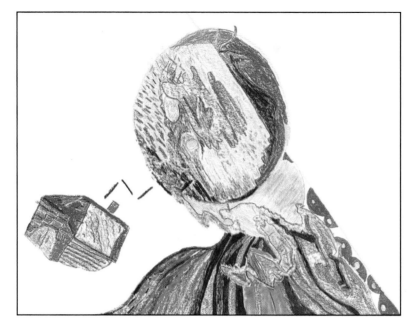

The thoughts and feelings of people with schizophrenia can be so chaotic that their world may seem to be disintegrating or hurtling out of control. Patients may require years of treatment to regain a sense of control over their lives.

Clozapine (marketed as Clozaril), a neuroleptic long available in Europe and approved for prescription use in the United States in October 1989, apparently helps many patients who do not respond to conventional neuroleptics. A 1987 study directed by psychiatrist Herbert Y. Meltzer of Case Western Reserve University in Cleveland found that 38 of 125 schizophrenia patients who had not responded to other drugs improved markedly on clozapine. However, about 1 per cent of Clozaril users can develop a potentially fatal reduction in infection-fighting blood cells. For this reason, anyone taking the drug must have their blood checked once a week.

Although neuroleptic drugs are the cornerstone of schizophrenia treatment, mental health professionals agree that medication is not the cure-all for the disorder. Research indicates that patients who show the most improvement receive drug treatment along with supervised care that emphasizes social skills and other practical living skills, such as vocational training.

Studies suggest that some psychological treatments are less successful. Psychotherapy, in which a patient and a therapist engage in an in-depth discussion and analysis of the patient's problems, lost favor in the 1980's as a treatment for schizophrenia. Many psychiatrists found that the complex examination of feelings and motivations psychotherapy requires offers little benefit and may even delay recovery by confusing some patients with schizophrenia.

Most treatment programs today combine medication along with counseling and supervised care within a structured living arrangement. Although many schizophrenia sufferers show

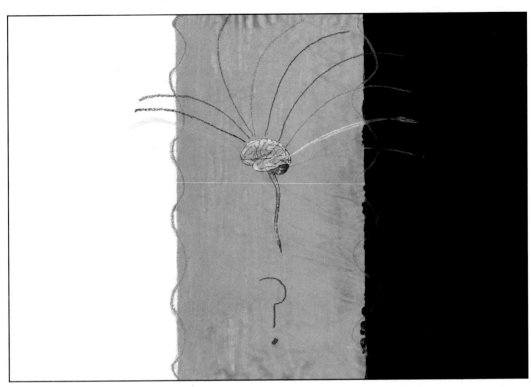

Through a drawing, a person suffering from schizophrenia tries to visualize and make sense of imaginary voices invading the brain. Visual and auditory hallucinations ("seeing" or "hearing" sights and sounds that are not present) are common symptoms of schizophrenia.

marked improvement with this kind of program, it may take years for a patient to find the best kind and dosage level of medication and a living arrangement most appropriate to his or her needs.

Outlook for recovery

The long-term outlook for recovery from schizophrenia provides room for cautious optimism. Mental health officials report that approximately 25 per cent of schizophrenia patients recover fully with no recurring symptoms, but 10 to 15 per cent show no improvement. The remainder can expect slow, fluctuating progress over a period of up to 30 years, depending on the individual. Although they may always need some degree of medical treatment, approximately 25 per cent of patients in this middle group usually recover enough to live independently with a minimum of supervision, according to mental health professionals.

Time is the biggest factor in recovery. Patients who recover fully generally do so within two years of the onset of the illness, according to Torrey. The time it takes others to recover enough to again lead relatively normal lives varies greatly, however.

Five studies involving more than 1,300 people hospitalized for schizophrenia in the United States and Europe indicate it took 20 years or more for about half the patients to recover or substantially improve after leaving the hospital. After 10 to 20 years, even people with the most severe, chronic schizophrenia may show remarkable progress, says psychiatrist Courtenay M. Harding of Yale University, who directed a 30-year study of former Vermont state mental hospital patients.

Effects on families

For families with a member affected by the illness, schizophrenia is extremely disruptive. When a family member develops the disorder, many families feel as if they are falling apart under the stress of their new problems. These problems touch nearly all aspects of daily life, causing financial, emotional, and physical strains.

Families suffer denial, anger, confusion, and grief. Some respond by blaming one another for somehow causing the illness. Others may try to hide the patient from friends, neighbors, and relatives, creating hostility and resentment in the affected family member. Parents sometimes devote so much energy and time to the patient that other family members feel slighted.

Most mental health experts, as well as many families who have lived with an individual who suffers from schizophrenia, agree that acceptance of the condition as an illness that may have changed their loved one forever is important. By working together with mental health professionals to understand the illness, a family can agree on realistic, uniform expectations for the patient. Experts note that if family members have varying expectations of the patient, this can confuse the patient and stifle progress toward recovery.

Accepting a family member's schizophrenia as a disorder that requires medical attention is also vital. Understanding that this is not simply rebellion or willful behavior ensures that the patient will be given medical treatment quickly.

Families can also save time and money by seeing a psychiatrist with a good knowledge of the latest drug treatments for schizophrenia. Mental health experts suggest that the psychiatric department of a large university hospital may be a good place to start. Such expertise is important, because drug treatments must be tailored to the individual. Unfortunately, trial and error is the only way to find the right drug or combination of drugs for each individual, a process that can be stressful for the patient, family, and physician.

Many families faced with the difficulties of living and caring for someone with schizophrenia find that other families in the same situation have a unique understanding of their problems. In 1979, families in the United States with mentally ill members established a self-help network, the National Alliance for the Mentally Ill (NAMI), headquartered in Arlington, Va. The organization now has approximately 1,000 offices with 130,000

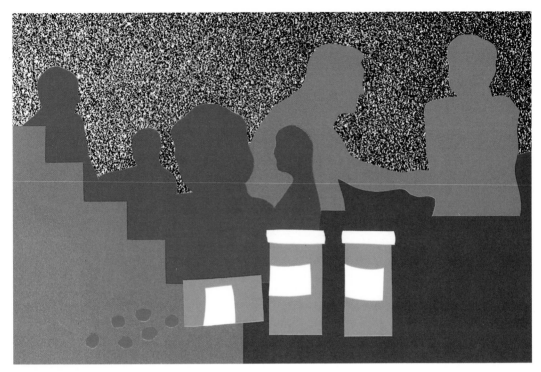

Drug therapy
Medication can help reduce the hallucinations some schizophrenia patients experience. These drugs, called *neuroleptics*, are often part of treatment for people with schizophrenia.

members in all 50 states and several other countries. Family members, relatives, and friends of people afflicted with schizophrenia share common experiences and problems through local support groups, which are usually led by family members. Local offices of NAMI are also valuable sources of information for handling all problems associated with schizophrenia, including where to find housing, treatment centers, and doctors with expertise in the disorder.

Many private or university psychiatric hospitals also run coping-skills workshops to educate families about the nature of schizophrenia and offer practical advice on how to help the patient and family live together. Families learn to establish clear, consistently enforced rules of behavior and to set limited, realistic goals for the patient—including, when appropriate, easing the patient into a regular job and independent living.

Schizophrenia's burden on society
Schizophrenia poses as daunting a challenge for society as it does for families. According to the NIMH's Torrey, public care for serious mental illnesses "is bad and getting worse." Approximately 360,000 people with schizophrenia reside in state hospitals, halfway houses, hotels, or group homes. But as many as 200,000 people with schizophrenia may live on the streets or in homeless shelters. Perhaps another 50,000 are in jails and pris-

ons, although those afflicted with schizophrenia commit no more crime than the general population, according to Torrey.

The problem of homelessness among people with schizophrenia started in the late 1950's, when the states began releasing patients from state mental health facilities in large numbers. Between 1965 and 1980, 358,000 people were released from state hospitals to live in local communities, according to Torrey. A number of factors spurred these releases, including public outrage at reported neglect and mistreatment of patients in some institutions and the bankruptcy of many state mental health systems. There was also an optimism among psychiatrists that people with the disorder would receive antipsychotic medication and counseling at community mental health centers, but these centers generally ended up as treatment facilities for less severe mental problems.

While public care for people suffering from schizophrenia is woefully inadequate, the outlook for research is brighter. Federal money for schizophrenia research continues to rise, up from $18.4 million in fiscal year 1985 (Oct. 1, 1984-Sept. 30, 1985) to an estimated $95.7 million in fiscal year 1990. Experts caution, however, against expecting a cure or chemical "magic bullet" for schizophrenia any time soon. Nevertheless, with the help of medication, supportive care, and time, patients can make remarkable progress.

"If you have schizophrenia, you don't have to be a burned-out shell," says Yale University's Harding. "You can be a phoenix."

For more information:

The National Alliance for the Mentally Ill, 2101 Wilson Boulevard, Suite 302, Arlington, VA 22201 (703-524-7600).

National Mental Health Association, 1021 Prince Street, Alexandria, VA 22314 (703-684-7722).

For further reading:

Fuller, E. Torrey. *Surviving Schizophrenia: A Family Manual.* Rev. ed. Harper & Row, 1988.

Gottesman, Irving I. *Schizophrenia Genesis: The Origins of Madness.* W. H. Freeman and Company, 1991.

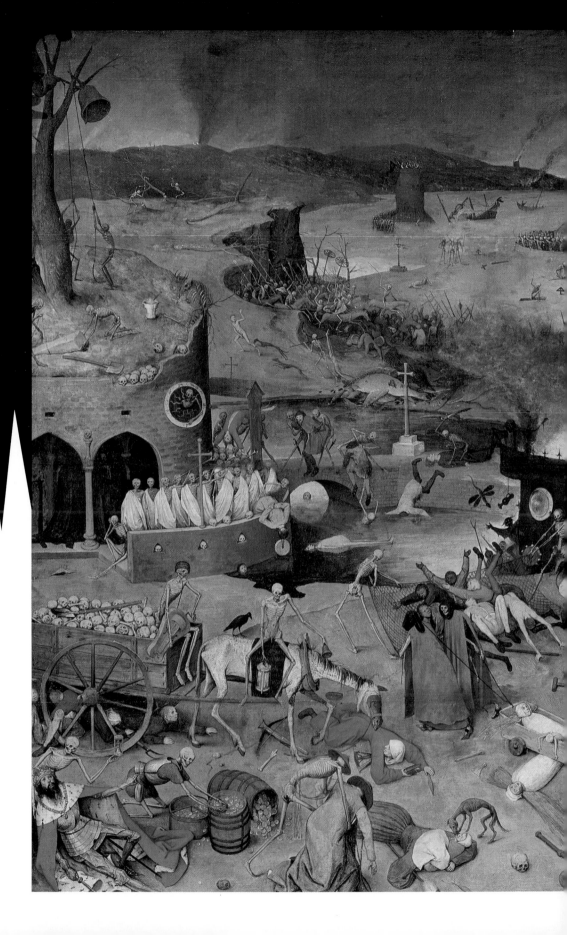

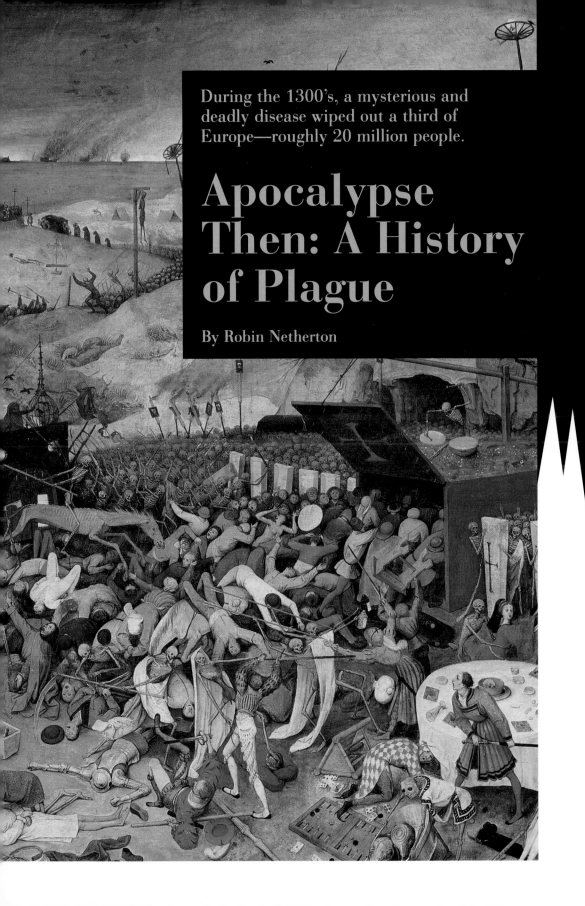

During the 1300's, a mysterious and deadly disease wiped out a third of Europe—roughly 20 million people.

Apocalypse Then: A History of Plague

By Robin Netherton

"How will posterity believe that there has been a time, without lightnings of heaven or fires of earth, without wars or other visible slaughter, [when] well nigh the whole world has been left without inhabitants? When before has been seen houses left vacant, cities deserted, fields too small for the dead, and a fearful and universal solitude over the whole earth?"

From a letter of May 19, 1348, written by the Italian poet Petrarch (1304-1374)

Previous pages: Death in the form of skeletons stalked the land, striking down the living in Pieter Bruegel's *Triumph of Death* painted in the 1500's. Images of death grew common in European art after the ravages of the plague.

The images of many terrible diseases haunt modern memory, but the one described by the Italian poet Petrarch was worst of all: deadlier than smallpox, more infectious than polio, more mysterious than AIDS. While all these illnesses have been called plagues, only one disease bears the name plague as its own.

When the disease swept like a brush fire across Europe in the 1300's, people called it by other names: the Great Mortality, the Pestilence, or simply, the Death. Later writers referred to that epidemic as the Black Death, perhaps recalling the black spots that covered victims' skin.

In only four years, from 1347 to 1351, plague killed as many as one of every three people in Europe, devastating families, communities, and society. Since then, scholars have routinely acknowledged the epidemic as the greatest single disaster in European history.

Looking back over a safe distance of 600 years, scientists find it easy to see how the epidemic cut its deadly path through Europe. They now know that plague is caused by bacteria—tiny one-celled organisms that were unknown to medieval physicians—and that the plague-causing bacteria normally infect rats and other rodents. They also know that fleas can transmit the bacteria to people by leaping onto—and biting—warm human skin after their rat hosts die.

But medieval people never suspected that victims were infected by the bites of common fleas. Nor did they realize that the disease owed its swift spread to the movement of flea-bearing rats from town to town. Perhaps most terrifying of all, people had no way of knowing when—or even if—the mysterious pestilence would end.

Even though that devastating outbreak finally did subside, plague is still with us. The disease strikes hundreds of people around the world each year, including some in the United States. Although plague today is hardly harmless, it can now be controlled and even cured.

The plague-causing bacterium, *Yersinia pestis*, is named after French bacteriologist Alexandre Yersin, one of the scientists who discovered it in 1894. At least 200 species of rodents carry *Yersinia pestis* today, including many types of rats, mice, squirrels, prairie dogs, gophers, and chipmunks. The bacteria move from one rodent to another by riding in the guts of fleas that live on animal blood. When one rodent dies of plague, its fleas hop to

The author:

Robin Netherton is a freelance writer and editor.

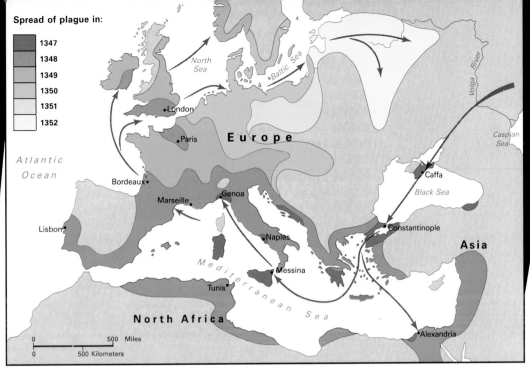

Spread of plague in:

- 1347
- 1348
- 1349
- 1350
- 1351
- 1352

North Sea

Baltic Sea

Volga River

North Sea

Europe

London

Paris

Atlantic Ocean

Bordeaux

Marseille

Genoa

Lisbon

Naples

Tunis

Messina

Mediterranean Sea

North Africa

Caffa

Black Sea

Caspian Sea

Constantinople

Asia

Alexandria

0   500 Miles
0   500 Kilometers

another, injecting the bacteria into the new host when they feed.

Plague does not automatically destroy every animal colony it infects, however. Rodents can often tolerate some plague bacteria in their systems without falling ill, and some rodents survive the disease and become *immune* (permanently protected against a disease). Most of the time, in fact, the disease stays within closed communities of animals, as the populations of rodents, fleas, and bacteria rise and fall in response to one another. When a disease becomes established in a community, it is said to be *endemic*. *Yersinia pestis* has been endemic among wild rodents in various parts of the world for centuries.

Sometimes, however, for reasons that scientists do not completely understand, an outbreak of plague will kill off an entire rodent colony. When a hungry flea can find no rodents left to bite, it seeks other sources of food—which might include human beings.

The bacteria responsible for the Black Death most likely came from central Asia, though scholars still debate the exact origin of that outbreak. In the mid-1340's, the bacteria reached the caravan route that ran between China and Europe—perhaps when trappers picked up dead animals for their furs. Via this busy trade route, plague could spread west to the Black Sea.

Plague in the 1300's: the path of the Black Death

Fleas infected with plague bacteria probably brought the infection to Europe from Central Asia. By 1348, rats on ships sailing from Caffa (on the Black Sea) had carried the disease to major ports on the Mediterranean Sea. From there, the disease spread rapidly. Before the epidemic subsided in 1352, it had afflicted most of Europe.

There, at the port city of Caffa (now Feodosiya in the Soviet Union), Italian merchant ships docked to pick up silks and spices from the Orient.

The ships were a haven for black rats, which hid by day and scavenged by night. In a crowded port, the rats could easily leap from ship to ship or climb ropes from ship to shore. A single infected rat might carry dozens of fleas, each of which could bear millions of bacteria. And the fleas themselves could live amid bales of fur or cloth for weeks without a meal, waiting to leap upon a new warm-blooded body.

Because surviving records are unclear, historians cannot be sure exactly when plague reached various Asian cities. They do know that by late 1347, the disease had struck the chain of ports along the shipping route from the Black Sea to Italy. It entered Europe in October when it struck Messina, the chief port of the Mediterranean island of Sicily.

The Sicilians had heard rumors of a dreadful pestilence sweeping the Orient. Realizing that the new disease might be this Eastern scourge, Messina's townspeople closed the port. Their efforts came too late: The entire island was soon infected. Meanwhile, the ships—and the plague—proceeded to other port cities, crossing the Mediterranean to Egypt, northern Africa, and Spain.

The epidemic reached Marseille, in southern France, in January 1348. Within a year, it had swept across France by land, and ships carrying French wine north to England carried infected rats as well. English wool merchants probably transported plague to Scandinavia in 1349. It swept through Denmark and Germany in 1350 and touched Poland in 1351 before reentering central Asia from the west.

Wherever the disease traveled, it brought a hideous, repulsive death. Written accounts tell of shivering fits, bloody vomit, and an intolerable stench radiating from a victim's breath, body, and wastes. Other symptoms were stranger. Italian author Giovanni Boccaccio (1313?-1375), who lived at the time of the epidemic, described the disease's hallmarks:

"It began both in men and women with certain swellings in the groin or under the armpit. They grew to the size of a small apple or an egg. . . . In a short space of time these tumors spread from the two parts named to all over the body. Soon after this the symptoms changed and black or purple spots appeared on the arms or thighs or elsewhere on the body, sometimes a few large ones, sometimes many little ones. These spots were a certain sign of death."

Gui de Chauliac, then physician to the pope, noted that while the illness Boccaccio described usually caused death in five days, some people recovered—as Gui himself did. But he also

How plague is transmitted

The plague bacterium, *Yersinia pestis*, primarily infects rats and other rodents. The bacteria are spread from rodent to rodent by fleas. If the rodents should die off, their fleas may bite human beings. Bacteria from an infected rodent can also enter the human body through a cut in the skin. An infected person can sometimes transmit the bacteria by sneezing or coughing.

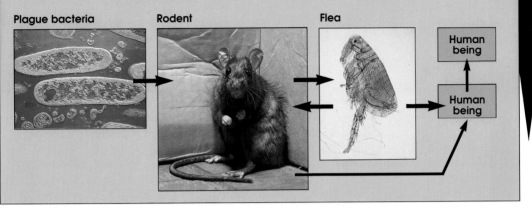

Plague bacteria **Rodent** **Flea** Human being Human being

recognized a more deadly form, with "continuous fever and spitting of blood," which invariably killed in three days. Other writings suggest yet a third form that struck so suddenly—and without warning symptoms—that people who went to bed healthy were found dead in the morning.

The medieval descriptions reflect quite clearly the three forms of plague known today: bubonic, pneumonic, and septicemic. Bubonic and septicemic plague most commonly result from flea bites, which inject *Yersinia pestis* directly into the body. These forms of plague can also be acquired by absorbing body fluids, such as blood or saliva, of an infected person through a break in the skin. Pneumonic plague is contracted from coughing plague victims whose lungs are infected.

Bubonic plague, the predominant form of the disease, takes its name from the lumps it causes in the neck, armpits, or—most often—the groin. Medieval doctors called the lumps *buboes*, from the Greek word for groin, *boubon*. A bubo is actually a mass of swollen *lymph nodes*, small bean-shaped structures clustered in bunches in the body. Fluids that bathe the body's cells circulate through the lymph nodes, which filter out harmful microorganisms. The presence of an infection causes the lymph nodes to swell.

When *Yersinia pestis* enters the body through a bite or break in the skin, it incubates for an average of two to five days before causing symptoms. Then come headache and weakness, followed by fever, aches, chills, rapid pulse, and vomiting.

The cluster of lymph nodes closest to the site of infection

swells to an extreme, forming the first bubo. Infection through the skin of the torso, arm, or head can cause buboes in the armpits or throat. But because fleas usually bite on the legs, the buboes most often appear in the groin. The lumps can grow up to 2 inches (5 centimeters) across. After a few days, the swollen nodes may burst, breaking the skin, and drain.

As the plague bacteria multiply in the body, the patient becomes listless and uncoordinated and may have trouble walking and talking. The bacteria often invade the lungs, causing pneumonia. Bacterial *toxins* (poisonous wastes) in the bloodstream produce clotting. The clots cause blood vessels to burst under the skin, creating the disease's characteristic dark blotches. Finally, the toxins attack nerve cells, producing agonizing pain, delirium, and despair. Death occurs in 60 to 80 per cent of untreated cases, usually within a week of the first symptoms. (By comparison, untreated smallpox killed up to 20 per cent of those it infected.)

Pneumonic plague develops when a person inhales the tiny, infected droplets coughed up by a bubonic plague patient who has pneumonia. Contracted this way, the bacteria invade the victim's lungs immediately, causing rapidly progressing pneumonia marked by high fever, chills, headache, and a cough that brings up blood. The patient's coughed-up fluids can infect others in turn. If untreated, pneumonic plague usually kills within two or three days.

Septicemic plague, which is almost always fatal, occurs when the bacteria overwhelm the bloodstream instead of congregating in the lymph nodes. The bacteria and their toxins invade and destroy tissues throughout the body, and the victim dies within a day or less.

Although septicemic plague generally kills before a diagnosis can be made, doctors today can cure bubonic and some pneumonic cases by administering antibiotic drugs as soon as they suspect plague. Delay can be fatal: With enough of a head start, the bacteria can fill the blood with so much toxin that the patient may die even after drug treatment controls the bacteria themselves.

Medieval doctors had no miracle drugs, however, and their treatments—which typically involved bloodletting, enemas, and a bland diet—proved powerless against the plague. Unaware of the true cause of the disease, some theorized that earthquakes or unseasonable winds had poisoned the air. Others blamed cataclysms in the Orient—rains of frogs and serpents, massive clouds of foul smoke—that were rumored to have preceded the plague. Scholars at the University of Paris cited a conjunction of the planets Saturn, Mars, and Jupiter on March 20, 1345, as having caused "pernicious corruption of the surrounding air."

Spiritual leaders saw a different reason for the plague: punishment for human sins. Yet prayer, penance, fasting, and other religious observances did nothing to stop the epidemic. Some people, observing that priests were struck down as often as others, abandoned the organized church for alternative cults. Many chroniclers describe cults of *flagellants*—groups who traveled from town to town, publicly whipping themselves in bizarre religious ceremonies.

Because no other means of transmission was apparent, many people readily accepted the explanation that the air itself had become contaminated. They wore masks to avoid evil vapors, carried herbs and perfumes to nullify them, or inhaled the stench from public latrines to drive the tainted air from their lungs. The pope, at his palace in Avignon in southern France, sat between two huge fires meant to purify the air.

Elsewhere, people banished or burned foreigners, Gypsies, beggars, or lepers for supposedly bringing the disease. Most often, the blame fell on the Jews—even though plague struck them as well—and many thousands of Jews were slaughtered throughout Europe.

Some people, faced with seemingly certain death, embraced wild living, drinking, gambling, and merrymaking. Most, however, closed themselves in their homes, marking crosses on the

Useless treatments
Treatments for plague in the 1300's included lancing and draining painful lumps that formed in the neck, armpit, and groin. The lumps, called *buboes*, were actually lymph nodes, swollen from fighting the infection that had overtaken the body. But lancing buboes proved useless against the disease.

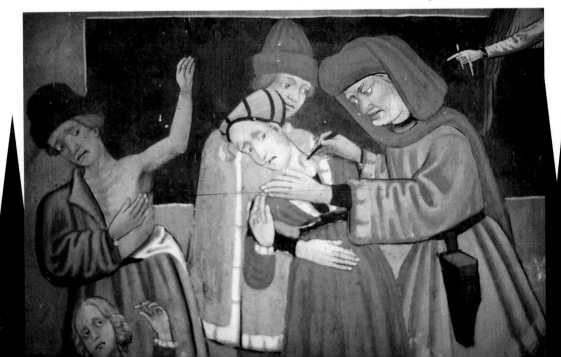

doors in the hope they would be spared. Many towns shut their gates to travelers and traders. In the Italian city of Milan, the archbishop ordered townspeople to brick up victims' houses, with any remaining occupants, sick or not, left inside. Such efforts at quarantine invariably failed, however, because rats still ran freely, and unnoticed, from house to house.

Ultimately, people fled, seeking refuge in regions yet untouched by plague. Many of those who ran merely carried the disease with them, infecting new communities. Those who left the cities for rural mountains seem to have survived in greater numbers, probably because rats and fleas dislike cool, dry climates. Yet survivors credited any of a hundred other rituals: bathing, or avoiding bathing; eating strange concoctions of herbs, or fasting; sleeping on one side or the other, or only sleeping at certain hours.

Cities, crowded and easily infected, suffered the worst losses. Major cities such as Paris and Rome saw hundreds of deaths daily at the epidemic's height. Oppressed by the ceaseless tolling of funeral bells, authorities in many cities forbade their ringing, along with large funerals or mourning clothes.

As the death count rose, so did the piles of rotting corpses. Before long, the dead began to overwhelm the living. Bodies were dragged out to doorsteps each morning, alongside the piles

Coping with catastrophe

Helpless against the epidemic's spread, people sought divine aid or at least a temporary escape from the devastation. A manuscript from about 1420, *below*, records how they participated in religious processions and prayed for an end to the misery. Wealthy city-dwellers sought relief by fleeing to countryside retreats, *opposite page, top,* and engaging in story-telling or other diverting pleasures.

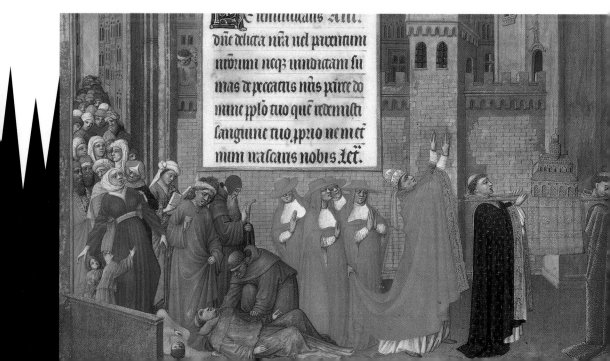

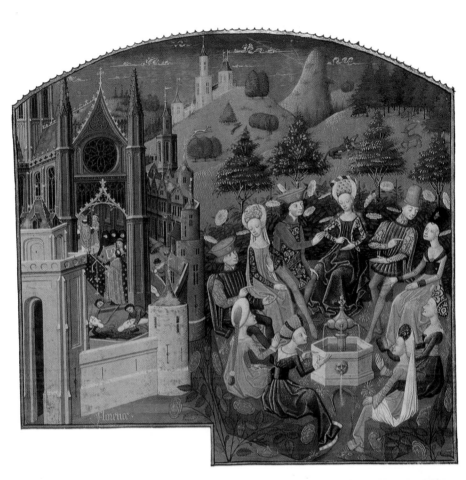

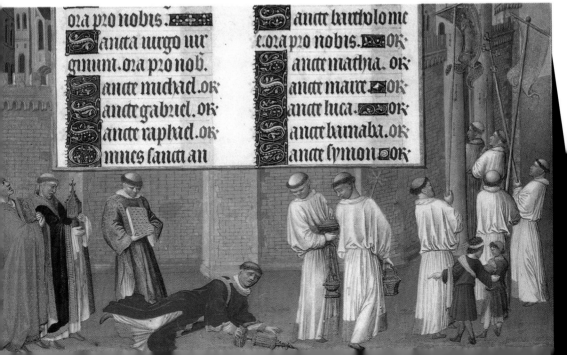

ora pro nobis.
Sancta uirgo uir-
ginum. ora pro nob.
Sancte michael. or.
Sancte gabriel. or.
Sancte raphael. or.
mnes sancti an

Sancte bartholome
e. ora pro nobis. or.
ancte mathia. or.
ancte maure. or.
ancte luca. or.
ancte barnaba. or.
ancte symon or.

of uncarted garbage. Convicted criminals, country laborers, or members of religious orders hauled the remains away until they, too, died.

When cemeteries filled, officials opened nearby fields for mass graves. In fact, the scene of a foul pit of ravaged or burning bodies, tended by doomed workers, became so universal a symbol of terror and despair that preachers and painters for centuries afterward were to summon it up as an image of hell.

Along with funeral customs, other trappings of civilized life were shed during the months and years of plague. An English bishop complained in a letter of 1349 about the lack of priests to hear confession or administer last rites for plague victims. Civil courts and meetings of governmental bodies were suspended. The streets were left to thieves, "for, like other men, the ministers and the executors of the laws were all dead or sick or shut up with their families," Boccaccio wrote.

In retrospect, the time of chaos in any one place was brief. A village might have suffered for six months, a large city for a year or two, before the plague moved on. But during that time, industry and trade all but ceased as many laborers lay sick or dying and the rest avoided contact with others. In Siena, Italy, work on a great cathedral halted, never to be resumed.

Mortality may well have reached 90 to 100 per cent in some communities, such as monasteries where many men shared crowded dormitories infested with rats. But the death rate throughout Europe was certainly far less. Estimates today, based on such evidence as wills and tax records, vary widely by region. Overall, modern scholars generally come up with the same rough estimate recorded by the French historian Jean Froissart (1337-1410): "At least a third of all the people" of Europe—perhaps 20 million or more—died in the Black Death.

Even after the initial wave burned itself out in 1352, plague reappeared in lesser epidemics every 10 years or so for the rest of the 1300's. In England, the second wave, in 1361, was called the "Pestilence of the Children" because it proved especially fatal to the young. That is probably because the adults who had survived the earlier outbreak of the disease were immune, while children born after it had no such protection.

After 1400 or so, plague's recurrences, while common, were far less severe and more localized. Experts suggest that by this time the European populations of rats, fleas, and *Yersinia pestis* had achieved some sort of balance.

But even as the plague moved toward a biological balance among animals, it destroyed the social balance among human beings. In Europe, a major effect was economic upheaval. The deaths of so many people produced an abundance of land and a shortage of labor, upsetting the old order. For example, peasants

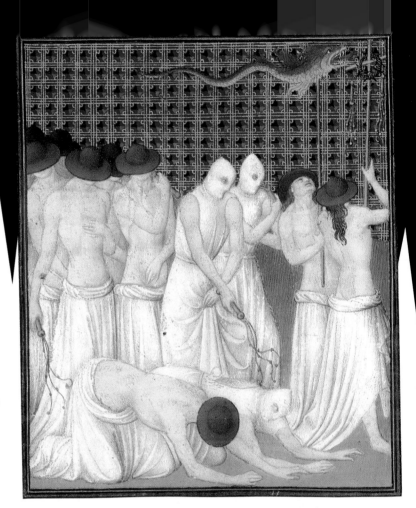

Casting blame

Unaware of the cause of the plague, people sought scapegoats. Thousands of Jews were put to death, often by burning, *below*. Some Christians, believing the plague was a punishment for their own sins, whipped each other or themselves as they prayed for mercy, *right*.

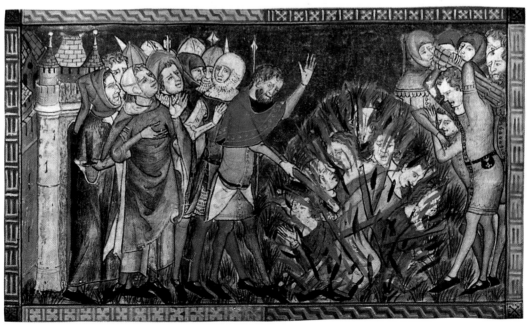

were able to demand higher wages and to take control of farms whose owners had died of plague, breaking down the centuries-old class distinction between laborers and landowners.

At the same time, the sudden deaths of so many of Europe's established scholars left a large gap in the world of learning, eventually filled by young thinkers with new ideas. And a disillusioned public began to question the overarching power of the medieval Church and the obedience it demanded. Defiance soon turned to revolt against Church and civil authorities. During the English Peasants' Revolt of 1381, for example, mobs stormed London to protest laws that protected the class structure. Many historians believe that the changes provoked by the Black Death laid the groundwork for the social revolutions of the next two centuries, including both the Protestant Reformation and the Renaissance.

The Black Death was without doubt plague's most devastating appearance. But it was by no means its last—or even its first.

Various epidemics called "plagues" have been recorded since ancient times, but historians believe bubonic plague made its first major showing in the mid-500's, when an epidemic crippled the city of Constantinople (now Istanbul, Turkey), capital of the Byzantine Empire. Plague recurred periodically throughout the Mediterranean region before subsiding in the 700's. After its reappearance in the 1300's, however, plague remained entrenched for four centuries before disappearing completely from western Europe around 1720.

In China in 1855, soldiers carried plague out of an isolated area where it was endemic, leading to a series of outbreaks throughout the Chinese interior. The disease gained international attention only when it reached the populous centers of Canton and Hong Kong in 1894. From there, the bacteria were transported by steamship to previously untouched areas, including North America. The first U.S. outbreak—in 1900 in San Francisco—was quickly contained, but the bacteria established a home in California's rodent communities. By then, however, scientists had discovered *Yersinia pestis* and identified its means of infection.

Today, plague is found in every part of the world except Australia and the islands nearby and western Europe. More than 80 per cent of reported cases occur in Africa, mostly in Kenya, Uganda, Tanzania, and Zaire, and analysts believe many more African cases go unreported. In South America, plague cases regularly are reported in Brazil, Ecuador, Peru, and Bolivia. In Asia, plague has appeared recently in Indonesia, Burma, Vietnam, and occasionally China. Health experts know that plague is endemic among rodents in the Soviet Union, but no human cases have officially been reported there in many years.

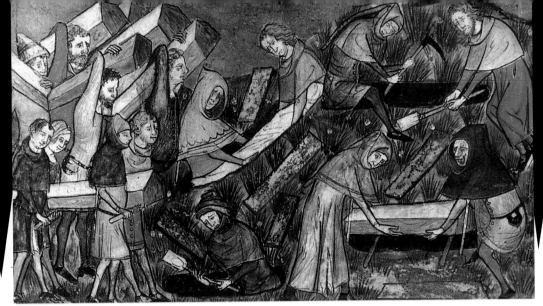

Scientists are still studying why plague no longer exists in western Europe. One current theory stems from the discovery of another strain of *Yersinia* bacteria there. This strain does not kill its host animals but does seem to make them immune to the deadlier *Yersinia pestis*. Scientists suspect such milder strains may have displaced the plague bacterium—not only in Europe, but also in the eastern United States, where plague is unknown.

Plague is well established, however, in host animals in the American Southwest. More than half of all U.S. cases occur in New Mexico, where plague-carrying rodents, especially ground squirrels, are plentiful. Most other U.S. cases are contracted in Arizona, California, and Colorado. The number of human cases peaks every five to eight years, reflecting cycles of plague in animal populations. The most recent peak was in 1983, with 40 cases and 6 deaths. Since then, the numbers have gradually fallen, with only 1 case reported in 1990—a nonfatal infection contracted in Colorado.

Human infection depends in part on the presence of the right kind of flea. To infect human beings with plague, fleas must be able to carry *Yersinia pestis* from host to host, and they must be willing to bite people. The species of fleas that live on California ground squirrels and rock squirrels meet both these criteria, but most other species of American fleas do not. The fleas that normally bite dogs and cats, for example, cannot transmit plague bacteria. Even so, a household pet may occasionally pick up an infected rodent flea and pass it to a human being.

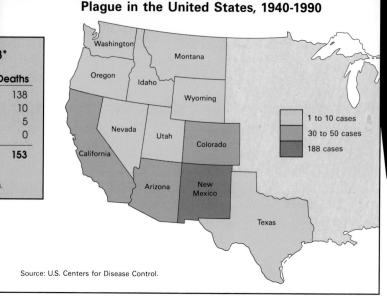

Plague in the United States, 1940-1990

	1 to 10 cases
	30 to 50 cases
	188 cases

Source: U.S. Centers for Disease Control.

Plague worldwide, 1988*	Cases	Deaths
Africa	1,109	138
Asia	202	10
South America	37	5
North America	15	0
World total	**1,363**	**153**

*Latest available statistics.
Source: World Health Organization.

Plague today

Plague still strikes hundreds of people each year. More than 80 per cent of reported cases occur in Africa. In the United States, plague is known only in the West. More than half of all U.S. cases occur in New Mexico, where infected rodents are plentiful. Deaths are rare because health officials know how to treat the disease and prevent its spread.

People can also catch plague by handling an infected animal. Hunters of ground squirrels, rabbits, and similar game, for example, can contract the disease if an infected animal's bodily fluids enter through a break in the skin. And because cats can contract plague by eating an infected rodent, cat owners sometimes become infected by the saliva or blood of their sick pet. Dogs rarely become ill from plague.

Plague is curable only if treated early with streptomycin or certain other antibiotics, so those who catch it are most at risk if diagnosis is delayed. And because plague is so rare, doctors outside plague-endemic areas often do not recognize it at once. Plague deaths are thus most common among travelers who become infected in the Southwest or a foreign country and fall ill after returning home.

Even when an unwary traveler carries the disease to a city, however, there's little danger of it spreading like the epidemics of old. Villagewide outbreaks do occur in underdeveloped countries, often because medical treatment does not arrive in time to prevent the first victim from developing pneumonia and infecting others. But U.S. cities are unlikely to experience an epidemic of plague for several reasons.

First, Americans rarely live in close quarters with the large numbers of rodents needed to spread the disease and cause an epidemic. And fleas that transmit the bacteria from rodents to people are not abundant in North America.

Second, plague is rarely transmitted from one human being

to another in the United States. Patients are generally diagnosed early and monitored closely to avoid contagion. And while fleas whose host of choice is people are an important means of human-to-human transmission in some countries, such fleas are not generally found among Americans.

Yet health officials still fear that someone will return from a trip with plague and develop secondary pneumonia, infecting both family and medical staff before a diagnosis is made. Says Allan Barnes, a research biologist who directs the plague laboratory at the federal Centers for Disease Control (CDC) in Fort Collins, Colo.: "We still worry about a plague pneumonia epidemic, even though the last time that happened in this country was 1924." About 40 people in Los Angeles contracted plague during that outbreak. And because antibiotic treatment was not yet known, nearly all died.

A vaccine for plague exists, but because shots must be repeated every few months, it is given only to people at high risk of contracting plague. These include certain animal control workers, laboratory researchers working with plague, travelers to plague-ridden areas, and some military personnel.

Preventive measures instead focus on monitoring animal populations and educating the public. In areas where plague is endemic, officials test dead rodents for the disease and spray rodent holes with insecticide to control fleas. Area residents are encouraged to report dead wild rodents. And the CDC monitors the nation's plague cases and informs doctors in plague-endemic areas of animal epidemics that might endanger people.

In the midst of the Black Death, the poet Petrarch envisioned a time in the distant future when the story of that epidemic would seem an unbelievable exaggeration. "Oh, happy posterity," he wrote, "which will not experience such abysmal woe and will look upon our testimony as a fable!" His prediction has proved close to the truth. While plague is still with us, scientists now understand its workings and know how to prevent its spread. Only accounts of its terrible history remind us of the devastation it once inflicted.

For further reading:

McEvedy, Colin. "The Bubonic Plague." *Scientific American*, February 1988.

Mee, Charles L, Jr. "How a mysterious disease laid low Europe's masses." *Smithsonian*, February 1990.

Tuchman, Barbara. *A Distant Mirror: The Calamitous 14th Century*. Knopf, 1978.

Ziegler, Philip. *The Black Death*. Harper, 1971. First published in 1969.

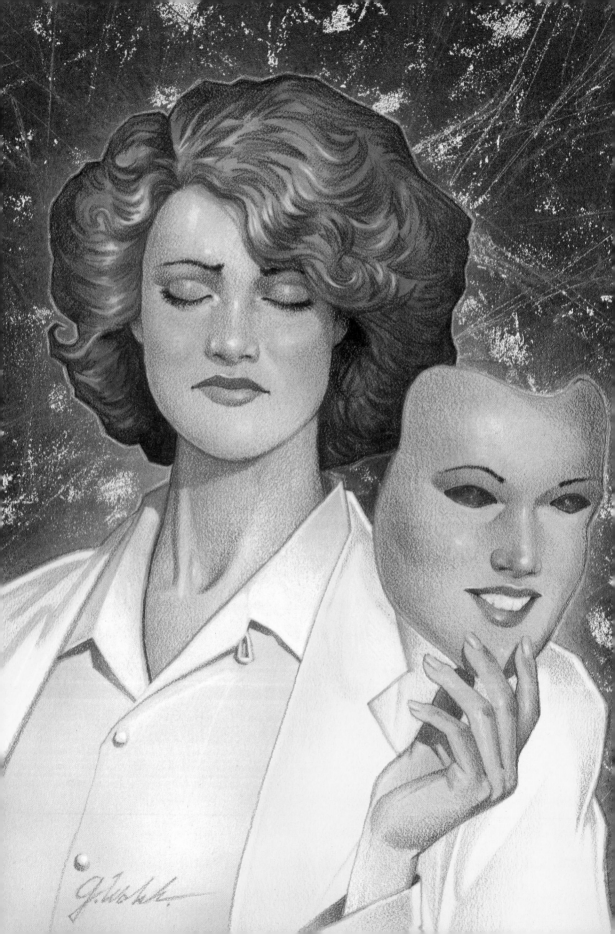

Psychologists say that some people are born with a tendency to be inhibited and shy. Many learn to cope with and even conquer their shyness—and parents can help.

What's Behind Shyness?

By Richard Saltus

Sarah, a journalist and feature writer, is well respected in her field for her candid profiles of important people. But when she's not doing her job, Sarah is a victim of extreme, lifelong shyness.

"I was terribly, terribly shy as a child," she says. "I'll bet you most of my elementary school teachers wouldn't even remember me. I was one of those kids who sat in the back and never raised their hand." Sarah's pals were the pet animals she kept. Even when her mother invited playmates to her house, Sarah was slow to warm up. "I always felt better if I had one of my animals with me, like a security blanket," she says, smiling. "I remember very clearly meeting a girlfriend at the front door clutching a pet skunk in my arms."

Although she can meet all kinds of people without anxiety as long as she is performing the role of interviewer, Sarah is miserable if made the center of attention. In social situations, her stomach flip-flops and her mouth becomes dry—signs of what may well be an inborn tendency to freeze up among strangers.

Gathering in social groups is one of the most common of human activities, yet for millions of people, mingling with strangers can cause unpleasant emotional responses, ranging from nervousness to panic. Today, research on shyness is helping people like Sarah lose some of their fears, but for many, the battle against shyness is never over.

What is shyness?

Shyness can range from a temporary fearful reaction in a specific situation to a fear of all social situations that pervades a person's entire life. Most people can recall having at least fleeting moments of shyness that caused momentary discomfort but little lasting distress. But extreme and persistent shyness can be so troublesome for those who experience it that many feel it ruins their personal and professional lives.

Psychologists distinguish between people who have feelings of apprehension only with strangers and people who not only exhibit shy behavior with others but also show fearful behavior when confronted with a variety of unfamiliar events and experiences. Psychologists define the former group as *shy* and the latter group as *anxious*. Some of these shyer, anxious people acquired their tendency as a result of stressful life experiences. Others, however, were born with a temperamental bias that predisposed them to become shy and fearful. Psychologists and psychiatrists have also identified a third category of behavior called *social phobia*, an extreme form of fear and anxiety to novel social situations, particularly speaking in public.

Since the early 1970's, many psychologists and other mental health experts have thus come to regard shyness as a potentially lasting problem, rather than a mere phase of childhood or a harmless eccentricity. Fortunately, this increased recognition of such consequences has prompted more and more people who suffer from shyness, especially in their adult years, to seek treatment in hopes of easing their distress.

How common is shyness?

Psychologists find it difficult to say how prevalent shyness is, because the definition of shyness is far from exact, and because surveys generally rely on questionnaires that ask people to rate themselves for shyness. According to some surveys, the prevalence may be as high as 40 per cent among people in their late teens or early 20's. Psychologist Philip G. Zimbardo of Stanford University in California, who carried out one such survey in the late 1970's among Stanford students, reported that some 80 per cent of respondents in the survey said they had once been shy. But some critics say that figure is suspect because people often remember themselves as being shyer than they probably were.

Studies suggest that shyness peaks in the adolescent years—generally between ages 13 and 18—and that the problem is less common in older adults. According to Paul Pilkonis, a psycholo-

The author:

Richard Saltus is a science writer for *The Boston Globe*.

Learning about shyness

Studies by Harvard University psychologist Jerome Kagan show that children who have an inborn tendency to be shy and inhibited are fearful in unfamiliar settings and slow to warm up to strangers.

As Kagan observes from an adjoining room, a child who is prone to shyness clings to his mother for comfort when they enter a laboratory "playroom" that is unfamiliar to him.

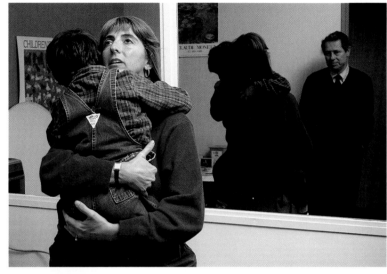

After a while, the child becomes less fearful and plays with toys while his mother stays reassuringly nearby.

Eventually, this shy child is able to talk and play with a stranger in the playroom. The study found that shy children took at least 20 minutes to chat with the stranger, compared with nonshy children, who showed no fear of the unfamiliar setting and who talked with the stranger within minutes.

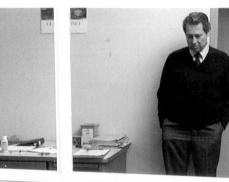

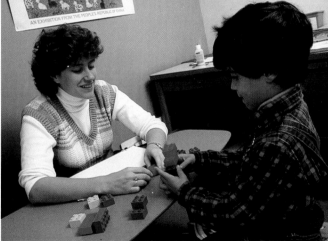

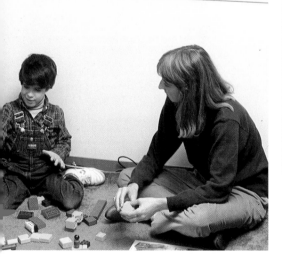

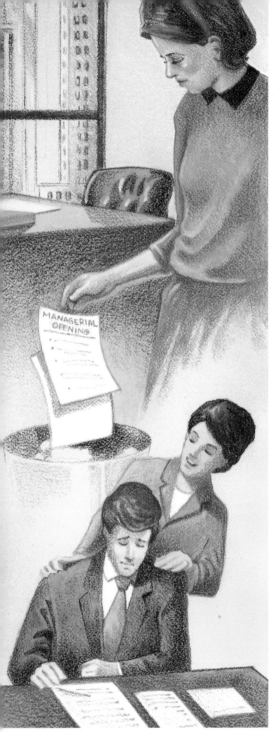

When shyness is a problem

Extreme shyness can pose many problems for a person's professional or personal life. For example, a very shy person may not apply for a promotion to a managerial job to avoid being put in a position of high visibility. Or such a person may be too reluctant to begin a romantic relationship.

gist at the University of Pittsburgh who formerly worked with Zimbardo at Stanford, 31 per cent of a sample of 216 adults described themselves as shy. Of those self-proclaimed shy people, nearly two-thirds rated this tendency as a moderate to extreme problem.

Psychologist Jerome Kagan of Harvard University in Cambridge, Mass., estimates that 10 to 15 per cent of young children have a temperamental tendency to be shy. These children not only are predisposed to shy behavior with strangers but also are restrained and timid in a variety of unfamiliar situations, even those that do not involve unfamiliar people. Kagan believes that these children should be categorized as *inhibited*, rather than shy. He notes that inhibited children may eventually overcome their shy behavior with strangers but remain restrained and timid throughout life when faced with unfamiliar situations or new kinds of challenges.

Seeking a scientific definition

Shyness is an old concept among human beings, but a relatively new subject for scientific study. The Oxford English Dictionary dates the word *shy* to an Anglo-Saxon poem of about the year 1000, in which it meant "easily frightened." But psychologists did not begin using the term until the early 1900's when the Swiss psychiatrist and psychologist Carl G. Jung cited shyness as an important characteristic of the *introvert*, or withdrawn and self-preoccupied personality. In a landmark work published in 1924, Jung said that all people could be classified as being either mainly introverted, or the opposite, extroverted.

Since the late 1900's, psychologists have formulated various definitions of shyness. Kagan regards some shy people as being biologically prone to this condition, and he views this type of shyness as a *trait* (characteristic) that can be observed in children from about age 1 onward. Kagan calls these children *behaviorally inhibited*. In a series of studies on shyness, he and his colleagues placed children in unfamiliar rooms with their mothers and observed the youngsters' behavior when a stranger entered or when unfamiliar events occurred. If the child was markedly shy with the stranger, withdrew, refused to approach an unfamiliar toy, and sought out the mother, while ignoring invitations to approach the stranger or to play with the unfamiliar toy, the psychologists regarded that child as inhibited.

Another expert, psychologist Jonathan M. Cheek of Wellesley College in Wellesley, Mass., defines shyness as a *syndrome* (a collection of symptoms) in which people are predisposed to feeling tense, worried, or awkward in social situations, especially those where most other people are strangers. Physical symptoms may include shaking, blushing, or a quickened heartbeat during a social encounter.

Besides causing such physical symptoms, shyness also affects a person's thoughts and behaviors, says Cheek. Shy people may be preoccupied with the notion that others are unfavorably scrutinizing them. As a consequence, shy people often appear physically awkward, shrink from other people, and avoid making eye contact.

A shy disposition, however, may not always manifest itself outwardly. Some people can disguise their fears of social situations and, to other people, may seem in control—even outgoing and sociable. But inwardly, these people experience distress.

A link to low self-esteem

Psychologists have linked shyness to other frequently occurring behavioral traits, such as extreme pessimism and poor self-esteem. Shyness sometimes leads to depression and severe anxiety. Many experts have observed that shyness and low self-esteem go hand in hand, but which is the cause and which is the effect is controversial.

Cheek and other experts say that shy people tend to blame themselves for social failures but attribute any social successes to luck or factors beyond their control. As Cheek put it, "shy people are their own worst critics." With all their fears, avoidance of social situations, and awkward style in public, the shy create their own obstacles to success in life. Failure in ro-

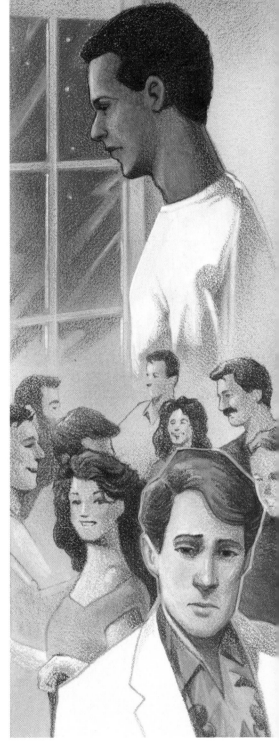

Some shy people will avoid social situations, even if it means feeling lonely. Others may participate in social gatherings, but such settings cause them emotional distress, making it difficult to establish friendships.

mantic relationships, holding jobs, and career advancement are common even when the person has intelligence and talent, says Cheek. Chronically shy adults tend to be lonely and have difficulties forming romantic relationships with the opposite sex, he notes.

Environmental causes of shyness

Psychologists believe there is no single cause of shyness but that a variety of factors work together to cause this trait. Such factors can be categorized as either *environmental* (involving surroundings and upbringing) or *genetic* (traits passed from parents to offspring in the genes). Psychologists have long thought that environmental factors play a role in shyness.

Environmental factors include everything that happens to an individual after conception, from exposure to the mother's hormones in the womb, to life experiences such as relationships with family members and peers. For many shy people, the problem is rooted in family interactions or life events that influenced their personality development. "There are at least six published studies that show that the more inhibited the emotional expressiveness and warmth in a family, the higher the level of the shyness and self-esteem problem," notes Cheek.

Other environmental factors influence the development of shyness. Failure to learn social skills can play a major part in contributing to shyness, according to psychologists, because the individual feels either uncomfortable or inadequate during social interactions. If an individual's family moved frequently, the child may have found it difficult to develop a core group of friends because he or she was always shunned as the "new kid on the block." Failure to develop close friendships can reinforce a tendency to shyness.

Inherited causes of shyness

There is also increasing evidence that, in some cases, people are born with an inherited tendency to shyness. Since the early 1970's, Kagan and other scientists have accumulated convincing evidence that early-appearing shyness often reflects some genetic influence. For example, studies have shown that identical twins are far more likely to share a tendency to be shy than are fraternal twins. Since identical twins have 100 per cent of the same genetic material and fraternal twins have only 50 per cent of the same genes (the same as any two nonidentical siblings), this finding suggests that certain genes predispose some individuals to be shy.

The notion that a tendency to be shy or inhibited can be inborn has been supported by animal studies conducted by researcher Stephen Suomi of the National Institutes of Health in

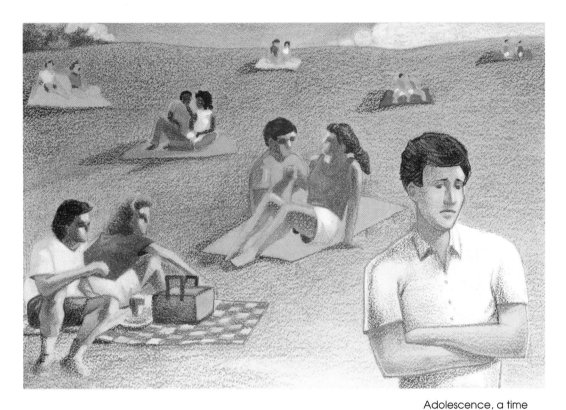

Bethesda, Md. Suomi studied how infant monkeys responded to being separated from their mothers and placed in unfamiliar situations early in life. During research conducted in the 1960's and 1970's, Suomi found that some monkeys, whom he labeled "uptight," were more prone to inhibition and showed certain physiological reactions to novelty, such as increased heart rate, that Kagan also observed in children. Breeding studies revealed that the "uptight" temperament is inherited, Suomi reported. Environment and interactions with other monkeys, however, can modify the "uptight" tendency, he said.

Kagan's most recent research, which he began in the late 1980's, suggests that some infants as young as 4 months show special behavioral signs of their inherited tendency to develop shyness, though they do not appear distressed in the presence of strangers or exhibit other expressions of shyness until at least 1 year of age. In a continuing series of experiments at Harvard, Kagan and his colleagues presented various stimuli—sights, sounds, and smells—to some 250 babies, 4-months-old, in a 40-minute session. About 20 per cent of the infants flexed their limbs with unusual vigor, arched their backs, showed unusual tension with their bodies, and fretted or cried while they were aroused.

Kagan theorizes that the combination of extreme motor arousal and crying indicates that these babies had unusually

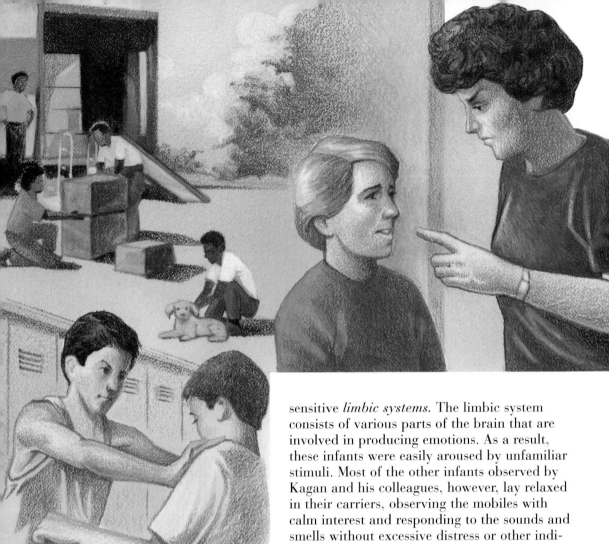

Experiences contribute to shyness

Experiences in childhood can greatly influence a child already genetically predisposed to shyness. Such experiences include being the target of a bully, as well as moving frequently and always being the "new kid on the block." Parents who are overcritical and lower a child's self-esteem also may intensify a child's tendency to be shy.

sensitive *limbic systems.* The limbic system consists of various parts of the brain that are involved in producing emotions. As a result, these infants were easily aroused by unfamiliar stimuli. Most of the other infants observed by Kagan and his colleagues, however, lay relaxed in their carriers, observing the mobiles with calm interest and responding to the sounds and smells without excessive distress or other indications of bodily tension.

When researchers tested the infants for shyness and fear at 14 and 21 months, two-thirds of those who had reacted to new stimuli with distress and crying when they were 4 months old were now the most fearful with strangers and timid with unfamiliar objects. In contrast, the formerly relaxed babies tended to be unafraid, explored their new environments, and were quite willing to play with a stranger.

According to Kagan, these results suggest that the 4-month-old babies with sensitive, overreactive limbic systems were predisposed to become shy later on. Further studies revealed that "temperamentally shy" children have physical responses to new situations that differ from those of the relaxed babies. Research by Kagan and psychologist J. Steven Reznick at Harvard and psychologist Nancy

Snidman at Yale University in New Haven, Conn., showed that when temperamentally shy babies face unfamiliar stimuli, their hearts tend to beat faster, their pupils tend to *dilate* (widen), and the skin on the right side of their face tends to cool slightly—all signs of stress.

Kagan believes that genes—as yet unidentified—are the source of this physiological difference and represent the biological basis for shyness. Exactly what these genes do is not known, but experts generally assume that they somehow exert their effects on the brain. Kagan, for one, believes that the region of the brain most affected is the *amygdala*, a small, almond-shaped cluster of nerve cells that belongs to the limbic system. The amygdala appears to play a role in emotional behavior and seems to be involved in reactions to novelty and uncertainty. In experiments in which other researchers damaged the amygdalas of animals that were previously wary of new situations, those animals lost their fear of novelty.

The amygdala and the system of which it is a part may be unusually excitable in temperamentally shy children, Kagan suggests. Consequently, when faced with new situations and people, these children overreact. Whatever the physical basis, Kagan estimates that about 20 per cent of all children are born with this "bias" for shyness.

A persistent trait

By following large numbers of infants into late childhood, psychologists have found that the persistence, or stability, of the shyness trait is as strong or stronger than any other personality characteristic. Shyness may be among the most heritable and stable of all human traits, according to studies done by Robert Plomin, a *behavioral geneticist* (a scientist who studies how genes influence behavior) at Pennsylvania State University in University Park.

These same researchers, however, are careful to emphasize that an inborn tendency does not mean that a shy child is bound to be bashful all his or her life. The temperamental trait can be strongly modified by environment and experience. For example, Kagan's long-term

Are you shy?

Psychologist Jonathan Cheek includes this measure of shyness in his book, *Conquering Shyness* (1990). Using the scale below, assign a number value to each statement. Add up all the numbers for a "shyness" score.

1 very uncharacteristic; strongly disagree
2 uncharacteristic
3 neutral
4 characteristic
5 very characteristic; strongly agree

___ I'm tense when I'm with people I don't know well.

___ It's difficult for me to ask other people for information.

___ I'm often uncomfortable at parties and other social functions.

___ When in a group of people, I have trouble thinking of the right thing to say.

___ It takes me a long time to overcome my shyness in new situations.

___ It's hard for me to act natural when I'm meeting new people.

___ I'm nervous when speaking to someone in authority.

___ I have doubts about my social competence.

___ I have trouble looking someone right in the eye.

___ I feel inhibited in social situations.

___ I find it hard to talk to strangers.

___ I am more shy with members of the opposite sex.

Rating: If over 45, you're very shy. If between 31 and 45, you are somewhat shy. If you scored below 31, you're probably not a particularly shy person. Most shy people score over 35, and a few reach the highest possible score of 60.

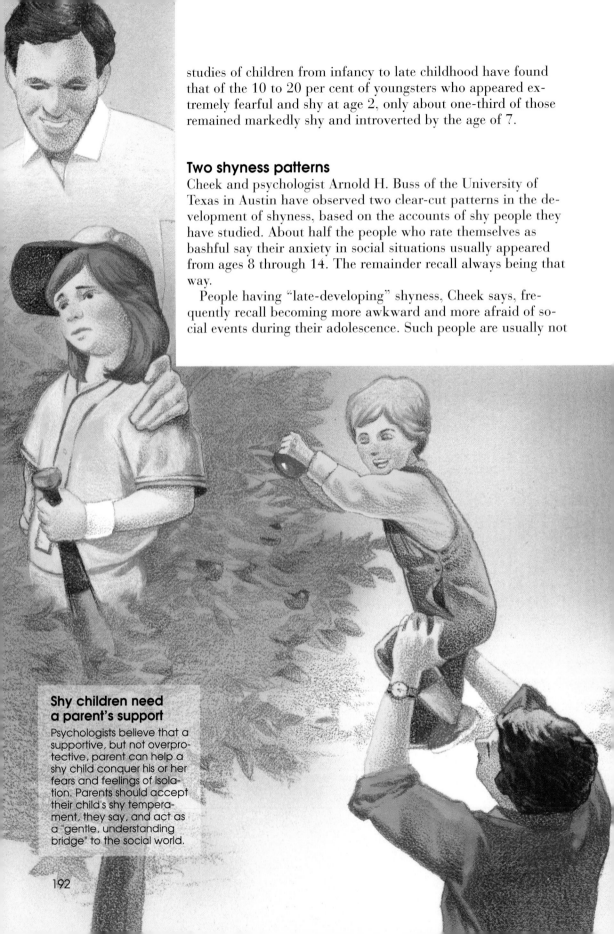

studies of children from infancy to late childhood have found that of the 10 to 20 per cent of youngsters who appeared extremely fearful and shy at age 2, only about one-third of those remained markedly shy and introverted by the age of 7.

Two shyness patterns

Cheek and psychologist Arnold H. Buss of the University of Texas in Austin have observed two clear-cut patterns in the development of shyness, based on the accounts of shy people they have studied. About half the people who rate themselves as bashful say their anxiety in social situations usually appeared from ages 8 through 14. The remainder recall always being that way.

People having "late-developing" shyness, Cheek says, frequently recall becoming more awkward and more afraid of social events during their adolescence. Such people are usually not

Shy children need a parent's support

Psychologists believe that a supportive, but not overprotective, parent can help a shy child conquer his or her fears and feelings of isolation. Parents should accept their child's shy temperament, they say, and act as a "gentle, understanding bridge" to the social world.

192

bothered by physical symptoms engendered by shyness, such as a racing heart and upset stomach, and more frequently find that their shyness lessens as they become adults. On the other hand, people with "early-developing shyness" are more likely to experience physical symptoms, and their shyness is more likely to persist into adulthood.

Therapy for shyness

Clearly, not all shy children grow up to be temperamentally inhibited and withdrawn adults. Some learn to cope with and even conquer their problem—and parents can help with this process. Psychologists say that parents can avoid blaming themselves for their child's fearful behavior if they recognize that their child may be temperamentally shy.

Kagan says research indicates that temperamentally shy children do best when they are neither forced into social situations nor are overprotected by their parents. A fearful and shy child needs to learn to put up with some anxiety and frustration. Parents can help a child become accustomed to new situations or people at his or her own pace. For example, Kagan recommends inviting playmates to the child's house so that the child can make new friends on familiar turf.

Cheek says that parents should be tolerant of children's differing temperaments. For example, they should not goad a timid, sensitive boy into rough-and-tumble play. If their child is shy, parents should "be a gentle, understanding bridge" to the social world, Cheek says.

Experts note that treating adults with severe shyness can be

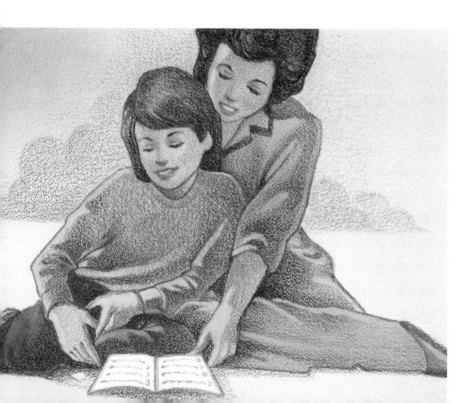

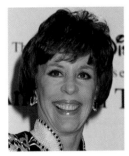

Carol Burnett

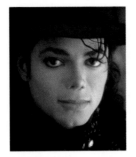

Michael Jackson

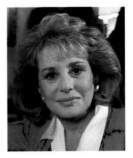

Barbara Walters

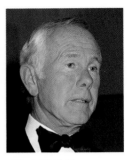

Johnny Carson

Shyness among celebrities is not uncommon, demonstrating that shyness need not be a barrier to success. These celebrities all confess to being shy but find that they can conquer their shyness while performing in public.

more difficult. Shyness therapies involve a combination of strategies: esteem-building to counteract low self-esteem; relaxation exercises to help cope with physical symptoms; and role-playing sessions in group therapy to prepare shy people for being more outgoing in the real world.

At the Palo Alto Shyness Clinic in California, therapist Lynne Henderson first evaluates patients by giving them psychological tests and questioning them closely about the types of situations that bring on attacks of shyness. She also administers a "self-esteem inventory," because Henderson believes that changing negative views of self-worth is crucial if the patient is going to overcome his or her shyness.

Henderson and the patient agree on a list of goals, such as asking a member of the opposite sex for a date, attending a social event, or being able to speak in public. She then assigns the patient various types of "homework," including relaxation exercises, ways to improve social skills, and instructions to watch people who are successful in social situations. If the shy person can copy some of the successful behavior they see in other people, this can help instill a sense of social confidence. "What we find is that people who do the homework improve; the others don't," she says.

Role playing aids adult therapy

Group role-playing sessions are another critical part of therapy. For example, a man who was terrified of asking a woman at his office for a date practiced various ways of starting up a conversation, then moved on to asking her out for coffee. Armed with these role-playing experiences, he was able to befriend the woman and take her to a movie. Henderson also encourages patients to take up an interesting hobby, or a sport, or to become familiar with events reported in newspapers or on television. Such activities should provide a person with a means of having something to contribute in a conversation.

"We're not talking about making incredible personality changes here," cautions Henderson. "But we have men dating who haven't dated before and people making speeches and accepting promotions"—situations that in the past they might have avoided.

Drugs for extreme shyness

Some psychiatrists are also finding drug therapy helpful in reducing social anxiety in particularly extreme cases of shyness. They are reporting good success with antidepressants, tranquilizers, and *beta-blockers* (drugs that block certain nerve messages involved with stress). Psychiatrist Michael Liebowitz of the New York State Psychiatric Institute in New York City reported in 1986 that an antidepressant called *phenelzine* was effective in treating patients with social anxiety or its most severe form, social phobia. Other researchers report good results with a tranquilizer called *alprazolam.*

Liebowitz reported that a number of patients, some of them severely anxious about such things as signing their name in public, dating the opposite sex, or having any social contacts at all, benefited markedly from the phenelzine treatment. One man, who had worked only at night in order to avoid other people, was able to work the day shift after taking the antidepressant. Others lost their fear of signing their name in public. A saleswoman had previously felt stark terror when her boss watched over her shoulder as she typed. With the drug treatment, her attitude changed, and she became much more relaxed and much less fearful.

Research on shyness has brought many rewards. For people whose social anxiety would previously have been ignored or regarded as trivial, there is now recognition that their problem is real, that it is more common than had been previously thought, and that in many cases it is treatable. For parents, research has relieved them of unnecessary guilt by showing that their shy and fearful child may have an inherited tendency to withdraw from social situations, not because of anything the parent did. At the same time, research has shown how parents can help their bashful child achieve a meaningful and happy life.

For further reading:

Cheek, Jonathan. *Conquering Shyness: The Battle Anyone Can Win.* Dell, 1990.

Kagan, Jerome. "Temperamental contributions to social behavior," *American Psychologist,* April 1989.

Zimbardo, Philip G. *Shyness: What It Is; What to Do About It.* Addison-Wesley, 1977.

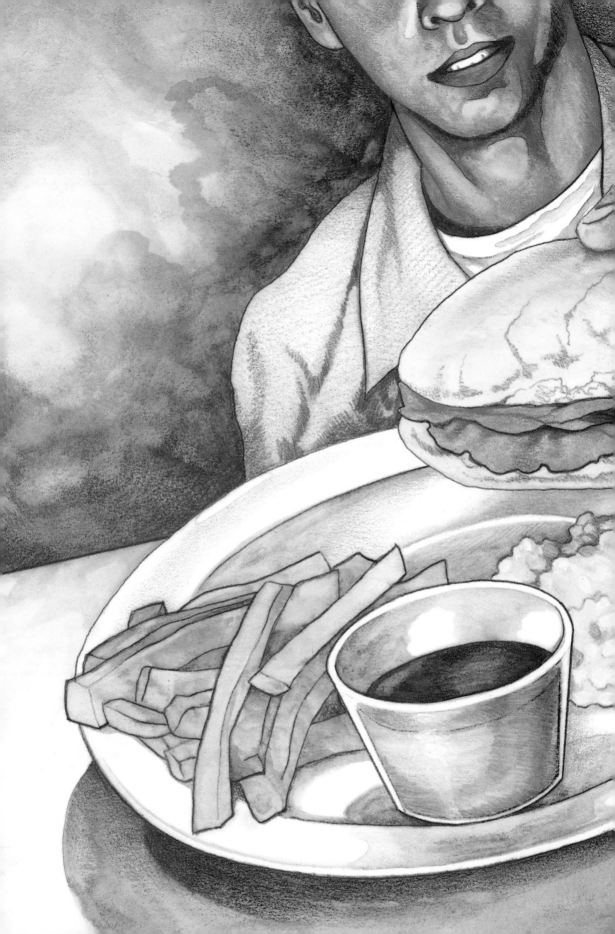

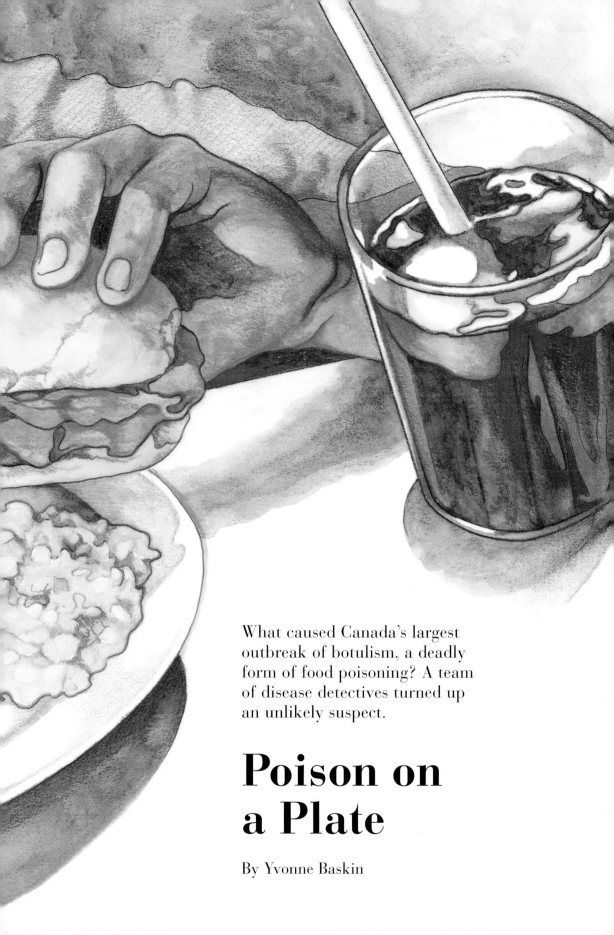

What caused Canada's largest outbreak of botulism, a deadly form of food poisoning? A team of disease detectives turned up an unlikely suspect.

Poison on a Plate

By Yvonne Baskin

Glossary

Botulism: A potentially deadly type of poisoning usually transmitted through food that has been improperly canned.

Clostridium botulinum: A bacterium that lives in the air, water, and soil and usually causes no harm. But under certain conditions, it can produce a life-threatening toxin.

Epidemiologist: Person who studies the cause, distribution, and control of diseases in a community.

Neurotransmitter: A chemical messenger released by a nerve cell that acts on a second nerve cell or a gland or muscle cell.

Spores: Dormant cells of an organism, such as bacteria, that can survive high temperatures and germinate into active microbes under less stressful conditions.

Toxin: Poison produced by a living organism such as a bacterium.

The author:

Yvonne Baskin is a San Diego-based writer who has written a book on genetics and published a variety of science articles.

At first, the physicians at Montreal Children's Hospital were at a loss to identify the mysterious illness that brought two teenage sisters into their care. The girls were weak and showed signs of paralysis. Worse yet, their breathing was becoming labored. Their muscles, including those used in breathing, were becoming paralyzed—and no one knew why.

Only hours earlier, hospital physicians had sent the girls home from the emergency room because they found nothing wrong with them other than nausea. Just a few days before, the sisters were feeling fine and had traveled with their family from Hong Kong to Vancouver and then to Montreal. Now, the girls were hooked up to *respirators*, machines that kept them breathing.

The next day, the girls' mother also became ill. The symptoms of the three patients—nausea, weakness, paralysis, and breathing difficulties—led the doctors to suspect that they were dealing with one of nature's deadliest forms of poisoning: botulism. The three cases, which occurred in September 1985, signaled what was to be Canada's largest outbreak of botulism.

Botulism is a type of food poisoning caused by the *Clostridium botulinum* bacterium. The term "food poisoning" usually refers to illnesses caused by eating food contaminated by bacteria or *toxins* (poisons) they produce. The most common types of food poisoning usually result only in vomiting or diarrhea. But botulism poisoning is far more dangerous because *botulinus toxin* (the poison made by *C. botulinum*) attacks the nervous system and can cause long-term health problems or death.

C. botulinum live all around us in air, soil, and water. We regularly consume this bacteria in fruits, vegetables, and seafood, and it normally does not harm us. But the bacteria produce dormant spores that can survive in boiling water for hours then germinate to produce a deadly toxin in an environment that lacks oxygen, such as a sealed can or bottle. Proper canning techniques make food safe by exposing the spores to high temperatures for a long enough period of time to kill them. Most botulism cases result when people consume food that was improperly canned at home.

When a person eats food contaminated with botulinus toxin, the toxin is slowly absorbed by the intestines and then moves into the bloodstream. Some of the initial symptoms—nausea, vomiting, or diarrhea—are similar to those seen in other types of food poisoning. Other symptoms—headache, dizziness, or blurred or double vision—are caused by the toxin's effects on the nervous system. The toxin finds its way to the places where nerve endings meet muscle fibers. These microscopic junctions, or *synapses*, are the points at which the nervous system controls the body's movements, from walking to breathing. Nerve cells signal the muscles to contract by releasing chemical messengers called *neurotransmitters* at the synapses.

In botulism, nerve signals are blocked when toxin molecules

attach themselves to nerve endings and prevent the release of neurotransmitters. If enough toxin is present, muscles become paralyzed, causing weakness, difficulty swallowing, and hoarseness. If breathing muscles are paralyzed, the poisoned person will die unless he or she is helped to breathe with a respirator.

Even before doctors confirmed that the teen-agers from Hong Kong were suffering from botulism, they gave them an injection of *antitoxin* (a substance that binds to the toxin and neutralizes it) specifically created for botulism. If antitoxin is administered soon enough, it can latch on to toxin molecules still circulating in the blood and prevent them from attaching to nerve endings. But because antitoxin cannot dislodge toxin molecules that have already bound to the nerves, some people never fully recover from botulism. The Montreal doctors could only hope that the girls' affected nerve endings would regrow around the toxin molecules—a process that could take weeks or months.

Meanwhile, hospital officials' concern extended beyond the lives of the Hong Kong family. They telephoned the Canadian Health Protection Branch in Ottawa to report the possible deadly botulism cases. The likelihood of a botulism outbreak always raises urgent questions for public health officials: What food harbored the toxin? Did other people eat it? Is any of the toxin-laden food still available to be eaten?

Health officials in Ottawa told the Montreal hospital to send samples of the girls' blood for testing. When the blood arrived three days later, technicians injected an extract of it into mice. If the blood contained the toxin, the mice would die in a few days. The Ottawa officials also ordered their agency's disease detectives, called *epidemiologists*, to begin an investigation.

When an unexplained outbreak of a rare illness occurs, epi-

The first victims
Two teen-age sisters, visiting Canada from Hong Kong, are connected to ventilators to help them breathe as they lay ill in a Montreal hospital. Suspecting that the girls are suffering from *botulism*, a form of food poisoning, doctors alert public health officials to verify the diagnosis and to determine the source of the poisoning.

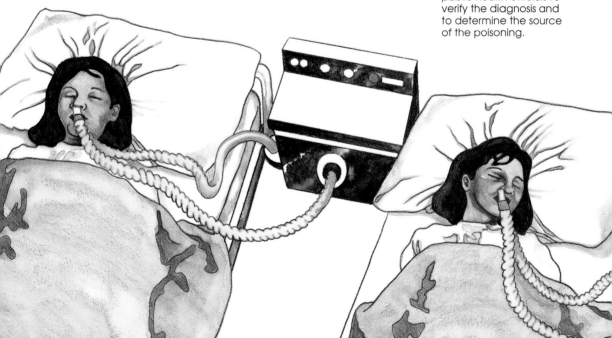

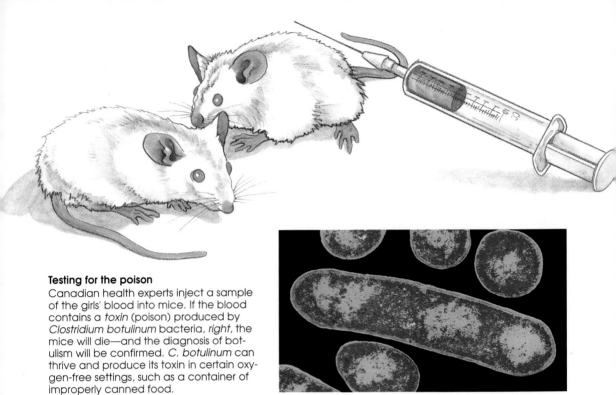

Testing for the poison
Canadian health experts inject a sample of the girls' blood into mice. If the blood contains a *toxin* (poison) produced by *Clostridium botulinum* bacteria, *right,* the mice will die—and the diagnosis of botulism will be confirmed. *C. botulinum* can thrive and produce its toxin in certain oxygen-free settings, such as a container of improperly canned food.

demiologists try to figure out what caused it, how to treat it, and how to prevent it in the future. In a food-poisoning case, they try to track down the poisonous food before other people eat it and become ill. If possible, they question the patients and their families to determine what they ate in recent days. To this end, epidemiologists from both the Canadian federal health department and from Montreal's health division began tracing the steps of the Hong Kong family.

When the investigators learned that the family had passed through Vancouver on their way to Montreal, they contacted Barry Morgan, chief of food inspection for the Health Protection Branch in Vancouver. Morgan, in turn, telephoned physician John Blatherwick, the chief medical officer for Vancouver.

But Morgan and Blatherwick could do little until a diagnosis of botulism was confirmed, which might take several days. Blatherwick, however, saw little cause for alarm. He assumed that if botulism was diagnosed, it was a one-family event, as is usually the case.

"There had never been a multiple outbreak of botulism in British Columbia," he said. "In fact, I'd only been involved in one case before—an accountant who loved his wife's home-canned corn. She had opened a can and thought that it smelled funny. She was going to throw it out, but he came in and ate the whole thing before she got to it. He was paralyzed for quite a while and never returned to more than 50 per cent capacity."

The information Blatherwick and Morgan were expecting

from the Ottawa lab arrived on Thursday, September 12, one week after the Hong Kong girls were admitted to the Montreal hospital. The mice had died; botulism was confirmed. Blatherwick notified area hospitals to be on the alert for more cases. Then he and Morgan and their inspectors began to try to track down the source of the poisoning.

The father of the teen-age girls could only provide an incomplete list of restaurants where the family had dined. It offered no clues.

Restaurant food was low on the list of suspects anyway. The classic culprit in botulism is home-canned food. However, botulism has occurred by other means, too. People have been poisoned by eating foods such as a beef stew containing potatoes and carrots, and a turkey loaf made with onions. These dishes contained soil-grown vegetables and were cooked and left at room temperature, in a relatively oxygen-free environment, for at least 12 hours.

Botulism has also been traced to baked potatoes that had been left unrefrigerated overnight and then covered with mayonnaise and made into potato salad. Mayonnaise, margarine, or oil can create the oxygen-free conditions the botulinum spores need to produce toxin.

The Canadian investigators soon learned that this episode was not a one-family event caused by tainted home preserves. A laboratory notified Blatherwick that a middle-aged man was in Vancouver's Shaughnessy Hospital, another potential botulism victim.

Blatherwick called the patient's brother, hoping he could supply a missing link that would tie all four victims in the two families together and lead inspectors to the source of the poison. But the epidemiologist was unable to speak with the brother.

Thursday had been a day of dead ends. On Friday, the case cracked wide open with two promising leads. First, the brother of the man in Shaughnessy Hospital was also admitted and interviewed.

The second lead surfaced at about 7:30 p.m. when Montreal investigators gave Blatherwick the name and address of a relative the Hong

Proper home-canning methods

Home canning can be an enjoyable and economical way to preserve fruits and vegetables. But do-it-yourself canning requires careful processing to avoid risking botulism.

Canning involves packing food in an airtight container and heating it in a vat of either boiling water (water-bath canning) or pressurized steam (pressure canning).

If proper measures are not used, *Clostridium botulinum* spores (a dormant form of the bacteria that is highly resistant to heat) may survive the canning process. In a low-acid environment and relatively oxygen-free surroundings, such as those provided by a jar, the spores germinate into active *C. botulinum* and produce toxin.

Safe canning requires specific cooking, storage, and handling techniques. Different foods require different processing times and temperatures. For example, high-acid foods, such as tomatoes and other fruits, usually can be prepared using a water-bath canner. Low-acid vegetables, such as corn, green beans, peas, and carrots, need pressure canning, which creates higher temperatures that destroy spores.

Some general rules apply for all types of home canning:

- Use current U.S. Department of Agriculture guidelines for canning. To order the *Complete Guide to Home Canning*, write to: USDA, Consumer Information Center, P.O. Box 100, Pueblo, CO 81002.

- Do not use a slow cooker or a conventional or microwave oven for processing; these methods cannot be relied on to kill all spores.

- Use containers that are specifically designed for home canning. Never use jars or cans that previously held another food, and do not reuse the lids of any container. Previously used containers may have tiny dents and other flaws that prevent an airtight seal.

- Leave the recommended space between the food and the lid. Packing food too tightly can prevent proper heating.

- Do not can overripe fruits or vegetables. As foods age, they lose the acidity that helps prevent toxin formation.

- If any can—whether processed commercially or at home—is bulging, leaking, or has a bad smell or appearance (foam or mold), discard it immediately. Never eat food in this condition because even the smallest amount might lead to botulism.

Kong family had stayed with in Vancouver. Morgan and one of Blatherwick's inspectors headed straight to the home of the relative, a nephew of the mother. "We sat with him and went through the schedule of everything they had done since the day the family arrived," Morgan said.

The aim of such exhaustive interviews in an epidemiological investigation is to uncover factors that all the victims have in common, such as exposure to a toxin or an infectious microbe. When the recitation got to Sunday noon of the visit, the nephew said the family had eaten at the White Spot restaurant in downtown Vancouver, one of a chain of such restaurants.

The name clicked. The brothers in Shaughnessy Hospital had eaten there, too. Both, in fact, had ordered the same meal: the "beef dip" sandwich plate consisting of a roast beef sandwich with a dipping sauce on the side, French fries, and coleslaw. The nephew recalled that his aunt and two cousins also had eaten beef dips. Now the investigators had five probable botulism cases, all connected by a restaurant and a specific meal.

Late that night, Blatherwick went to the White Spot and asked the restaurant staff to remove the beef dip sandwich from the menu. The restaurant complied immediately. Blatherwick considered ordering the restaurant to close but decided, with some misgivings, to let it remain open.

"I didn't sleep for six weeks wondering if I'd done the right thing," Blatherwick said. "Did I miss something? Was the culprit still on the menu?"

The next morning, at the Vancouver headquarters of the White Spot chain, Blatherwick huddled with provincial and federal health authorities and representatives of the restaurant. As they talked, they learned of other possible botulism cases, al-

Tracing the patients' actions
Public health officials interview a relative of the Hong Kong family to determine what the sisters ate in the days before they became ill. The relative recalls a meal the family ate at a restaurant in Vancouver. The sisters—and their mother, who had also become ill—had ordered the same entree, a "beef dip" sandwich plate.

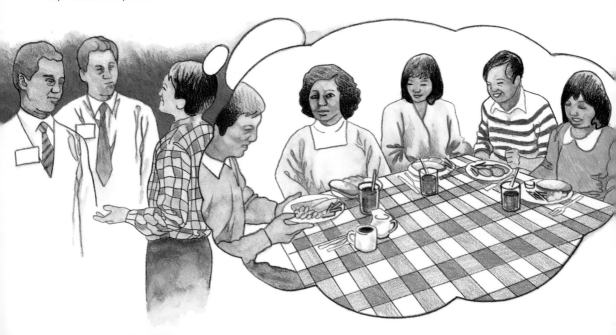

though all the victims apparently had been poisoned before Blatherwick had the beef dip meal removed from the menu. The manager of the suspect restaurant had been admitted to a hospital in North Vancouver. Another Vancouver hospital had admitted a husband and wife who had eaten at the White Spot and were showing symptoms of botulism. The husband needed a respirator.

Canadian federal officials decided to issue a national alert. Shortly before noon, they informed the news media of the botulism cases. When the news hit the airwaves, it brought a peculiar sense of relief to a few people.

Irene Mandarino, a 21-year-old waitress at the White Spot, was one person who welcomed information that would pinpoint the baffling illness that had left her dizzy, weak, and disoriented for 10 days. A hospital emergency room physician had diagnosed her condition as a slight ear infection, which can cause dizziness. Later, a family doctor said she probably had a viral infection and prescribed medication. By the time a cousin called to tell her about the radio report of food poisoning at the White Spot, Mandarino's illness was clearly serious—her right arm had become almost paralyzed.

Mandarino immediately went to Vancouver General Hospital, and a physician quickly diagnosed her ailments as possible botulism. It turned out that Mandarino, too, had recently eaten the White Spot's beef dip meal.

Having narrowed their search to the beef dip plate, the investigators tried to pinpoint the exact source of the toxin. They approached the meal like detectives sizing up suspects. Had the French fries or coleslaw done it? Improbable, they decided, since these foods were also served with many other menu items. What about the dipping sauce? This they ruled out because interviews with victims had revealed that not everyone who became ill had eaten the dip. They also doubted that the beef was to blame because all the sandwiches involved contained more meat than would have been available on one roast, and multiple poisonous roasts were highly unlikely. The investigators turned their attention to a garlic butter that was spread on the bread for the beef dip sandwiches. The preparation was mixed each day at the restaurants by combining butter with a commercial product of chopped garlic bottled in soybean oil.

The garlic was a reasonable suspect for several reasons. First, it grows in soil where *C. botulinum* bacteria may also reside. Second, it was bottled in oil, which provided the oxygen-free environment required for the bacteria's spores to produce toxin. And third, despite instructions on the garlic bottle to store the product in the refrigerator (cold temperatures help prevent the formation of toxin), unopened bottles had been unrefrigerated

Other types of food poisoning

A variety of microorganisms can cause food poisoning. Thorough cooking and good hygiene can prevent most cases of illness.

Salmonellosis is a common type of food poisoning caused by *salmonella* bacteria. According to the U.S. Centers for Disease Control (CDC) in Atlanta, Ga., every year as many as 4 million Americans may be affected by this food poisoning, and at least 500 of them die.

Salmonella bacteria are found on raw meats, poultry, eggs, and dairy products, and on kitchen utensils that have been in contact with such foods. In food, these microbes cannot be detected by smell, taste, or appearance.

The symptoms of salmonella poisoning usually begin 12 to 48 hours after eating contaminated food and include abdominal cramps, diarrhea, nausea, vomiting, and fever. Chills and a headache may also occur. Although doctors normally do not recommend medication, they do advise patients to frequently drink small amounts of clear liquids as soon as the stomach will tolerate it. This helps prevent dehydration that diarrhea and vomiting can cause. They also note that other food should be limited to bland items, such as dry toast or crackers, until the stomach and intestines return to normal. Most cases clear up within one to four days.

People can prevent acquiring salmonellosis at home by thoroughly cooking meats and poultry. Eggs should never be eaten raw, even in cookie batter, eggnog, or homemade ice cream. Clean hands and scrubbed work surfaces in the kitchen are important. Utensils, cutting boards, or dishes that have been in contact with raw meat should be thoroughly cleaned before being used for preparation of other food, and raw foods should be kept separate from cooked items.

Shigellosis is caused by a bacterium found in the feces of infected people. It is spread when individuals handle food without properly washing their hands after using the toilet or changing a diaper. Incidences of this type of food poisoning afflict as many as 450,000 Americans annually, yet it is easily prevented by taking the simple precaution of thoroughly washing hands before preparing food.

Symptoms, which include diarrhea (sometimes bloody), cramps, fever, vomiting, and headache, usually appear within 24 to 48 hours of exposure. The illness may last a few hours or a few days and can clear up without treatment. But severe cases require antibiotics.

Ciguatera, a seafood poisoning, is caused by a toxin produced by *dinoflagellates* (single-celled microorganisms). This toxin accumulates in the flesh of many species of fish from tropical waters. Larger, predatory fish tend to be the most hazardous, because they have accumulated the most toxin. The toxin cannot be detected by taste, and no methods of preparing the fish can guarantee its safety. Health experts estimate that ciguatera occurs in about 10,000 Americans per year, a much higher number than for any other type of seafood poisoning.

The best way to avoid ciguatera is to avoid eating species of fish that accumulate the toxin. These include types of barracuda, grouper, snapper, jack, mackerel, parrotfish, surgeonfish, and wrasse. Experts believe that true red snapper is safe. But they note that some snapperlike fish are sold under this name, and this can confuse the consumer.

Ciguatera's symptoms usually begin within one hour after eating tainted fish. The symptoms include such typical signs of food poisoning as nausea, vomiting, and diarrhea, but other symptoms may be present. Many people experience a tingling feeling—like an electrical shock—in the fingers, toes, lips, or tongue. Hot items can feel cold, and cold items hot. Ciguatera victims may also experience muscle weakness and pain and a lack of coordination. Symptoms can last 6 to 18 months but may persist longer. There is no known cure.

Listeriosis is caused by *Listeria monocytogenes* bacteria, found in a variety of foods. This rarer type of food poisoning affects an estimated 1,700 people yearly, killing about 450 and causing about 100 stillbirths. Three major outbreaks of listeriosis occurred in North America in the 1980's, when transmission via food was documented for the first time. In these outbreaks, health officials traced the bacteria to soft cheese, unpasteurized milk, and coleslaw made from tainted cabbage.

Most people experience either no symptoms or mild, flulike symptoms from listeriosis. But in fetuses, newborns, the elderly, and people who are sick from other illnesses, the poisoning can be deadly. Listeriosis can cause *meningitis* (inflammation of the membranes surrounding the brain and spinal cord) and other neurological problems, as well as inflammation of the heart.

Health experts know of no certain preventive measures. The organisms have a high tolerance for heat, salt, and acidity and cannot be destroyed easily. The bacteria are difficult to detect, and, in most cases, the source of the poisoning is unknown. Doctors treat seriously ill victims with antibiotics.

for about eight months, according to White Spot employees.

As far as anyone knew, garlic-in-oil had never before caused botulism. But the outbreak resembled another one in October 1983 when 28 people in Peoria, Ill., acquired botulism after eating contaminated onions in a patty-melt sandwich from a local restaurant. The onions had been cooked in margarine, held at room temperature, and served without reheating.

In Vancouver, investigators took samples of the garlic oil to test in the laboratory. First, they checked its acid content. If *C. botulinum* spores are kept in an acidic substance, they cannot produce toxin. The lab technicians found that the garlic oil's acid level was low enough to allow toxin production.

Despite this observation, the evidence pointing to the garlic was not conclusive—especially since the same garlic spread had also been used on the White Spot's steak sandwich, which so far appeared not to have poisoned anyone. Nevertheless, the chain pulled the garlic-in-oil product from all of its restaurants.

By the next day, the number of botulism reports had grown to 16. Because one victim who had eaten at the White Spot was hospitalized in Seattle, Wash., officials sounded an alert across North America. Ten physicians-in-training also began reviewing records of patients recently treated at local emergency rooms. This search, followed by interviews with patients, produced several overlooked victims.

The noose of evidence encircling the garlic oil drew tighter when doctors confirmed botulism in a child who had eaten a steak sandwich prepared with garlic butter at the White Spot.

The search narrows
After learning that other people had been poisoned and that they also ate the beef dip sandwich plate at the same restaurant, investigators target the meal as the probable source of the botulinum toxin. The entree includes a roast beef sandwich, dipping sauce, coleslaw, and French fries. But which item carries the deadly poison?

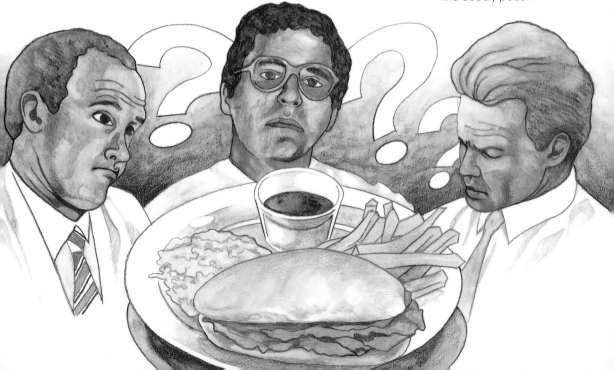

On a wall chart in Blatherwick's office, the investigators logged all the cases according to when the patients ate at the White Spot, when their symptoms began, what symptoms they experienced, and when they were hospitalized. The chart revealed a startling surprise. An unrecognized outbreak had begun about six weeks before doctors diagnosed the Hong Kong girls' cases.

In the end, the investigators pinned down two eight-day periods—one from late July to early August and the other from late August to early September—during which all the known victims ate at the White Spot. But they could not account for the gap in August when no one who ate at the White Spot became ill.

The investigation also uncovered another seeming contradiction. When health workers had first targeted the White Spot, they had samples of all the suspect food tested for *C. botulinum* bacteria and its toxin. Technicians injected a sample of the bacteria's spores into bottled garlic and confirmed that the spores could produce toxin at room temperature. Yet they found no other toxin in any jars of garlic-in-oil, opened or not.

A logical explanation for both puzzles finally emerged. "We learned weeks later that someone at the restaurant had thrown out one jar of garlic that they said 'didn't seem right,'" Blatherwick recalled. "They had used it for a while, then it got pushed to the rear of the refrigerator for some time. It was put into use again later and finally discarded." These events could explain the three-week gap in August and why the lab did not find the toxin. The probable culprit had been thrown out before investigators arrived on the scene.

About two weeks into the investigation, Canadian health officials called the United States Centers for Disease Control (CDC) in Atlanta, Ga., for help. The CDC, like its counterpart in Ottawa, investigates disease trends and assists state and local officials in handling epidemics. The CDC undertook the task of surveying large numbers of healthy people who had dined at the White Spot on the same dates of the poisonings and had eaten, in some cases, the same type of meal that the victims had.

The studies showed that the majority of people who ate the sandwiches did not fall ill. The ratio of botulism cases to beef dips served fluctuated day to day, from a high of 1 illness to 3 beef dips served to a low of 1 illness to 18 beef dips served. Several factors could account for this. Some diners may have consumed more toxin than others did. Also, the differences in people's digestive systems, such as the amount of acid in the stomach or the efficiency with which nutrients are absorbed into the bloodstream, could explain why not everyone became sick.

The interval between eating the sandwich and the onset of symptoms varied widely, too, ranging from 19 hours to 10 days.

The extent of the illness differed from person to person as well. The researchers could not explain why, but ethnic background seemed to affect the severity of the poisoning. For example, 60 per cent of Chinese patients, but only 4 per cent of other patients, required respirator treatment.

Although no new cases occurred after early September—presumably after the contaminated garlic was discarded—three months passed before reports of botulism cases slowed to a trickle and stopped. Like Irene Mandarino, many of those poisoned had initially received an incorrect diagnosis, which delayed the reporting of their cases.

The final botulism tally included 36 people—4 employees and 32 patrons of a single restaurant. As of 1991, this botulism outbreak remained the second largest in North America, exceeded only by an outbreak in Pontiac, Mich., in 1977, which struck 59 people. None of the victims of the Vancouver outbreak died, but the disease changed some of their lives. "We did a survey a year later, and 50 per cent of the patients we contacted still had [neurological] problems," Blatherwick said. "After three years, we found that many still had significant problems, especially those who had had the most severe symptoms initially."

Other researchers who performed follow-up studies on the victims of the 1983 Peoria outbreak also reported similar long-term effects from botulism. Three years after contracting botulism, half the Peoria patients still became easily fatigued, and some still had muscle weakness, headaches, and blurred vision.

The rate of food-borne botulism reported in the United States is fairly stable—about 25 cases annually—according to the CDC's Botulism Laboratory. However, as Blatherwick's team pointed out, some cases of botulism may go unrecognized and

The villain is revealed
Circumstantial evidence points to the probable source of the poison: a garlic-in-oil product used on the beef dip sandwich. Although investigators fail to find tainted garlic-in-oil at the restaurant, workers there recall disposing of a bottle that seemed spoiled.

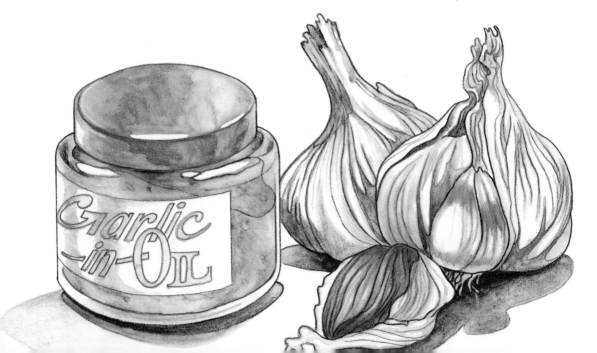

A deadly poison serves some patients

Could there possibly be a good side to the deadliest natural poison known? Since the late 1970's, the answer to this question has been yes. People suffering from abnormal tics, twitches, and spasms called *dystonias* can find relief in the botulinus toxin. Doctors found that injecting tiny doses of the *C. botulinum* toxin—which researchers have nicknamed *botox*—directly into malfunctioning muscles can paralyze them temporarily and stop spasms that can be distressing and even disabling.

The first to try this daring therapy was ophthalmologist Alan B. Scott of the Smith-Kettlewell Eye Research Institute in San Francisco. In 1976, Scott began experimenting with botox injections to disable muscles that cause cross-eye, squinting, and *walleye* (an eye that turns out). Scott's successes led others to begin testing botox on patients suffering from dystonias affecting the mouth, jaw, eyelids, neck, feet, or hands. Such spasms are caused by malfunctioning nerves that release abnormal bursts of chemical messengers called *neurotransmitters*, which then cause certain muscles to contract. The nerves' excessive "firing" makes the muscles move in jerky spasms.

When a doctor injects botox at the site of the problem nerves, the toxin molecules attach themselves to the nerve endings and prevent the nerve cells from sending signals to muscles. This is exactly what happens when a person becomes poisoned after eating the botulinus toxin. The trick for the doctor is to inject just enough poison to stop the spasm without paralyzing other muscles.

Botox does not cure whatever defect is causing the nerves to misfire, nor does it provide permanent relief. The nerves eventually grow new ends around the toxin molecules and start firing their messenger chemicals to the muscles once again. Thus, the patient must receive injections every few months to remain free of the spasms. Scientists are experimenting with ways to alter botox so that it would provide a one-shot cure.

For now, surgery that severs or destroys malfunctioning nerves offers the only permanent solution to most people who have dystonias. But such a radical approach is not always effective or even possible. For example, surgeons cannot reach nerves located deep in the neck without cutting and injuring other muscles, nerves, or blood vessels. Surgical cutting can also permanently damage the wrong nerves and cause such disfiguring complications as a sagging eyelid or drooping mouth. So far, botox injections have not resulted in any such serious or long-term side effects.

In February 1990, the United States Food and Drug Administration (FDA) decided that the evidence showing the benefits of botox was strong enough to approve the toxin as standard treatment for three conditions. These include *strabismus* (cross-eye, squints, and walleye); *blepharospasm* (uncontrollable blinking or winking due to involuntary muscle contractions in the eyelids); and *hemifacial spasm* (involuntary grimacing and muscle contraction on one side of the face).

Successful research in other areas of botox use led the FDA to declare in February 1991 that the therapy was safe and effective, but still experimental, for three more conditions. The first is the most common form of dystonia, called *spasmodic torticollis*. This condition produces painful spasms in the neck and causes the head to twist to one side. The second type of problem, called *oromandibular dystonia*, causes the jaw to open and close spasmodically, making it difficult to speak or swallow. The third type is known as *adductor spasmodic dystonia*. This condition constricts the vocal cords, interferes with the flow of air, and leaves the afflicted person with a hoarse and choppy voice.

Researchers are testing botox as a possible type of therapy for other sorts of speech disorders, including some cases of stuttering. Botox may also be used in the future to relieve conditions caused by overuse of the hand, such as writer's cramp. If all these uses turn out to be effective, the poison that *C. botulinum* produces may soon be helping far more people than it harms. [Y.B.]

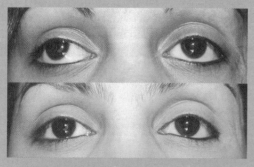

In *strabismus* (walleye), spasmodic eye muscles cause the eye or eyes to turn out, *top*. Tiny doses of botulinus toxin injected into these muscles paralyzes them, relieving the condition, *bottom*.

unreported if the symptoms are mild and progress slowly, and if other more severe cases don't show up to provide a connection.

Physicians may not suspect botulism for a number of reasons. First, botulism is a rare disease with symptoms that are also found in a variety of other illnesses or disorders. "Especially in the mild cases, the symptoms are so general they often sound like a hypochondriac's complaints," Blatherwick noted.

In the Vancouver outbreak, doctors initially misdiagnosed even some severe cases. They concluded that their patients were suffering from *myasthenia gravis* (a muscle-weakening disease); psychiatric disorders; viral diseases; stroke; *Guillain-Barre* syndrome (an inflammatory nerve disease); and other conditions.

The outbreak was also made less visible because many of the cases involved travelers who became ill in Vancouver but sought treatment back in their hometowns. This situation prevented health-care workers from seeing a cluster of cases, which is the usual way a botulism outbreak presents itself. Finally, the poisonings did not have the usual cause—home-canned food.

Although the epidemiologists in Vancouver never acquired proof positive that bottled garlic was the source of the deadly toxin, garlic-in-oil was finally caught in the act in February 1989. At a dinner at a home in Kingston, N.Y., a man served his guests bread prepared with a bottled garlic product. Within four days, he and two of his guests were hospitalized with botulism. The man recalled storing the jar of garlic at room temperature for about three months before he opened and refrigerated it. Investigators isolated both the botulinus toxin and live *C. botulinum* bacteria from the leftover garlic.

This development led the U.S. Food and Drug Administration (FDA) to announce that garlic-in-oil products are inherently unsafe if left unrefrigerated. Since it was clear that not everyone follows label instructions to refrigerate, the FDA also ruled in April 1989 that all companies making these products must add ingredients to prevent bacterial growth or toxin production.

The experience Blatherwick's team had with the 1985 botulism outbreak helped them crack another food poisoning case two years later. In February 1987, 11 cases of botulism were reported among people who had eaten at the Five Sails Restaurant in the Pan Pacific Hotel on the Vancouver waterfront. The culprit was quickly pinpointed: mushrooms picked in the forests on Vancouver Island and bottled at the restaurant.

"That second epidemic took us all of 12 hours to solve," Blatherwick noted. "I shut the restaurant down the night the outbreak started. It's the fanciest restaurant in town. The queen of England stayed at that hotel. But I shut it down. And this time I slept a lot easier."

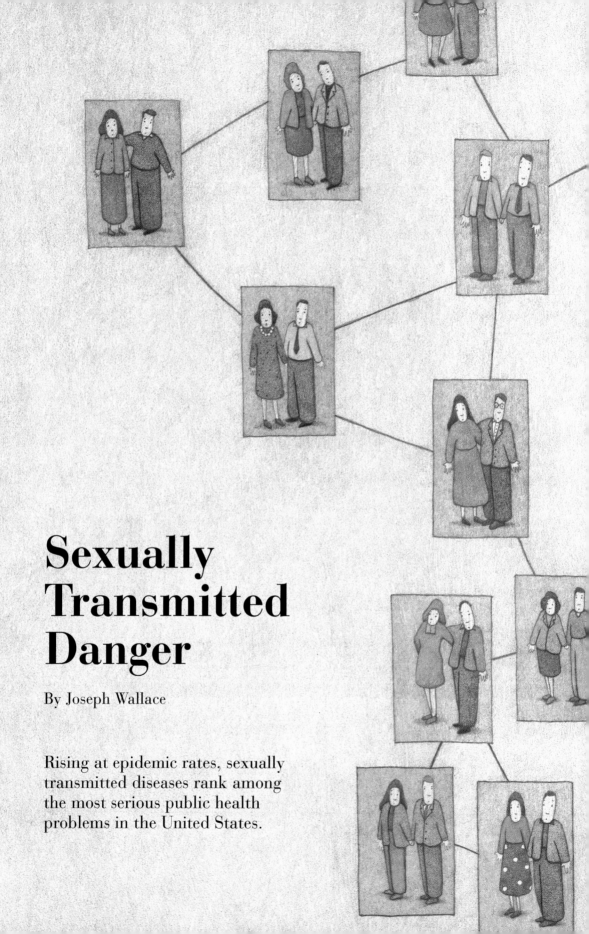

Sexually Transmitted Danger

By Joseph Wallace

Rising at epidemic rates, sexually
transmitted diseases rank among
the most serious public health
problems in the United States.

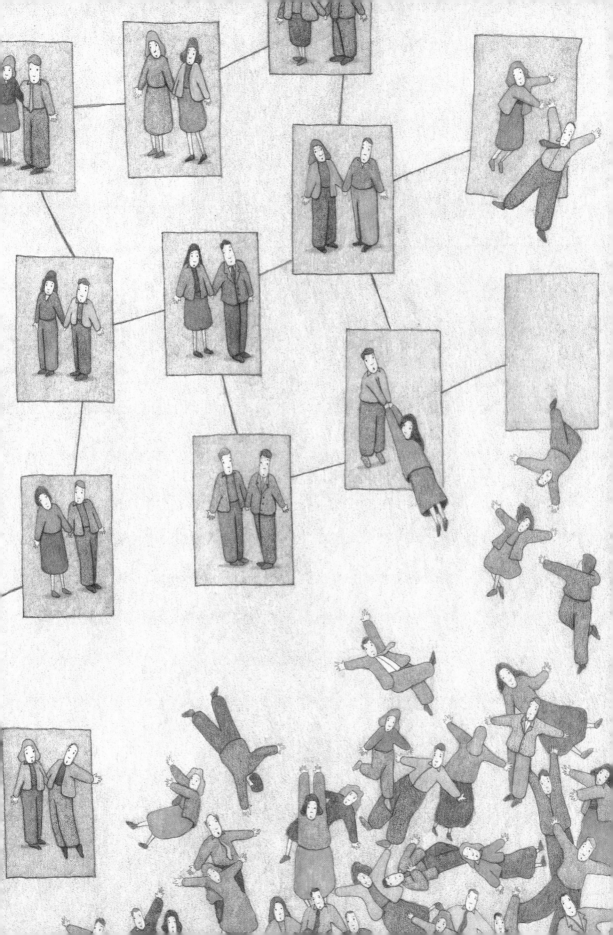

Sexually transmitted diseases (STD's) have been a source of human misery throughout history. Despite medical advances in understanding and treating STD's (formerly called venereal diseases), these diseases continue to be a significant public health threat. Millions of new cases are reported to U.S. public health authorities each year. According to one 1991 study, three STD's—*gonorrhea*, *syphilis*, and *chancroid*—are rising at epidemic rates in the United States, particularly among urban minority populations.

Since the 1970's, attitudes in the United States toward sexual relationships have become much freer than ever before, and cases of STD's have risen dramatically. The exchange of sex for drugs is a significant underlying cause of spreading STD infections among drug abusers, according to many health experts. Other behaviors may also increase risks of contracting STD's. Smoking cigarettes, for example, seems to increase the risk of genital wart infections, possibly because smoking impairs the immune system. Use of drugs and alcohol may impair a person's judgment so that they participate in unsafe sexual behavior.

Doctors warn that a single sexual encounter with an infected partner can be enough to transmit an organism that causes an STD. Syphilis, *genital herpes*, *chlamydia*, and other infections can strike any sexually active person, even someone who rarely engages in sexual activities. And the rise of STD's has taken on a deadlier aspect in light of the spread of AIDS (*acquired immune deficiency syndrome*).

Although most STD's (with the exception of AIDS) do not usually lead to death, they can give rise to serious health problems. In women, for example, chlamydia can cause *pelvic inflammatory disease*, which itself can cause infertility. Having one STD also can make it easier to contract another—including deadly AIDS.

The precise number of new STD cases in the United States each year is unknown. There are a number of reasons for this, including a lack of uniform regulations among the states for formally reporting cases of STD's to health authorities. Chlamydia, for example, is not a "reportable" disease but gonorrhea, syphilis, and chancroid are reportable, and the Centers for Disease Control (CDC) in Atlanta, Ga., says that these are now rising at epidemic rates in the United States, particularly among urban teen-agers and young adults.

The CDC estimates that as many as 4 million to 5 million Americans contract chlamydia infections each year, making it the most common STD. More than 690,000 cases of gonorrhea were reported in 1990, and experts believe the true number of new cases may actually approach 2.5 million. Genital herpes may now affect 30 million Americans, with an additional 800,000 new cases being reported each year. And more than 50,000 new cases of syphilis were diagnosed in 1990, its highest

The author:

Joseph Wallace is a free-lance writer specializing in medical and scientific topics.

212

level since the 1950's. Chancroid, rare in the United States since World War II (1939-1945), rose from 665 cases in 1984 to 4,215 cases in 1990.

Some STD's, including chlamydia, gonorrhea, and syphilis, are caused by bacteria. Others are caused by viruses or other organisms such as one-celled animals. STD's caused by viruses are more difficult to treat; antibiotics do not kill viruses. Vaccines can prevent some viral infections by stimulating the body's immune system to resist the viruses that cause those diseases. But no vaccines or drug cures exist for three important viruses that cause STD's: *herpes simplex virus type 2*, which causes genital herpes; *human papillomavirus*, which causes genital warts; and *human immunodeficiency virus*, which causes AIDS.

Chlamydia

Chlamydia is caused by the bacteria *Chlamydia trachomatis*. In both sexes, chlamydia is frequently *asymptomatic*—that is, producing no symptoms. Medical researchers have found that a person can harbor an asymptomatic chlamydial infection for years, and then discover the infection only when symptoms appear. Therefore, even people in *monogamous* (one-partner) relationships can suddenly seem to "catch" chlamydia when actually something triggered a previous asymptomatic infection.

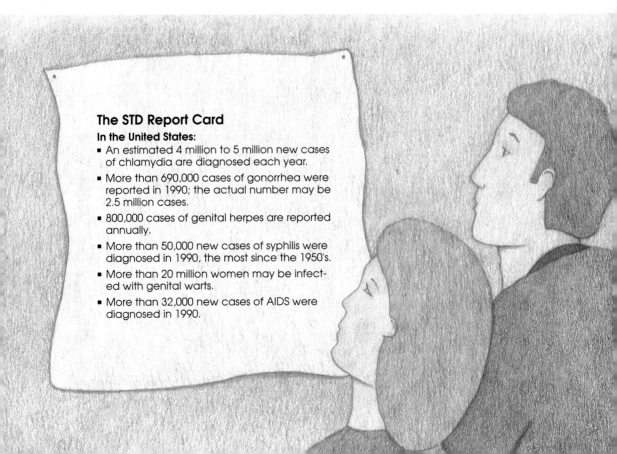

The STD Report Card

In the United States:
- An estimated 4 million to 5 million new cases of chlamydia are diagnosed each year.
- More than 690,000 cases of gonorrhea were reported in 1990; the actual number may be 2.5 million cases.
- 800,000 cases of genital herpes are reported annually.
- More than 50,000 new cases of syphilis were diagnosed in 1990, the most since the 1950's.
- More than 20 million women may be infected with genital warts.
- More than 32,000 new cases of AIDS were diagnosed in 1990.

Men with chlamydial infections can suffer from a variety of symptoms, including discharge from the *urethra* (the tube that carries urine from the bladder through the penis) and difficult, painful urination. In rare instances, men can suffer *epididymitis* (an inflammation of the structure located behind the testicles that stores sperm), *prostatitis* (an inflammation of the prostate gland), and perhaps even *Reiter's syndrome*, a form of arthritis.

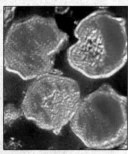

Chlamydia trachomatis bacteria (shown in red)

Disease:	**Chlamydia**
Cause:	*Chlamydia trachomatis* bacteria.
Symptoms:	Frequently none. In men, urethral discharge, painful urination. In women, cervical inflammation, vaginal discharge.
Treatment:	Antibiotics.
Complications:	Major cause of pelvic inflammatory disease in women, which can lead to sterility. Can infect newborns.

"Chlamydia bacteria can scar the Fallopian tubes, and this can cause sterility if the tubes are completely blocked by the scars."

Women's symptoms can include inflammation of the *cervix* (the lower opening of the uterus) and vaginal discharge. Doctors say that young women and women taking oral contraceptives seem more susceptible than others to infection of the cervix.

The complications for women can be severe. Chlamydia is the leading cause of pelvic inflammatory disease, a painful infection of the uterus and *Fallopian tubes* (the ducts that carry the eggs from the ovaries to the uterus). Symptoms include abnormal bleeding, vaginal discharge, or lower abdominal pain. Chlamydia bacteria can scar the Fallopian tubes, and this can cause sterility if the tubes are completely blocked by the scars.

Partially blocked tubes can prevent a fertilized egg from reaching the uterus and can result in a potentially fatal complication, an *ectopic*, or tubal, pregnancy. In this condition, an embryo, growing within one of the Fallopian tubes, can rupture the tube and cause life-threatening bleeding. The CDC reports that ectopic pregnancies increased from 18,000 in 1970 to 84,000 in 1986, with half of these caused by pelvic inflammatory disease.

In addition, as is the case with many STD's, obstetricians warn that an infected pregnant woman can infect her child during delivery. A chlamydial infection can lead to pneumonia in infants and threaten their lives. Chlamydial bacteria can also infect the eyes of newborns and is one of the causes of *conjunctivitis*, an inflammation of the membrane covering the eye.

Laboratory testing for chlamydia is not widely used. Diagnosis of chlamydial infections by *culturing* (in which bacteria from a sample of urethral or cervical discharge or urine are grown in the laboratory) can be expensive and difficult to obtain. Chlamydia, however, causes symptoms very similar to those of gonorrhea, a comparatively easy STD to diagnose. Doctors can therefore first test for and rule out gonorrhea as a possibility, then make the diagnosis of chlamydial infection based on the patient's symptoms.

Doctors treat diagnosed or suspected chlamydial infections with a seven-day course of an antibiotic, such as tetracycline or erythromycin. Health-care providers stress the importance of treating all sexual partners of an infected individual—even those without symptoms—to prevent reinfection of the treated individual or spreading the infection to others.

Gonorrhea

Gonorrhea, caused by a bacterium called *Neisseria gonorrhoea*, is the most commonly reported STD and has one of the longest recorded histories. References to the disease appear in ancient Chinese, Greek, and Roman literature, as well as in the Old Testament. Only about 100 years ago, however, did scientists discover that gonorrhea is caused by bacteria that thrive on the body's mucous membranes (moist linings of the genitals, mouth, throat, and other parts of the body).

Disease:	**Gonorrhea**
Cause:	*Neisseria gonorrhoea* bacteria.
Symptoms:	In men, urethral discharge, pus formations, painful urination. In women, vaginal discharge, abnormal bleeding, pain.
Treatment:	Antibiotics.
Complications:	Can cause pelvic inflammatory disease in women. Can infect infant during delivery, causing blindness.

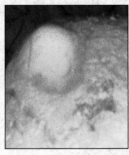

Pus formation caused by gonorrhea

"... gonorrhea can spread ... through the blood to the throat, rectum, eyes, heart, brain, skin, and other organs ...."

Gonorrhea bacteria can infect the rectum or throat, as well as the genitals. Anyone who has had sexual contact with an infected partner can contract the disease. Since 1984, the rate of gonorrhea for urban minority populations began a rapid rise.

In men, the most common symptoms include burning and pain during urination, along with an uncontrollable discharge of thick, puslike material from the tip of the penis. These symptoms usually occur within 2 to 10 days of infection, but infected men may show no signs of the disease for weeks or months. Some men may never develop symptoms.

Women infected with gonorrhea may have vaginal discharge and pain on urination. More frequently, the first signs of infection are the symptoms of pelvic inflammatory disease, which may occur within two weeks of first infection. About half the infected women may never show symptoms.

On rare occasions, gonorrhea can spread from the genitals through the blood to the throat, rectum, eyes, heart, brain, skin, and other organs as well as joints. Infected mothers can pass the disease to their infants during delivery, and this can cause blindness in the child.

To diagnose gonorrhea in men, a smear of urethral discharge is examined under a microscope for the presence of organisms that cause the disease. But in women, asymptomatic men, and patients with suspected gonorrhea of the throat or rectum, the microscopic examination of a smear may not provide proof of infection. In these cases, the doctor must collect a sample from the suspected area and send it to a laboratory for culturing.

Gonorrhea, like other bacterial STD's, is treated with antibiotics. Until 1976, a single large dose of penicillin or its relatives, ampicillin or amoxicillin, could cure the disease. But that year epidemiologists discovered a penicillin-resistant strain of *N. gonorrhoea*. At first, doctors prescribed larger and larger doses of penicillin to combat the bacteria. But the resistant strains spread. Five per cent of gonorrhea cases reported in the United States by 1989 were unaffected by the penicillins. *Ceftriaxone*, a cephalosporin antibiotic that is chemically related to penicillin, is the current drug of choice for treating resistant gonorrhea. Treatment failure is rare with this drug.

Chlamydial infection frequently coexists with gonorrhea. Thus, the CDC now recommends a single injection of a gonorrhea-eradicating drug, followed by a seven-day course of a tetracycline antibiotic to ensure that chlamydia, if present, is also eliminated.

Syphilis

Another bacterial STD with a long past is syphilis. Historians debate whether it originated in the Americas or Europe and Asia. Its existence was first documented in the late 1400's, and epidemics have raged periodically in many parts of the world since then. U.S. health authorities describe the current upsurge of syphilis as particularly explosive in urban black and Hispanic populations.

Syphilis is caused by a microscopic *spirochete* (a corkscrew-shaped bacterium) called *Treponema pallidum*. Infection with *T. pallidum* occurs when the spirochete passes from one person to another through a sore or a break in the mucous membranes of the body, usually during sexual activity. Infection is also pos-

Disease:	**Syphilis**
Cause:	*Treponema pallidum* bacteria.
Symptoms:	Primary stage: painless red lesions enlarge to form ulcers.
	Secondary stage: fever, fatigue, enlarged lymph nodes. Extremely infectious, flat ulcers; rash across most of the body, palms of the hands, and soles of the feet.
	Latent stage: no symptoms.
	Tertiary stage: infection of brain, nervous system, eyes, or heart. Can cause death.
Treatment:	Antibiotics for primary and secondary stages. Antibiotics for latent and tertiary stages arrest the disease, but cannot repair tissue damage.
Complications:	Tertiary stage can cause blindness, seizures, insanity, or death. Infant can be infected before birth and die at birth or be born with the disease.

"The earliest symptom of primary syphilis is the appearance of a small, painless red lesion called a *chancre*. . . ."

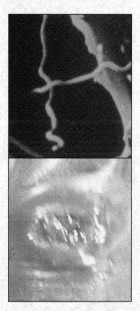

Top: Corkscrew-shaped *Treponema pallidum* bacteria. *Bottom:* Primary syphilis lesion.

sible through cuts in the skin. Transmission can occur even if the sore is so small that it is virtually unnoticeable. A pregnant woman can also pass syphilis to her developing fetus through the placenta.

Physicians classify the symptoms of syphilis into four stages: primary, secondary, latent, and tertiary. The earliest symptom of primary syphilis is the appearance of a small, painless red lesion called a *chancre* (pronounced *shangker*) on the site where the bacteria entered the body, usually about three to four weeks after infection. The chancre appears as a small pimplelike *papule*, then gradually enlarges and erodes to form an ulcer with firm, raised edges. In women, the chancre may occur internally and escape notice. This ulcer heals without treatment in about three to six weeks, often leaving a scar.

About six to eight weeks (sometimes as long as six months) after the chancre disappears, the symptoms of secondary syphilis begin. These can include fever, fatigue, and enlargement of the *lymph nodes* (small, bean-shaped structures located in the neck, under the arms, and in the groin region). Extremely infectious, large papules or flat sores may appear, especially where mucous membranes meet the skin. Almost everyone with secondary syphilis develops a rash across much of the body. The rash is particularly apparent on the palms of the hands and soles of the feet.

The signs of secondary syphilis will usually disappear within several weeks, though they may recur. The disease then progresses to the latent stage, which has no obvious symptoms. About two-thirds of patients never suffer any other symptoms of syphilis; researchers believe that in such cases, the body's own defenses succeed in overcoming or keeping the *T. pallidum* organism under control.

After a symptom-free period, which may last from several months to 30 years, the remaining third of patients develop symptoms of the tertiary stage. This stage produces the most life-threatening symptoms of syphilis, including damage to the heart, brain, spinal cord, and other parts of the nervous system. A patient can suffer blindness, stroke, seizures, severe mental impairment, or even death.

To test for primary or secondary syphilis, a doctor examines some fluid from a chancre or lesion under a microscope to search for the easily recognizable corkscrew shape of *T. pallidum*. In addition, the doctor will send a blood sample to a laboratory to test for signs of the disease.

Once diagnosed, primary and secondary syphilis can be cured with an antibiotic, usually penicillin. Patients who are allergic to penicillin receive tetracycline or erythromycin.

Long-term latent syphilis and tertiary syphilis require higher doses and longer courses of antibiotic therapy than do earlier stages of the disease. The outlook for patients treated for latent syphilis is good; unfortunately, treatment can arrest, but not repair, the often devastating tissue damage of tertiary syphilis. In all cases, doctors must test frequently after treatment to ensure that *T. pallidum* is eradicated.

Trichomoniasis

Trichomoniasis, or trichomonal vaginitis, is caused by a *protozoan*, a microscopic one-celled animal called *Trichomonas vaginalis*. Trichomoniasis, which is confined to the genitals and urinary tract, can remain silent for many years and then suddenly manifest symptoms for no apparent reason.

Symptoms of trichomoniasis appear far more often in infected women than they do in infected men. One of the clearest signs of the disease in women is a grayish or yellow, watery vaginal discharge, sometimes tinged with blood, that has a foul odor. Other symptoms include vaginal itching, pain on intercourse, and a burning sensation during urination.

The majority of men with trichomoniasis infection have no symptoms. When symptoms do occur, they include pain on urination, difficulty in urinating, and, occasionally, a slight discharge from the tip of the urethra.

Disease:	**Trichomoniasis**
Cause:	*Trichomonas vaginalis* protozoa.
Symptoms:	In men, usually no symptoms. In women, grayish, watery vaginal discharge tinged with blood.
Treatment:	Metronidazole pills. Vaginal cream for a pregnant woman.
Complications:	Pain during intercourse.

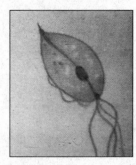

Trichomonas vaginalis protozoa

"Symptoms of trichomoniasis appear far more often in infected women than . . . men."

Doctors diagnose trichomoniasis by examining a sample of vaginal or urethral discharge under a microscope. For about 80 per cent of patients, large protozoa concentrations are present on the slide. For asymptomatic patients with suspected trichomoniasis (such as a sexual partner of a confirmed patient), doctors can send samples to a laboratory to culture *T. vaginalis*.

The best current treatment for trichomoniasis is a drug called *metronidazole*, usually given in a single dose in pill form. When both sexual partners are treated (to prevent reinfection), the drug's cure rate is greater than 95 per cent.

Doctors do not prescribe metronidazole for women who are pregnant (particularly during the first three months). Research has shown that the drug may cause birth defects or premature birth. Instead, many doctors prescribe vaginal creams containing metronidazolelike drugs, or vinegar and water douches (solutions for washing the vagina). These rarely cure the disease, but at least they ease the symptoms.

Genital herpes

Although not life-threatening, genital herpes is one of the most widespread of all STD's, affecting more than 30 million people in the United States alone. Most genital herpes is caused by the *herpes simplex virus type 2*. But *herpes simplex virus type 1*, which commonly produces cold sores around the mouth, can also infect the genital area. Genital herpes was first mentioned by a French physician in 1736, but undoubtedly existed long before that time. Public attention did not focus on this disease until the 1970's, when there was an explosion in the number of cases in the United States.

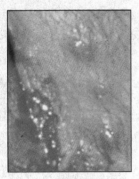

Genital herpes blisters

Disease:	**Genital herpes**
Cause:	*Herpes simplex virus type 2.*
Symptoms:	Small blisters appear, fill with fluid, and eventually rupture into rounded, red ulcers. Ulcers are painful, but crust over and heal in a few days, leaving scars. Fatigue, fever, and headache are common. Latent stage follows, which lasts indefinitely or as short as two weeks. Blisters may reappear when latent stage ends.
Treatment:	Incurable, but acyclovir shortens period of outbreak.
Complications:	Sensitivity to light, inflammation of the lining around the brain. Can cause brain damage or be fatal to newborns infected during birth.

"Public attention did not focus on this disease until the 1970's, when there was an explosion in the number of cases in the United States."

An individual with genital herpes can transmit the infection even when he or she shows no signs of the disease. Within one to three weeks of exposure to a partner who has genital herpes, the newly infected individual develops small blisters at the point of contact, which can increase to 30 or more blisters over the course of about two weeks. The blisters become filled with fluid and rupture, then crust over and heal in about another 10 days.

During the episodes of infection, the area around the outbreak also may be tender or painful. In addition, during the first attacks, nearly half of all patients will suffer such flulike symptoms as fatigue, fever, muscle aches, and headache. More serious complications can include eye infections and *aseptic meningitis* (an inflammation of the lining around the brain).

Symptoms subside without treatment, but the virus survives in certain nerve cells until stress, physical injury, or other diseases bring on another outbreak of the painful sores, usually less severe than the first.

Although such outbreaks may be unpleasant, the chief risk of genital herpes is infecting certain individuals who are vulnerable to more serious complications. Such people include newborns, who can become infected during the birth process, and people who have difficulty fighting infections, such as AIDS and cancer patients.

Physicians can usually diagnose genital herpes by the presence of the fluid-filled sores and by examining the fluid under a microscope for infected tissue cells. Although the disease remains incurable, the antiviral drug *acyclovir*, taken orally, appears to reduce the duration of symptoms and speed healing in first episodes. A study published in February 1991 found that daily doses of acyclovir appear to suppress the blisters for at least three years.

Some physicians have suggested that acyclovir may reduce a pregnant woman's risk of infecting her baby. But most health experts do not recommend this course of action because the drug's potential adverse effects on the fetus are unknown. Instead, women with herpes outbreaks around the time of delivery may limit risk to their babies by undergoing a *Caesarean section*, a surgical procedure in which the baby is removed through an incision in the abdomen and uterus.

Genital warts

Genital warts are the most common STD caused by a virus. According to the CDC, three times as many cases of genital warts are diagnosed in the United States each year as are cases of genital herpes.

Human papillomavirus (HPV), which causes genital wart infections, is usually transmitted by direct sexual contact, often by individuals with either a hidden infection (such as a woman with warts inside the reproductive tract) or with no symptoms. Genital warts also can occur on the anus, lips, tongue, or palate.

These warts vary in appearance from a single small, flat wart, to a "carpet" of large, protruding warts. In rare cases, a huge wart (called a *giant condyloma*) may appear, usually on the penis, and then grow and spread.

Some HPV strains—ones that do not usually cause visible warts—have been linked to cancers of the reproductive organs. In particular, evidence now indicates that infection by certain strains of HPV increase a woman's risk of developing cancer of the cervix.

Diagnosis of genital warts involves ruling out the possibility that cancer, syphilis, or another condition caused the warts. To eliminate such a possibility, a doctor performs a biopsy in which a small part of the wart is snipped off and studied in the laboratory. In addition, doctors can test for the presence of strains of HPV linked with cervical cancer.

After a positive diagnosis of HPV infection, a physician can remove warts by applying a chemical, freezing them with liquid

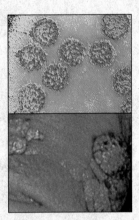

Top: Human papilomavirus. Bottom: genital warts.

Disease:	**Genital warts**
Cause:	*Human papilomavirus.*
Symptoms:	Single, flat wart or carpet of warts. In women, warts can be unnoticed in the vagina. Warts can also occur on the anus, lips, tongue, or palate.
Treatment:	Removal of warts by cryotherapy (freezing), electrocautery (burning), laser therapy, or painting on an acid. Warts can return after removal.
Complications:	Evidence indicates that certain strains of papilomavirus increase a woman's risk of developing cervical cancer.

"According to the CDC, three times as many cases of genital warts are diagnosed in the United States each year as are cases of genital herpes."

nitrogen, burning them away with electric current, or vaporizing them with an intense beam of laser light. These procedures can be done on an outpatient basis. If the procedure does not remove all the viruses, however, HPV can return.

AIDS

The most deadly viral sexually transmitted disease is AIDS, which is spreading at an alarming rate in the United States and throughout the world. There currently is no cure for AIDS. For more information about AIDS, see THE SPECTER OF AIDS in the Special Reports section.

There is growing evidence that a person who has an active STD infection has a greater risk of becoming infected with the virus that causes AIDS than someone who does not—perhaps because sores or breaks in the skin help the virus invade the body. According to some researchers, STD's that cause genital ulcers—syphilis and genital herpes—have been associated with an increased risk of acquiring HIV infection in people in the

Disease:	**AIDS**
Cause:	*Human immunodeficiency virus.*
Symptoms:	Fever, chills, night sweats, fatigue, unexplained weight loss, dry cough, diarrhea, pink to purple blotches on or under the skin, swollen lymph nodes.
Treatment:	AZT and treatment for opportunistic infections may prolong life.
Complications:	Opportunistic infections, such as pneumonia, meningitis, encephalitis.

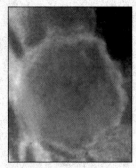

AIDS virus (shown in purple)

"The most deadly viral [STD] is AIDS, which is spreading at an alarming rate in the United States. . . ."

United States and Africa. But many health experts are even more concerned about the AIDS association with another STD that causes genital ulcers, chancroid.

Chancroid

Chancroid is a bacterial infection caused by *Hemophilus ducreyi*. The patient develops a small, ulcerating (and highly infectious) sore on the genitals. More ulcers may develop and the

Disease:	**Chancroid**
Cause:	*Hemophilus ducreyi* bacteria.
Symptoms:	In men, painful sores, becoming open ulcers or infected abscesses. Groin lymph nodes become swollen. In women, sore can be painless and unnoticed.
Treatment:	Antibiotics.
Complications:	Evidence mounting that chancroid causes increased risk for infection by the AIDS virus.

Chancroid ulcers

"Today, health experts advise, prompt diagnosis and treatment of any genital sore is absolutely essential."

lymph nodes in the groin become tender and swollen. The infection poses no harm to a fetus or a newborn and is curable with antibiotics.

The disease's inability to harm a fetus or a newborn child and its comparatively mild effects once led many experts to dub chancroid a "minor" STD. Now that opinion has changed. Doctors regard chancroid as a serious public health threat because research indicates that it significantly raises the risk of acquiring AIDS. Studies suggest that chancroid has reached epidemic proportions in Africa and is a chief cause of the rampant spread of AIDS among heterosexuals there.

Chancroid is much less common in the United States; between the late 1940's and the early 1980's, there were fewer than 0.6 cases per 100,000 population. But beginning in 1985, the infection rebounded, rising to about 1 case per 100,000 population in 1990. Most of the reported cases involved black or Hispanic men who frequented female prostitutes. Chancroid's reputation as a "minor" STD is a thing of the past. Today, health experts advise, prompt diagnosis and treatment of any genital sore is absolutely essential.

Combating STD's

The federal government, CDC, and state health departments are engaged in ongoing programs to limit the spread of STD's. These efforts involve education programs, advertising, and a strategy called contact tracing to reach everyone who may have contracted an STD from an infected person.

Contact tracing begins when an individual is diagnosed with a

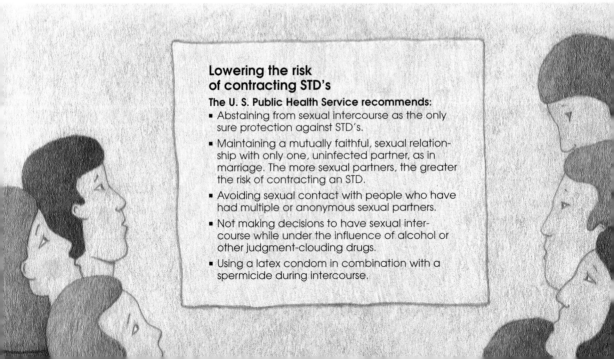

Lowering the risk of contracting STD's

The U. S. Public Health Service recommends:
- Abstaining from sexual intercourse as the only sure protection against STD's.
- Maintaining a mutually faithful, sexual relationship with only one, uninfected partner, as in marriage. The more sexual partners, the greater the risk of contracting an STD.
- Avoiding sexual contact with people who have had multiple or anonymous sexual partners.
- Not making decisions to have sexual intercourse while under the influence of alcohol or other judgment-clouding drugs.
- Using a latex condom in combination with a spermicide during intercourse.

reportable STD. The local health department asks this person to reveal the names of any sexual partners, and a health worker notifies those individuals that they may have been infected with an STD and should seek treatment.

There is nationwide contact tracing for syphilis and gonorrhea. In addition, local health-care clinics—including those at colleges—try to inform people who may have been infected with other nonreportable STD's such as chlamydia.

Despite such efforts, millions of new cases of STD's are diagnosed every year. Clearly then, the primary responsibility for halting the spread of STD's rests with the individual.

Health professionals say that the only way to guarantee that people remain free of STD's is for them to abstain from sex. Short of abstinence, they say, or a monogamous sexual relationship between uninfected individuals, people should avoid sexual contact until they and their partners are tested and declared STD-free. People who are sexually active should limit their number of sexual partners to reduce the chance of coming in contact with an STD-infected person.

Most doctors agree that, for people who are sexually active, using latex condoms combined with a virus-killing spermicide during intercourse will lessen chances of becoming infected with an STD. But because condoms tear, they cannot offer foolproof protection. Diaphragms, used with a spermicide, seem to provide some protection against bacterial STD's, but are ineffective against viral STD's.

Health professionals emphasize that the first line of defense against STD's requires seeking information about symptoms, long-term effects, and treatments. But, most important, people should take preventive measures against these diseases by being responsible about their own conduct. Public health officials warn that those who do not adopt risk-lowering behaviors are taking unnecessary chances with their own health and the health of others.

For further reading:

Landau, Elaine. *Sexually Transmitted Diseases.* Enslow Publishers, Inc., 1986.

Health & Medical News Update

In 41 alphabetically arranged articles, Health & Medical News Update contributors report on the year's major developments in health and medicine.

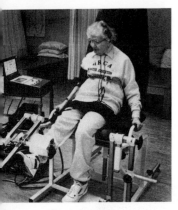

Aging 228
Aging research
Drug treatments

AIDS 230
Policy issues
AIDS research

Alcohol and Drug Abuse 233
Health effects of substance abuse
Substance abuse research

Allergies and Immunology 236
Asthma
Transplantation research
Food allergies research
Close-Up:
 Chronic fatigue syndrome

**Arthritis and
Connective Tissue** 240
Arthritis research

Birth Control 243
Contraceptives
Abortion-counseling restrictions

Blood 244
Blood supply safety measures
New treatments

Bone Disorders 246
Falls and fractures
Carpal tunnel syndrome

Books of Health and Medicine 248

Brain and Nervous System 250
Brain research
Alzheimer's disease
Lou Gehrig's disease (ALS)

Cancer 254
Cancer research
Preventive measures
New treatments

Child Development 258
Language development
Self-esteem and teen-agers

Dentistry 262
Safety of fillings
Fluoride in drinking water
Smoking and gum disease

Diabetes 263
Diabetes research
Effects of exercise

Digestive System 265
Gene for colon cancer
New diagnostics, treatments

Drugs 267
New drugs

Ear and Hearing 271
Ear infections
Exercise and hearing loss
Laser surgery

Emergency Medicine 272
Motorcycle helmets and safety
New emergency techniques

Environmental Health 273
Radiation
Air pollution
Lead poisoning

Exercise and Fitness 276
Health benefits of exercise
Exercise screening test

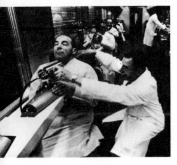

See page 229.

See page 274.

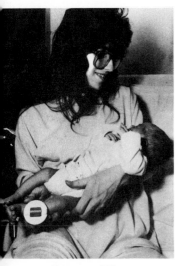

See page 293.

Eye and Vision 279
Eye disorders and injuries

Financing Health Care 283
Medicare, Medicaid
Private insurance

Genetics 285
Genetics research
Close-Up:
    Gene therapy

Glands and Hormones 290
Effects of exercise
Estrogen therapy
High blood pressure
Close-Up:
    Graves' disease

Health-Care Facilities 293
Hospitals
Nursing homes

Health Policy 295
The uninsured
AIDS testing and disclosure
Abortion counseling
Right-to-die issues
Close-Up:
    The legacy of Nancy Cruzan

Heart and Blood Vessels 299
Mechanical heart pump
Heart disease research

Infectious Diseases 303
Drug for blood poisoning
Vaccines
Bacteria and stomach cancer
Close-Up:
    Cholera epidemic

Kidney 306
Dialysis risk
Diet
Transplants

Mental Health 308
Research on mental disorders

Nutrition and Food 311
Nutrition research

Pregnancy and Childbirth 314
Video display terminals
Prenatal care

Respiratory System 316
Asthma
Lung diseases

Safety 318
Accidents and accident prevention
Seafood safety
Electromagnetic fields

**Sexually
Transmitted Diseases** 322
Syphilis and genital warts
Health effects on women
Contraceptive devices and STD's

Skin 324
Tattoo removal
Tanning salons, "tanning" pills

Smoking 326
Health risks
Benefits of quitting

Stroke 329
Prevention
Stroke research

Urology 331
Prostate treatments

Veterinary Medicine 332
Lyme disease vaccine
Rabies hazard
Neutering pets

Weight Control 335
Obesity in children
Dieting
Surgery
Close-Up:
    New weight guidelines

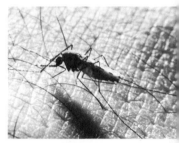

See page 305.

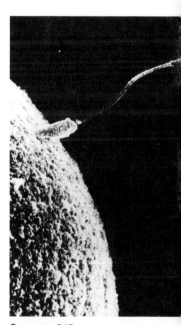

See page 315.

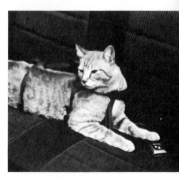

See page 333.

Aging

Hip pads cushion falls
Pads placed in the pockets of special shorts may help prevent hip fractures due to falls, a common injury among the elderly. The pads, created by engineer Jeffrey Huston of Iowa State University in Ames, will be tested on nursing home residents starting in January 1992. The shorts are worn under other clothing.

Researchers studying longevity reported in November 1990 that in order for the average life expectancy of newborns to increase to 85 years, overall mortality rates must decrease by 55 per cent. Mortality rates must decline by 60 per cent if people over age 50 are to achieve a life expectancy of 85, the report further noted. The current life expectancy of newborns averages about 75 years of age.

To increase the life span of the general population, scientists would have to eliminate the major fatal diseases, such as heart disease, diabetes, and cancer, that afflict people older than age 50. But even then, the average

life expectancy at birth would not exceed 90 years, because the aging process itself imposes a natural limit to life, according to the researchers.

The study noted that unless scientists make major breakthroughs in understanding and controlling the aging process, future medical advances will only modestly extend longevity. Thus, the researchers proposed that scientists shift their focus from lengthening life to improving the quality of life by relieving older people of symptoms of arthritis, *osteoporosis* (loss of bone tissue), and other conditions that are debilitating but not fatal.

Estrogen helps women live longer.
Women who receive treatment with the hormone estrogen after they have passed the age of *menopause* (the time of life when menstruation ceases) generally live longer than women who do not take the hormone. Women's bodies produce *estrogen,* a sex hormone, only in small amounts after menopause. Synthetic estrogen treatments to replace the hormone result in a decreased risk of heart attack, stroke, and osteoporosis, according to a study published in January 1991 by researchers at the University of Southern California in Los Angeles.

The researchers studied 8,853 residents of a retirement community for more than seven years. During this time, 1,447 of the women died.

About half of all the women had received estrogen replacement therapy at some point after menopause. The overall death rate for these women was 20 per cent lower than for those who had never received estrogen. The death rate for women who had used estrogen for at least the past 15 years was 40 per cent lower than for women who had never taken the hormone. These figures indicated that the longer the women took estrogen, the more the mortality rate declined.

Researchers suggested that estrogen probably helps prevent deaths from heart disease and stroke by lowering cholesterol levels. Although previous research showed that estrogen therapy increases the risk of cancer of the breast and *endometrium* (uterine lining), this study indicates that estrogen's benefits may outweigh its risks.

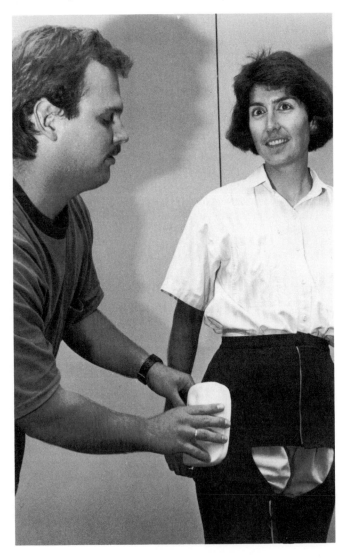

Stress and brain aging. Chronic stress may hasten aging, at least in the brains of rats. This finding was reported in a study published in May 1991 by researchers at Wake Forest University in Winston-Salem, N.C.

For six months, the scientists subjected three groups of rats aged 4, 12, and 18 months to a stressful task. Three similar groups were maintained under comparable conditions but not subjected to stress.

Then the researchers examined the rats for neurological changes that are associated with aging, such as slower chemical reactions in the brain. When compared with unstressed rats of the same ages, the rats in the two younger groups showed brain changes. The oldest group of stressed rats did not show a decline in brain-chemical function compared with the oldest unstressed rats. But the study suggested that such brain functions might have already declined and not be susceptible to further stress-related loss.

However, the older stressed rats did show an accelerated loss of brain cells compared with their unstressed counterparts. This effect was not seen in the two younger groups.

The researchers suggest that chronic stress in the young or middle-aged might hasten some brain changes associated with aging. And stress experienced later in life might deplete brain cells. Whether such findings are relevant to human beings is unproven.

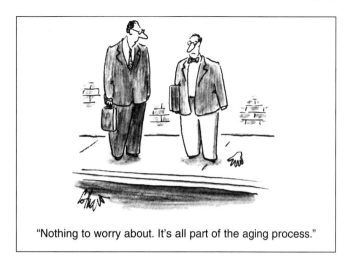

"Nothing to worry about. It's all part of the aging process."

Lower blood pressure helps heart. Controlling a type of high blood pressure in the elderly helps prevent stroke and heart attack, according to a study published in June 1991.The research was carried out at 16 medical centers in the United States. It found that among 2,365 elderly patients taking low doses of inexpensive drugs to reduce *systolic pressure* (the first number in a blood pressure reading that measures the strength of the heart's contractions), the risk of stroke decreased by 36 per cent. The risk of heart attack declined by 27 per cent in patients taking the drugs.

☐ Denham Harman

In WORLD BOOK, see AGING; HEART.

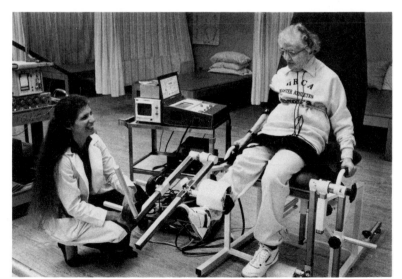

Weight training boosts strength and mobility
A 92-year-old woman exercises with weight-training equipment as a researcher measures her muscle strength. Medical researchers based in Boston in 1990 and 1991 were studying the effects of strength training in people over age 90. They reported that nine frail elderly men and women increased leg strength and walking speed after performing muscle-strengthening exercises for eight weeks.

AIDS

Physicians, medical ethicists, and the public during 1990 and 1991 debated whether health-care professionals infected with the virus that causes AIDS should inform their patients and be restricted from performing surgery and other invasive procedures. The debate began in August 1990, after the Centers for Disease Control (CDC) in Atlanta, Ga., announced that a dentist had infected one of his patients with the AIDS-causing human immunodeficiency virus (HIV). Then in September, a Florida newspaper printed a letter from the dentist, David J. Acer, asking that his patients be tested for AIDS.

Acer died of AIDS on Sept. 3, 1990. By August 1991, four more of Acer's patients were diagnosed with HIV.

Kimberly Bergalis, the first of Acer's patients diagnosed as having AIDS, received national attention when she campaigned for improved patient protection against HIV-infected health-care professionals. In a letter published in June 1991, she said, "If laws are not formed to provide protection, then my death was in vain." By August 1991, Bergalis was gravely ill.

Doctors were uncertain exactly how the virus was transmitted from Acer to Bergalis and the other patients. Acer had removed two wisdom teeth from Bergalis in 1987. One theory was that Acer had used HIV-contaminated instruments.

The American Dental Association in January 1991 recommended that dentists infected with AIDS inform their patients or stop doing procedures that could infect patients. And in June 1991, the American Medical Association (AMA) urged voluntary AIDS testing for both doctors and patients. The AMA recommended that HIV-infected doctors should stop performing invasive procedures or inform their patients that they are *HIV positive* (infected with HIV).

A Gallup Organization survey published in July 1991 showed that 94 per cent of those surveyed in the United States believe that physicians and dentists should be required to inform their patients if they are infected with the AIDS virus. That same survey found that 65 per cent of respondents would discontinue all treatment with a physician, dentist, or other health-care worker who was HIV positive.

AIDS from tissue transplants. In May 1991, federal health officials disclosed that at least six individuals had contracted the AIDS virus from tissue, organ, or bone transplants that they had received in 1985 from a 22-year-old Virginia man, who was killed during a robbery. Three of the infected transplant recipients had already died of AIDS at the time of the announcement. Although tests had suggested that the donor was *HIV negative* (free of HIV infection) before the transplants

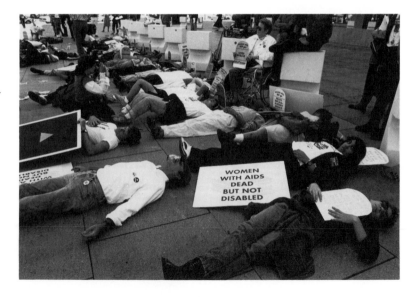

Women and AIDS
Protesters demanding more attention for women with AIDS demonstrate in front of the U.S. Department of Health and Human Services in Washington, D.C., in October 1990. AIDS activists say that women have been underrepresented in studies involving AIDS drugs and ignored in other research concerning AIDS.

took place, officials believed that he had been infected so soon before his death that the presence of the virus did not show up in tests.

AIDS statistics. The CDC reported that as of June 30, 1991, there were 182,834 cases of AIDS in the United States (including 3,140 children ages 12 and under). Of these individuals with AIDS, 115,984 (including 1,646 children) had died.

In January 1991, the CDC reported that AIDS had become the nation's second-leading killer of young men (ages 25 to 44), exceeding deaths caused by heart disease, cancer, and suicide, and surpassed only by "unintentional injuries" (including homicides). Also, about 1 in 500 college students in the United States were infected with the virus in 1990, according to a CDC study published in November 1990. Researchers studied the prevalence of HIV infection on 19 university campuses.

Lowering AZT doses. In October 1990, two studies were published indicating that low doses of the drug zidovudine (AZT) were as effective and less toxic than the higher standard doses. AZT has been the primary treatment for people infected with HIV. Side effects such as *anemia* (low levels of red blood cells) and *neutropenia* (low levels of white blood cells) are associated with AZT. Thus, doctors welcomed the news that patients may do just as well on a dose as low as 300 milligrams, compared with doses of 1,500 milligrams typically prescribed since March 1987, when AZT was first approved in the United States.

Expanding the AIDS drug arsenal. The drug erythropoietin received U.S. Food and Drug Administration (FDA) approval in January 1991 for use by AIDS patients who are taking AZT. Erythropoietin stimulates bone marrow to make red blood cells and can help counteract AZT-caused anemia.

Researchers found that another drug, a relatively inexpensive antibiotic combining trimethoprim and sulfamethoxazole (marketed under the brand names Bactrim and Septra), effectively staves off the onset of *Pneumocystis carinii* pneumonia (PCP), a

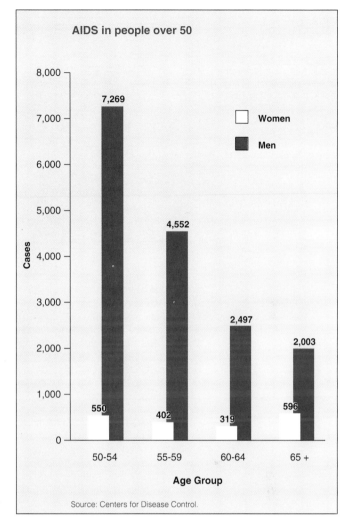

AIDS in people over 50

Source: Centers for Disease Control.

life-threatening infection that commonly afflicts AIDS patients. In a study published in February 1991, researchers at Kaiser Permanente Medical Center in Los Angeles reported that none of 116 patients taking Bactrim or Septra for three days a week developed PCP over periods ranging from 3 to 42 months. More than 60 per cent of patients had previously had one or more episodes of PCP. Although another drug, *pentamidine* (taken in an aerosol form) is FDA-approved for the prevention of the AIDS-related pneumonia, patients taking this agent sometimes acquire the infection anyway.

The rates of respiratory failure and death from PCP in AIDS patients are reduced when the patients are treated

More than 18,000 people in the United States aged 50 years and over reportedly had AIDS as of May 1991. Evidence suggests that the disease progresses at a faster rate in older people than in younger ones. But health experts say that it may take longer to diagnose AIDS in older people, because some symptoms of AIDS, such as muscle weakness and a weakened immune system, also are signs of normal aging.

AIDS coloring book

Some of San Antonio's children in kindergarten through third grade learn about AIDS with the help of an eight-page coloring book, introduced in 1991 by the University of Texas Health Science Center. Public health experts stress the importance of educating children about the disease as soon as possible.

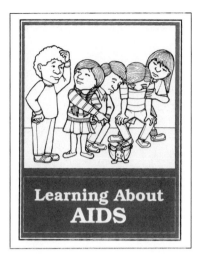

Learning About AIDS

with drugs called *corticosteroids,* according to two studies published in November 1990. A University of Miami (Fla.) study of 23 AIDS patients found that 9 of the 12 patients who received corticosteroids survived a bout of PCP and were released from the hospital. Only 2 of 11 patients who received a *placebo* (a pill containing an inactive substance) survived an episode of PCP and were released from the hospital. Researchers at the University of California at San Diego found that patients who received corticosteroids in addition to standard treatment had a death rate after 31 days only one-half that of patients receiving standard therapy alone.

An FDA advisory panel in July 1991 recommended approval for *dideoxyinosine* (DDI) for AIDS patients who cannot tolerate AZT. Health experts believed that the FDA would approve the drug within a few months, probably in the autumn of 1991.

Transmitting the AIDS virus. *Dendritic cells* (a type of white blood cell) in the mouth and genitals could be a path for the entrance of HIV into the body. Pathologist William A. Haseltine, chief of AIDS research at the Dana Farber Cancer Institute in Boston, reported this finding at the Seventh International Conference on AIDS, held in Florence, Italy, in June 1991. He said that HIV can enter and reproduce in these cells, and noted that this finding suggests that, theoretically, the virus could be transmitted in saliva via

deep kissing. But there is no other evidence to support this.

Initial vaccine results. The first AIDS vaccine tested on human beings was proven safe, according to a report published in January 1991. Researchers reported results from six hospitals that were part of a federal program. Each of the 36 healthy volunteers was injected in 1988 with three to four doses of a genetically engineered vaccine. The volunteers developed some immune response— that is, their disease-fighting immune systems showed signs of activity. Part of this activity included the development of *antibodies* to HIV. (Antibodies are disease-fighting proteins formed by the body in response to an "invader," such as a bacterium or virus.) The vaccine's side effects were minimal, but whether it actually gives protection against HIV infection is not known.

Barring HIV-infected foreigners. In a widely criticized decision, the Administration of President George Bush announced in May 1991 that the United States would continue to prevent HIV-infected foreigners from entering the country. That decision blocked a regulation scheduled to go into effect on June 1 that would have reversed a 1987 immigration policy barring HIV-positive persons from visiting or establishing residence in the United States. That policy had been attacked as discriminatory and medically unnecessary by public health officials.

France discovered HIV. An article by U.S. AIDS researcher Robert Gallo, published in May 1991, contained statements that some observers interpreted as an admission that the organism he had identified as HIV in 1984 was a contaminant from a virus specimen supplied by French scientists. Gallo, head of the U.S. National Cancer Institute's laboratory of tumor cell biology, was accused of intentionally or accidentally using a specimen sent to his lab by the French. In his article, Gallo appeared to accept that a mix-up had occurred.

☐ Richard Trubo

In the Special Reports section, see THE SPECTER OF AIDS. In WORLD BOOK, see AIDS.

Drug abuse may be linked to nearly 50 per cent of all strokes in people under age 35 and to 22 per cent of strokes in people under 45. This finding was reported in November 1990 by physicians at San Francisco General Hospital Medical Center and the University of California at San Francisco. The researchers, who studied the cases of 214 stroke patients admitted to San Francisco General Hospital, found double the number of drug-abuse related strokes that were reported three years earlier.

The physicians found that the risk of stroke among drug abusers under age 45 is six times higher than average for that age group. Drug-abuse related strokes were fatal in one-third of the patients studied and left many of the rest with physical or mental impairments.

According to the study, smoking was the most common risk factor for stroke in the under-45 group. But cocaine use was the second most common risk factor, followed by use of heroin, amphetamines, the stimulant methylphenidate, and phencyclidine (PCP). These five drugs were the direct cause of stroke in 22 per cent of the cases studied.

The physicians calculated that the risk of stroke is 50 times greater during the first six hours after a person takes drugs. The risk is especially high for users of cocaine—which can dangerously elevate blood pressure—and amphetamines—which can cause spasms and inflammation of the blood vessels. Four per cent of all strokes occur among people less than 45 years old, and stroke deaths for this age group total 10,000 per year in the United States.

Driving while intoxicated. The typical drunken driver is a male less than 24 years old, according to a 1991 report by the Center of Alcohol Studies at Rutgers The State University of New Jersey in New Brunswick. According to statistics compiled by the center, about twice as many men as women are involved in fatal car accidents in which the driver's blood alcohol level is above 0.10 per cent (the percentage required for a drunken driving conviction in most states).

The Center of Alcohol Studies also reported that the risk of automobile accidents is clearly linked to the driver's blood alcohol level. With a level of 0.10 per cent, the risk of accidents is about 6 times greater than when the driver is sober. At a blood alcohol level of 0.15 per cent, the risk is nearly 20 times greater.

Rise in alcohol-related deaths. After declining in the 1980's, the number of deaths related to alcohol use in California has begun to rise again. This finding, reported in January 1991 by the California Department of Health Services, reflects death-rate statistics

Alcohol and Drug Abuse

Drug abuse detection
A public service advertisement sponsored by Partnership for a Drug-Free America highlights some of the physical symptoms that may indicate a child is using drugs such as cocaine, crack, or marijuana.

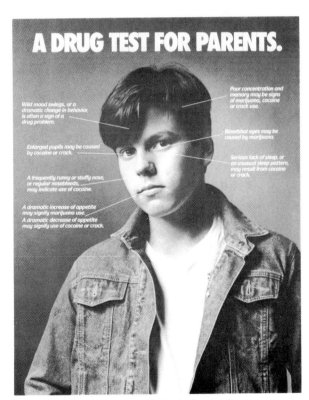

for 1979 through 1988. The National Center for Health Statistics in Hyattsville, Md., reported that national statistics show a similar, though less pronounced, trend.

According to James W. Sutocky, spokesperson for the California department, the deaths were caused by such medical problems as alcohol-related heart disease, alcohol poisoning, and alcohol-related liver disorders. Deaths due to impaired automobile driving were not included in the study.

Researchers mentioned several possible causes of the apparent upswing. For example, physicians may have become less reluctant to report alcohol abuse as a cause of death.

Another possible cause is an increase in liquor sales to young people. The researchers cited in particular the new popularity of wine coolers, alcoholic beverages usually marketed like soft drinks to young adults. Some experts believe that advertising of the wine coolers, as well as their display in stores near milk and other nonalcoholic beverages, may prompt young people who normally drink nonalcoholic beverages to switch to wine coolers.

Blocking alcohol craving. Drug researchers at Purdue University in West Lafayette, Ind., reported in autumn 1990 that molecular fragments of an important biochemical called *adrenocorticotropic hormone* (ACTH) seem to block the craving for alcohol in rats. The hormone, normally secreted by the pituitary gland, stimulates the body's production of other hormones.

The researchers first made alcohol-laced water available to the rats. After the scientists exposed the rats to stressful situations, the rats began drinking the alcohol-water mixture regularly. However, after the rats received injections of parts of the ACTH molecule, they stopped drinking the alcohol-laced water. The scientists reported that the rats did not appear impaired by the treatment and suggested that the finding might help in the search for a drug treatment for alcoholism.

Drug abuse among students. Drug abuse was less prevalent among U.S. high school seniors in 1990 than in 1989, according to a survey sponsored by the National Institute on Drug Abuse (NIDA) in Rockville, Md. The institute has sponsored annual surveys of drug and alcohol abuse among high school seniors for the past 16 years. The 1990 survey, conducted by social researchers at the University of Michigan in Ann Arbor, was released in January 1991.

More than half of those surveyed in 1990 reported that they had never used illegal drugs. Only one-third of the entire group of students reported using illicit drugs at any time during the previous year. In addition, the percentage of students who had used cocaine and marijuana during the

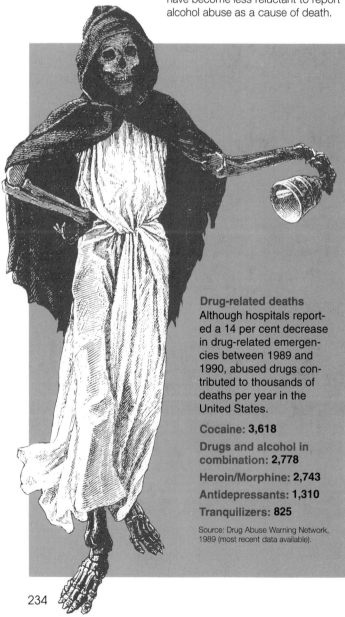

Drug-related deaths
Although hospitals reported a 14 per cent decrease in drug-related emergencies between 1989 and 1990, abused drugs contributed to thousands of deaths per year in the United States.

Cocaine: 3,618

Drugs and alcohol in combination: 2,778

Heroin/Morphine: 2,743

Antidepressants: 1,310

Tranquilizers: 825

Source: Drug Abuse Warning Network, 1989 (most recent data available).

month before the survey decreased in 1990.

Marijuana, the most widely used illegal drug among those polled, was nonetheless used less frequently than cigarettes and alcohol. The survey found no decline in the prevalence of cigarette smoking since 1989 and only a 3 per cent decrease in the use of alcohol since 1989. Nineteen per cent of the high school seniors reported that they smoked cigarettes daily and 11 per cent smoked at least half a pack per day. Fifty-seven per cent of those surveyed had used alcohol during the previous month, and 4 per cent drank daily.

More alarming were the June 1991 results of another survey of alcohol use among teen-agers. Researchers at the U.S. Department of Health and Human Services examined the drinking habits of more than 20 million students in the 7th through 12th grades in eight states.

The government researchers found that 39 per cent of the students drank alcohol every week and that 2 per cent consumed an average of 15 drinks per week. Of those students who drank every week, 31 per cent reported drinking when alone; 41 per cent said they drank when they were upset to make themselves feel better; and 25 per cent said they drank to "get high."

Alcoholism gene? Throughout 1990 and 1991, scientists were searching, with mixed results, for evidence that a predisposition to alcoholism is linked to a gene described in 1990 by genetic researchers Kenneth Blum at the University of Texas in San Antonio and Ernest Noble at the University of California at Los Angeles. The geneticists had reported that alcoholism might be linked to the gene for a protein on the surface of brain cells. The protein, called the *dopamine D$_2$ receptor*, allows *dopamine* (a biochemical that transmits messages among brain cells) to enter the cell. Other scientists have linked dopamine to the pleasurable effects of alcohol and other substances.

Blum and Noble found the gene for the receptor in 69 per cent of 35 deceased alcoholics but in only 20 per cent of the same number of deceased

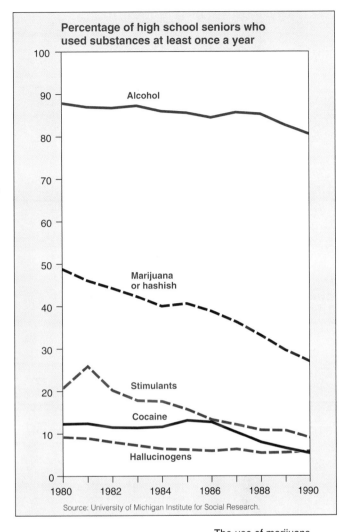

Percentage of high school seniors who used substances at least once a year

Source: University of Michigan Institute for Social Research.

subjects who were not alcoholic. But genetic researchers with the National Institute on Alcohol Abuse and Alcoholism in Rockville, Md., in December 1990 reported that they were unable to duplicate Blum and Noble's results.

The government scientists searched for the gene pattern in 40 alcoholics and 127 nonalcoholic subjects and among nonalcoholic and alcoholic members of two families. They did not find that the dopamine D$_2$ receptor gene was more prevalent among the alcoholic family members. In June 1991, a research group at the Veterans Administration Medical Center in Westhaven, Conn., reported similar results in a study of 44 alcoholics and 68 nonalcoholics.

However, Blum and Noble in July

The use of marijuana, cocaine, and stimulants among high school seniors declined in 1990, according to the latest results of an annual survey conducted by the University of Michigan Institute for Social Research in Ann Arbor. Experts were concerned about the continued prevalence of alcohol use, however.

1991 announced a second experiment in which 159 people were examined for the presence of the gene. The geneticists found the gene in half of the alcoholics but in only one-fifth of the nonalcoholic subjects. That same month, researchers at Washington University in St. Louis, Mo., reported evidence supporting some aspects of Blum and Noble's findings.

Even if the gene does play a role in alcoholism, other factors—such as other genes and aspects of a person's surroundings and upbringing—almost certainly contribute significantly to the disease, experts note. Other studies of the gene's role in addictive behavior—including drug abuse as well as alcoholism—were expected by the end of the year. In late 1990, the growing body of evidence supporting the theory led two of the field's leading organizations to revise their definitions of alcoholism. The National Council on Alcoholism and Drug Dependence, a public interest group, and the American Society of Addiction Medicine, a physician organization, both in New York City, now describe alcoholism as a "chronic disease with genetic, psychosocial, and environmental factors influencing its development. . . ."

☐ Gayle R. Hamilton

In the Special Reports section, see DEFEATING DRUG DEPENDENCY. In WORLD BOOK, see ALCOHOLISM; DRUG ABUSE.

Allergies and Immunology

People who develop mild asthma are better off taking *anti-inflammatory* (inflammation-reducing) drugs than drugs that act to widen breathing passages. That finding was reported in August 1991 by physicians at Helsinki University Central Hospital in Finland.

Research since the late 1980's has shown that asthma results from a still-unexplained inflammation of the airways in the lungs. In treating asthma patients, physicians have traditionally prescribed *bronchodilators*—medications designed to *dilate* (open) airways. Many physicians, especially in the United States, have not considered anti-inflammatory drugs to be a "first-line" defense against asthma.

Allergy experts expect the Finnish study to change that approach to asthma therapy. Over a two-year period, the Helsinki physicians studied 103 people who had recently been diagnosed with mild asthma. The patients were treated with either an inhaled bronchodilator or an inhaled anti-inflammatory drug. The doctors found that the anti-inflammatory medication—a type of drug called a *corticosteroid*—was superior to the bronchodilator in treating the underlying condition and, therefore, in relieving the patients' allergy symptoms.

Earlier in the year, a panel of asthma

For reasons yet to be determined, asthma death rates among people in the United States aged 5 to 34 have been rising sharply since the late 1970's. From a low of 1.6 deaths per 1 million population in 1977, the asthma death rate for young Americans had risen to 4.2 per million by 1987 (the most recent figures available). Health experts speculated that several factors, including declining access to medical care, have contributed to this increase.

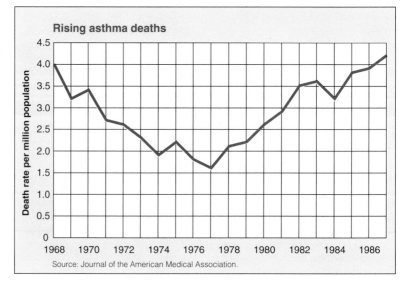

Rising asthma deaths

Source: Journal of the American Medical Association.

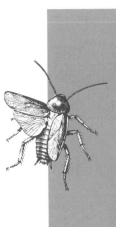

Allergic to cockroaches?
Most people want to keep cockroaches out of their homes. But this is especially important for people who are allergic to these pests. Researchers at the U.S. Department of Agriculture say that household cleanliness along with clean, dry air are keys to creating a roach-free living environment. The scientists recommend keeping kitchen counters and other surfaces free of food scraps, putting garbage outside as it accumulates, and ventilating and dehumidifying such spaces as attics and cabinets—places favored by roaches. For those with roach allergies, the experts recommend filtering household air to remove airborne body parts from dead roaches.

experts convened by the National Institutes of Health in Bethesda, Md., endorsed the use of anti-inflammatory therapy as a first-line treatment for patients with more severe asthma. The doctors recommended that such patients be treated with inhaled anti-inflammatory drugs.

Asthma in childhood. Frequent and thorough housecleaning might protect many children from developing asthma, physicians at Poole General Hospital in Great Britain reported in August 1990. Specifically, keeping a clean house reduces the presence of tiny organisms called mites that thrive in dust and to which many children become allergic.

The physicians studied a group of 42 children who had a history of asthma. Skin tests revealed that 26 of those children were allergic to mites.

The researchers concluded that exposure to dust mites in early childhood can contribute significantly to the development of asthma in individuals who are genetically susceptible to asthma. They recommended that people with small children make an effort to reduce the amount of dust in their homes.

Preventing tissue rejection. A new approach to tissue transplantation was reported in 1990 and 1991 by researchers at several institutions in the United States and Europe. All the studies were done with laboratory animals. Rather than using drugs to prevent the animals' immune systems from rejecting transplanted tissue, the scientists were experimenting with fooling the immune systems into accepting foreign tissue as a natural part of the body.

Transplanted tissue, such as a donated organ, normally provokes a reaction by the immune system, which attacks the tissue as it would an invading virus or bacterium. Transplant surgeons overcome this rejection mechanism with drugs that suppress the immune system. But the drug therapy also leaves the patient vulnerable to many infections and, in some cases, even to cancer.

The newer approach aims at preserving the transplant while leaving the immune system's disease-fighting abilities intact. At least two techniques were being investigated in 1990 and 1991 by medical scientists at the University of Pennsylvania in Philadelphia, Massachusetts General Hospital in Boston, and elsewhere.

At the University of Pennsylvania, researchers used a "priming" technique that involved introducing tiny bits of tissue from a donor rat into the *thymus gland* of a recipient rat. The thymus gland, located below the neck area, aids in the development of disease-fighting white blood cells.

The investigators injected small pieces of tissue from a donor rat's kidneys or pancreas into the thymus of the recipient rat. That rat's thymus then apparently "instructed" the immune system to accept the donor

Few Answers for Chronic Fatigue Sufferers

Researchers at several medical centers in 1990 and 1991 were studying puzzling cases of chronic fatigue, debating among themselves the nature of the illness as they searched for its cause. Severe, unexplained fatigue has virtually disabled hundreds of thousands—perhaps millions—of people in the United States.

Now called *chronic fatigue syndrome* (CFS), the disorder was first widely reported after about 100 previously healthy and active residents of a resort community in Nevada became ill in 1985. CFS quickly attracted widespread attention when thousands more apparent cases were diagnosed across the nation.

According to the U.S. Centers for Disease Control in Atlanta, Ga.—which has monitored the illness since the mid-1980's—CFS differs from the normal fatigue that most people experience at one time or another. The center's guidelines state that fatigue in CFS persists or recurs for at least six months and reduces the affected person's normal activity level by more than half.

The illness usually begins suddenly, with flulike symptoms such as sore throat, headache, fever, and pain in the muscles and joints. Some patients also experience psychological problems, including memory loss, confusion, difficulty concentrating, and depression.

Soon after the Nevada cases were reported, researchers thought they had evidence that a virus caused these mysterious symptoms. Tests for *antibodies* (disease-fighting proteins) in the blood of people with CFS showed that many were infected with *Epstein-Barr virus* (EBV), which causes infectious mononucleosis, a flulike viral infection that sometimes causes lingering fatigue.

But by late 1991, physicians had generally discarded the notion of a link between EBV and chronic fatigue. EBV infection is extremely common, and many people—whether they have CFS or not—have high levels of antibodies to the virus. In addition, a significant percentage of CFS sufferers have low EBV antibody levels.

With EBV virtually ruled out, some experts argued that most cases of CFS are actually related to psychological disorders, usually *clinical depression* (mood disorders that can cause fatigue, sleep disturbances, and other symptoms similar to those of CFS). Some studies lend support to this theory. A 1990 study by medical researcher Deborah Gold of the University of Washington School of Medicine in Seattle indicated that many CFS patients have a medical history of—or are currently suffering from—depression.

Yet the onset of CFS is often abrupt, while clinical depression tends to have no clearly defined start. It is also unclear which comes first: Does clinical depression cause the chronic fatigue? Or do CFS patients become depressed because of the frustrations and limitations of their illness?

Several other factors, including viruses other than EBV as well as disorders of the body's disease-fighting immune system, have come under suspicion as possible causes of CFS. For example, one of the ways the immune system combats microbes or other foreign

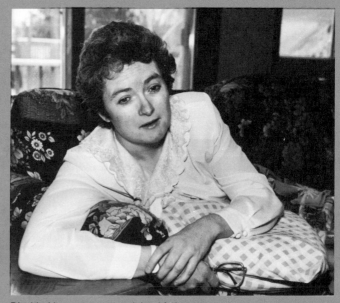

Disabled by severe, unexplained fatigue.

substances in the body is by producing *cytokines,* natural compounds that help destroy the invaders. Doctors using cytokines in cancer therapy have found that these biochemicals may cause side effects including fatigue, muscle aches, and other symptoms strikingly similar to CFS.

In most people, production of cytokines declines after an infection is over. But, according to many scientists, the immune system in CFS patients may remain activated for months or years, continuously producing cytokines and causing the CFS symptoms.

Other findings support the theory that some abnormality in the immune system causes CFS. For instance, a large percentage of CFS patients have allergies—which occur when the immune system overreacts to harmless substances such as plant pollen.

While researchers look for the cause of CFS, practicing physicians are limited in their ability to diagnose and treat the illness. Patients may benefit, however, from pain relievers or other medications that relieve individual symptoms.

Physicians generally encourage CFS sufferers to eat a balanced diet, get adequate rest, avoid stress, and remain as active as possible. And, as is often the case with poorly understood disorders, patients may benefit from the exchange of information and advice among members of a support group. In the six years since CFS was first noted, about 400 CFS support groups have been established throughout the United States. □ Michael Woods

rat's tissues as a normal part of the body rather than as foreign tissue. Thus, when other cells from the donor rat were transplanted into the recipient rat, no rejection response occurred. The scientists said they did not know how the thymus had "reeducated" the immune system.

At Massachusetts General Hospital, researchers reported success with a different technique. They camouflaged transplanted mouse pancreas cells so the immune system of the mouse receiving the cells would not recognize them as foreign tissue.

The scientists modified immune system molecules called *antibodies.* Antibodies normally attach to proteins on the surface of foreign cells or microorganisms and alert other elements of the immune system to join the attack. The modified antibodies were used to cover up the surface proteins of the pancreas cells in the donor mouse, making the proteins inaccessible to regular antibodies. When the cells were then transplanted into another mouse, they were "invisible" to that mouse's antibodies and so were not rejected. The researchers noted that such an approach may permit successful transplantation of pancreas cells—an outcome that could someday help millions of diabetics, whose pancreases do not function properly.

Food allergy test questioned. In many people thought to be allergic or sensitive to certain foods, the allergy test results may be more psychological than physical, physicians at the University of California at San Francisco reported in August 1990.

Some physicians believe that food allergies can be diagnosed with a *symptom provocation test,* in which the doctor injects a patient with an extract of a suspect food and notes any symptoms that occur in the next 10 minutes. Many physicians, however, doubt the technique's value, noting that patients' expectations can influence their physical and emotional responses in such a testing situation.

The researchers conducted a series of provocation tests on 18 patients who complained of various symptoms, including headaches, nausea, or nasal congestion, after eating certain foods. However, the scientists de-

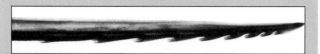

Sensitivity to insect stings: a potentially fatal allergy
For more than 25 million people in the United States, the stinger of a honey bee, *above,* can be a lethal weapon. An individual allergic to insect venom from the sting of a bee, wasp, or other insect is at risk of developing reactions ranging from hives to coma, and even death. Many people do not know they are sensitive to insect venom until they are stung for the first time and experience unpleasant symptoms. Often, that first sting is not life-threatening, but the next one may be. After getting a "warning sting," a person should consult with a physician about preventive treatment.

signed the tests in such a way that neither they nor the patients knew whether an injection contained a food substance or a harmless solution.

The tests revealed that the individuals were not really allergic to any of the foods they thought were causing the symptoms. The doctors concluded that symptom provocation, as well as treatments based on "neutralizing" such reactions, lack scientific validity.

Progress on myasthenia gravis.
Immunologists expressed optimism in 1991 that a successful treatment may soon be available for *myasthenia gravis*, a disease that causes progressive muscle weakness. Myasthenia gravis

is an *autoimmune disease*, a disorder in which the immune system attacks the body's own tissues.

Researchers have learned that myasthenia gravis results when certain cells of the immune system, called *B and T lymphocytes*, cease to recognize particular nerve-cell *receptors* as part of the body. Receptors are protein molecules on cells that serve as doorways into the cells. The affected receptors are for a *neurotransmitter* (a chemical that transmits signals from one nerve cell to another) called *acetylcholine*. The B and T cells form antibodies against the receptors, thereby inhibiting the flow of nerve impulses to the muscles. Without proper stimulation from the nervous system, the muscles cease to function properly and grow weaker.

Researchers at several U.S. institutions in 1991 were experimenting with modified antibodies that mimic the shape of the acetylcholine receptor. Those antibodies attach to molecules on the surface of B and T cells that enable the cells to latch onto the acetylcholine receptor. This prevents the B and T cells from linking up with the receptors on the cells.

Human trials of this new approach, which has proved successful in animal experiments, were underway at several U.S. medical centers in 1991.

☐ Robert A. Goldstein
In WORLD BOOK, see ALLERGY; ASTHMA; IMMUNITY.

Arthritis and Connective Tissue Disorders

A new *syndrome* (collection of symptoms) involving the joints and connective tissues was described by two physicians at St. Thomas' Hospital in London in April 1991. The physicians reported seeing a group of patients who had the following symptoms: arthritis or joint pain; recurrent *sinusitis* (inflammation of the nasal sinuses); wheezing or mild asthma; red eyes; tender, swollen fingertips; and a slight elevation in the white blood cell count. The patients had not responded to various treatments prescribed earlier by other physicians.

Like many forms of arthritis, the as-yet-unnamed syndrome seems to result from an *autoimmune disorder*, in which the body's immune system at-

tacks the body's own tissue. The St. Thomas' physicians found that some of the patients responded dramatically to treatment with *immunosuppressants* (drugs that suppress the body's immune response). The results underscore the importance of identifying a new syndrome: By recognizing that some or all of the symptoms are manifestations of a single medical condition, physicians are better able to learn about its underlying causes and develop effective treatments.

Fibromyalgia and chronic fatigue.
Two other syndromes of interest to *rheumatologists* (physicians who specialize in diseases of the joints, muscles, tendons, and other connective

tissues) received increased attention in 1991. One syndrome was *fibromyalgia,* a condition involving generalized muscle pain; the other was chronic fatigue, a disorder characterized by debilitating fatigue. Physicians at the University of Connecticut Health Center in Farmington looked at 39 patients whose chief complaint was chronic fatigue. They reported their findings to a meeting of rheumatologists in May.

Each patient was given a detailed examination. Of the group, 9 patients met the criteria for fibromyalgia—widespread muscle pain along with specific points of tenderness. Seven met the criteria for chronic fatigue syndrome, which include a mild fever, sore throat, and joint and muscle pain—along with prolonged fatigue. One patient met the criteria for both.

The important finding was that many patients who reported chronic fatigue actually had fibromyalgia, which can be treated, unlike chronic fatigue syndrome. Physicians treat fibromyalgia with small doses of tricyclic antidepressants, taken before bedtime. The drugs help adjust the patient's disturbed sleep patterns, which are part of the disorder. See ALLERGIES AND IMMUNOLOGY (Close-Up).

Gut reaction to spinal arthritis. Research reported in November 1990 by researchers in Texas strengthened the association between *ankylosing spondylitis* (AS)—spinal arthritis—and a gene found in 90 per cent of people with the disease. About 20 per cent of those who inherit this gene develop AS or a related condition. The disease strikes 3 to 10 times as many men as women. Many patients with AS also develop a related bowel disorder.

The gene, HLA-B27, was isolated from human cells and injected into fertilized rat eggs by a team at the University of Texas Southwestern Medical Center in Dallas. Some of the rats incorporated the human gene into their own genetic material. Of those so-called *transgenic* animals, 10 out of 14 males and 1 out of 9 females developed AS. Their symptoms—joint inflammation, thickening of the skin and nails—bore a striking resemblance to human symptoms of the disease.

In addition, all the rats with the in-

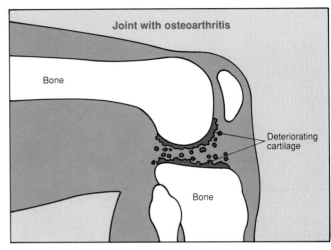

Joint with osteoarthritis

Bone

Deteriorating cartilage

Bone

corporated human gene developed diarrhea, and their intestinal tracts showed evidence of chronic inflammation. These symptoms commonly occur in a form of arthritis, known as *reactive arthritis* or *Reiter's syndrome,* that appears to result from a bacterial infection.

The rats thereby provided an important clue, suggesting that AS, like reactive arthritis, starts with a bacterial infection in the gastrointestinal tract of people who are genetically predisposed to the disease. Research on people with AS supports this association. Certain bacteria that can live in the intestinal tract trigger a strong response from the immune systems of

Scientists have found that a genetic defect underlies some cases of *osteoarthritis,* a condition in which the cartilage lining the joints breaks down. A faulty gene causes the production of cartilage that is too weak to take stress.

Mapping joints
Using a grid—projected with a spotlight onto a bone to provide reference points—and photographs taken from different angles, researchers can construct a three-dimensional computer model of a joint. The model helps them study joint disorders.

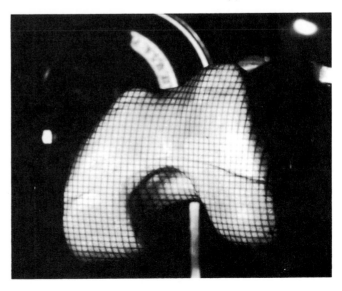

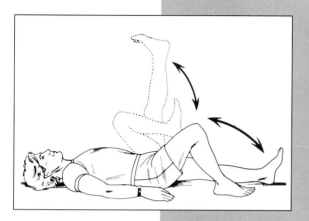

Keeping joints flexible
Proper exercise can help people with arthritis move their joints more easily. They may even feel less pain and stiffness as they perform daily tasks. A brochure available from the Arthritis Foundation offers suggestions on making exercise part of a daily routine and provides examples of exercises that help keep joints flexible. To obtain a free copy, send a stamped, self-addressed envelope to Exercise & Your Arthritis, Arthritis Foundation, P.O. Box 19000, Atlanta, GA 30326. Before undertaking any exercise program, however, it's important to consult your physician.

AS patients, while leaving other people unaffected.

Prior to the Texas research, the disease had no counterpart in animals. Transgenic rats may now provide a testing ground for likely triggers of AS and for new antibiotic treatments. For example, researchers might introduce different bacteria into the animals' intestines to see which bacteria most actively trigger the disease.

Genetic link to osteoarthritis. The first clear evidence that a gene may play a significant role in the most common form of arthritis was reported by researchers in September 1990. The disorder—*osteoarthritis*—involves the deterioration of *cartilage,* the tissue that cushions the joints. Although osteoarthritis can result from injuries and overuse of the joints, most cases have no known cause.

Research groups at Thomas Jefferson University in Philadelphia and at Case Western Reserve University in Cleveland studied an abnormal gene found in members of a single family who developed osteoarthritis at an early age. Because of the genetic defect, their cells produced an altered version of a protein that forms a major component of cartilage. This alteration apparently weakened the cartilage, setting the stage for osteoarthritis.

Ankle brace helps. A support brace around the ankle can substantially reduce the pain that people with rheumatoid arthritis (RA) experience while

walking. This finding was reported by physicians at Selly Oak Hospital in Birmingham, England, in April 1991. Rheumatoid arthritis causes crippling inflammation of the cartilage around the joints. In many cases, RA affects the joint just above the heel bone that allows the foot to move inward and outward. As a result, patients lose mobility and suffer pain when walking, especially on an uneven surface.

The Birmingham physicians reported that their support brace markedly reduced or even ended swelling and pain in 78 per cent of the RA patients who tried it. These patients had already received intensive drug therapy for RA.

Prednisone and bone loss. The drug prednisone is prescribed to reduce inflammation and improve mobility in patients with RA. But physicians have worried that the drug might also accelerate the loss of calcium from bones, particularly in women following *menopause* (the time of life when menstruation ceases).

They need no longer worry, according to a study published in March 1991 by researchers at the Brigham and Women's Hospital in Boston. The researchers measured the bone density of women taking an average dose of 6.6 milligrams of prednisone per day. They found no difference in bone density between that group and a group of women not taking the drug.

☐ John Baum

In WORLD BOOK, see ARTHRITIS.

Behavioral Disorders
See Mental Health

Research published in April 1991 challenged a 1981 study whose findings contributed to the withdrawal of most intrauterine devices (IUD's) from the market in the United States. The research was reported by a team headed by biostatistician Richard A. Kronmal of the University of Washington in Seattle. Kronmal once acted as a consultant to the company that manufactured the Dalkon Shield, one of the most popular IUD's at one time. The American College of Obstetricians and Gynecologists, however, said that the new study appeared to be "solid."

The 1981 study concluded that the rate of pelvic infections among women who used IUD's was 60 per cent higher than that among nonusers. Such infections can lead to sterility. A 1983 study, based on the same data, reported a similar conclusion.

These studies played a major role in lawsuits filed against A. H. Robins, the manufacturer of the Dalkon Shield, which was removed from the market in 1974. Health experts have suggested that the legal battle surrounding the Dalkon Shield also contributed to a decline in U.S. research into new contraceptive devices.

For their research, Kronmal and his team reanalyzed the data from the original study. They contended that

Birth Control

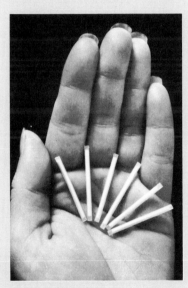

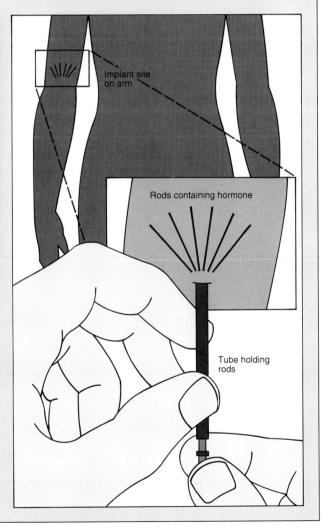

Implant site on arm

Rods containing hormone

Tube holding rods

Contraceptive implant
Norplant, a long-term birth control device that is surgically implanted under the skin of the upper arm, *right*, was approved for use in the United States in December 1990. The device provides effective contraceptive protection for five years. It consists of six soft rods, each about 1 inch (2.5 centimeters) long, *above*, that slowly release low doses of a synthetic female hormone that prevents ovulation. The hormone also thickens the mucus in the cervix, blocking the entry of sperm into the uterus. The rods can be surgically removed easily.

the original findings were inaccurate because of serious flaws in the statistical methods used by the researchers. According to Kronmal and his colleagues, the data suggest that the use of IUD's, in general, does not increase the risk of pelvic infection.

Like the original researchers, Kronmal's team found that Dalkon Shield users were more likely to develop pelvic infection than were users of other IUD's. But they said it was unclear whether the higher infection rate could be traced to the Dalkon Shield or whether errors in the study misled researchers into concluding that the rate was higher.

Abortion-counseling restrictions.
The government may bar doctors and counselors at federally funded family-planning clinics from providing patients with information about abortion, the Supreme Court of the United States ruled in May 1991. In *Rust v. Sullivan,* the court said that federal regulations forbidding the staff at such clinics from counseling women about abortion or referring them to an abortion clinic do not violate a woman's right to an abortion or a doctor's right to freedom of speech.

The regulations, issued in 1988 by the Administration of President Ronald Reagan, changed federal policy governing the enforcement of a 1970 law that provides federal funds to family-planning clinics run by state and local governments and private agencies. Under the 1970 law, such clinics may not perform abortions.

Before the regulations were issued, these family-planning clinics, which serve about 5 million women annually, were permitted to counsel women about the procedure and to refer them to an abortion clinic. The 1988 regulations, which were not implemented pending the court review that culminated in the May ruling, ban counselors from discussing abortion with their patients.

Under the regulations, the staff also would have been forbidden to tell patients where they might obtain an abortion, even if a patient's life was in danger. The court ruled, however, that doctors may provide an abortion referral to a patient whose pregnancy is life threatening.

Although antiabortion groups hailed the ruling, abortion-rights groups argued that the decision would restrict health care available to poor women and damage the relationship between doctors and their patients. Several medical associations also condemned the decision, contending that it sanctioned government interference in the doctor-patient relationship.

In June, the House of Representatives approved a bill that would overturn the restrictive regulations. In July, the Senate passed a similar measure.

☐ Barbara A. Mayes

In WORLD BOOK, see BIRTH CONTROL.

Birth Defects
See Genetics

Blood

The American Red Cross announced plans in May 1991 for sweeping changes in its procedures for collecting, processing, and distributing blood in the United States. The announcement was made a few weeks after the U.S. Food and Drug Administration (FDA) threatened to shut down a Red Cross blood center in Portland, Ore., because of numerous laboratory and record-keeping problems there. The FDA had previously cited other Red Cross centers for not adhering strictly to procedures that guard against receiving or dispensing blood that could be contaminated with viruses that cause AIDS or hepatitis.

The Red Cross, which handles half of the nation's blood supply, planned to temporarily close each of its 53 U.S. blood centers for eight weeks beginning early in 1992 while it replaces an inefficient computer system and trains employees in new procedures. Since 1984, when the FDA required blood suppliers to perform more tests to screen blood for infectious agents, the Red Cross has had to conduct almost 100 million additional tests.

Despite the decision to overhaul their system, Red Cross officials maintained that the U.S. blood supply was safer than it had ever been. Although the U.S. Centers for Disease Control in Atlanta, Ga., estimates that 1 million people in this country are infected with the AIDS-causing human immu-

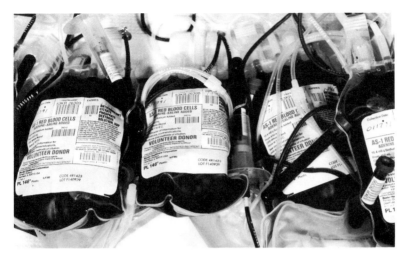

Making blood safer
Donated blood that may have been handled improperly led the American Red Cross to announce in May 1991 a plan to overhaul its blood collection and distribution methods. The agency, which handles half of the U.S. blood supply, will close each of its 53 centers beginning in early 1992 to update its record-keeping system and train employees in new procedures.

nodeficiency virus (HIV), only a few thousand cases have occurred via blood transfusions, and most of these were acquired before suppliers routinely screened blood for HIV.

Pigs produce human hemoglobin.
Biologists using genetic engineering methods created pigs that produce human *hemoglobin,* the substance in blood that carries oxygen throughout the body. Officials at DNX Incorporated of Princeton, N.J., announced in June 1991 that the firm's researchers had created three such pigs by injecting human hemoglobin genes into single-celled pig embryos. Fifteen per cent of the hemoglobin produced by

the pigs that developed from these embryos was of the human type.

Human hemoglobin from pigs could offer several benefits as an alternative to donated human blood. Unlike donated red blood cells, which must match a patient's blood type, purified human hemoglobin would be suitable for all human patients. Furthermore, while donated whole blood cannot be stored for more than several weeks, hemoglobin could be stored for several months. Hemoglobin is also free of such disease-causing microbes as HIV and the hepatitis virus, which can be carried in whole blood.

The pig-produced hemoglobin has not yet been tested in human beings.

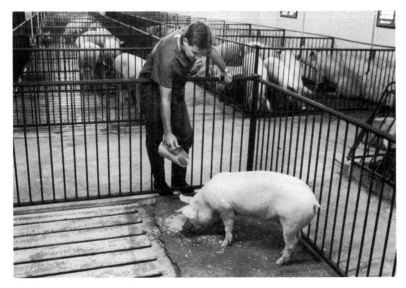

New hemoglobin in pigs
A worker feeds a pig that produces human *hemoglobin,* a component in blood that delivers oxygen throughout the body. Officials at DNX Incorporated in Princeton, N.J., reported in June 1991 that biologists there had used genetic engineering techniques to create three such pigs. About 15 per cent of the pigs' hemoglobin is of the human type, which, if proven safe and effective, could replace donated whole blood for use in human beings.

The company plans to apply by 1992 for FDA approval to begin such tests.

Treatment for cancer patients.
Cancer *chemotherapy* (drug treatment) destroys white blood cells and makes patients vulnerable to infections that could become life-threatening. But treatment with an agent that stimulates the growth of infection-fighting white blood cells can help decrease infections in such patients and reduce the need for hospitalization and antibiotics, according to oncologist (cancer specialist) John Glaspy at the University of California School of Medicine in Los Angeles.

Glaspy announced in December 1990 that lung cancer patients who received *granulocyte colony-stimulating factor* (G-CSF) while undergoing chemotherapy had more white blood cells and were twice as likely to avoid an infection as patients who did not receive G-CSF. Even patients who received high doses of chemotherapy had significantly more white blood cells with G-CSF than patients who did not receive the growth factor. The only side effect of G-CSF treatment was mild bone pain. Experts predict that G-CSF and other substances that stimulate white blood cell production may help chemotherapy patients to fight infections.

Treating hemophilia.
A team of researchers from several medical centers reported in December 1990 that a synthetic blood-clotting agent controlled bleeding in patients with Hemophilia A. Hemophilia A is a genetic disease that affects about 1 in 10,000 U.S. males. People with the disorder are unable to make a blood-clotting protein called *factor VIII* and are at risk for developing uncontrollable, life-threatening bleeding.

The researchers found that the clotting agent used in the study, a version of factor VIII, was a safe and effective alternative to the factor VIII derived from blood plasma, the traditional treatment for the disorder. Health experts note that synthetic factor VIII for hemophiliacs may be a safer treatment than the plasma-derived clotting agent because it avoids exposing the patient to infectious agents that may be present in donated blood.

New drug for AIDS anemia.
Many AIDS patients take AZT, a drug used to help keep the AIDS virus in check. But the drug often produces anemia. The FDA in January 1991 approved use of a drug to combat *anemia* (a shortage of red blood cells) in AIDS patients taking AZT. The drug, called *erythropoietin,* stimulates production of red blood cells. Erythropoietin has previously been used to treat patients with anemia due to kidney disease.

☐ David Roodman

In WORLD BOOK, see ANEMIA; BLOOD; HEMOPHILIA.

Bone Disorders

Many hip fractures in elderly women are caused by falls that could be prevented, according to a study published in May 1991. Researchers who studied 174 women who had fractured a hip as the result of a fall found several factors that seemed to put the women at risk for falling.

Compared with elderly women who had not broken a hip, the women with hip fractures were almost twice as likely to have weak legs; five times as likely to have poor vision; and nine times as likely to have *Parkinson's disease* (a neurological disorder that causes tremors, rigidity, and weakness). The women with hip fractures also tended to be thin. Fat may provide a protective layer around the hip and thus help prevent fractures, the researchers noted. Those who used sedatives or sleeping pills containing barbiturates, and women who had previously suffered a stroke, were also at increased risk for falling and breaking a hip.

More than 90 per cent of hip fractures are due to falls, and each year in the United States more than 200,000 elderly people—most of them women—fall and break a hip. Elderly women may be more prone to hip fractures because of *osteoporosis,* a condition in which bones become thin and brittle. But the researchers noted several measures that may help prevent falls.

The researchers recommended that for elderly patients, doctors should

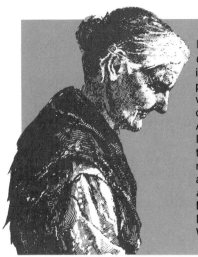

Keeping bones strong
Osteoporosis, or thinning of the bones, is a condition that strikes many older people, nearly 80 per cent of them women. Proper calcium intake throughout life can help prevent osteoporosis. Advice is available from the Calcium Information Center at New York Hospital/Cornell Medical Center; the toll-free number is 1-800-321-2681. In addition, a free booklet, *Osteoporosis: A Woman's Guide,* may be obtained from the National Osteoporosis Foundation, Dept. FC, 2100 M St., Suite 602, Washington, DC 20037.

aggressively treat eye problems; reevaluate the need for medications, such as barbiturates; and prescribe physical therapy to improve strength and balance. They also suggested home modifications, such as lowering the height of beds, installing wall-to-wall carpeting instead of area rugs that are easy to trip or slip on, and placing grab bars in bathrooms.

New test for hand and wrist pain.
A new test for diagnosing a painful condition of the hand and wrist called *carpal tunnel syndrome* may be more accurate than other standard tests for this ailment. A study published in April 1991 reported that the carpal com-

pression test was 90 per cent effective in determining carpal tunnel syndrome, while other tests have been 80 or 84 per cent accurate. The results were based on tests of 31 patients known to have carpal tunnel syndrome and 50 patients who did not.

Carpal tunnel syndrome can be caused by repeating the same hand movements—such as typing—over long periods of time. In this condition, the tendons that pass through the *carpal tunnel* (the bony channel in the wrist) become swollen and press on the wrist's main nerve, called the *median nerve,* resulting in disabling pain.

To perform the test, a physician applies direct pressure to the median

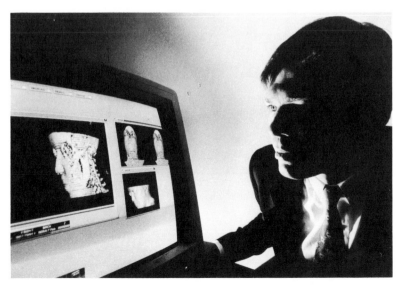

Computer allows surgeon to rehearse
A surgeon at Montefiore Medical Center in New York City practices reconstructive skull surgery on a three-dimensional computer image before performing an operation in February 1991. The computer creates the skull's image using dozens of X rays taken of the patient's head. The surgeon can rotate and "slice" the image to see the exact shape of the skull and to preview the results of various reconstructive strategies.

247

nerve for 30 seconds, using either the thumbs or a *manometer* (a device to measure pressure). The doctor then records the level of pain, numbness, or other sensations. Patients who have carpal tunnel syndrome may be treated conservatively (avoiding the repetitive movement or wearing a wrist splint) or with surgery.

Dental care and artificial joints. Dentists have long advised that people who have had a natural joint replaced by an artificial one should take antibiotics before receiving dental care. This advice is based on the belief that dental procedures can allow bacteria to enter the bloodstream, travel to the joint, and cause an infection that could result in loss of the joint and even death.

But after reviewing scientific reports on joint infections, researchers at the University of Otago in New Zealand reported in March 1991 that no convincing evidence exists to support this advice. However, the researchers recommend that dentists prescribe antibiotics before treating people with artificial joints who also have diabetes, a suppressed immune system, or rheumatoid arthritis; or who take steroids or have had more than one artificial-joint operation.   ☐ John J. Gartland

In WORLD BOOK, see BONE; CARPAL TUNNEL SYNDROME.

Books of Health and Medicine

Here are 21 outstanding new books in health and medicine written for the general reader. They have been selected from books published in 1990 and 1991.

Aging. *Biomarkers: The 10 Determinants of Aging You Can Control.* William Evans, chief of the Human Physiology Laboratory at Tufts University in Boston, and Irwin H. Rosenberg, director of the Human Nutrition Research Center on Aging, also at Tufts, discuss muscle mass, strength, body fat, cholesterol, and other factors that affect aging. (Simon & Schuster, 1991. 297 pp. $21.95)

Choosing a Nursing Home, by Seth B. Goldsmith, professor of health policy and management at the University of Massachusetts. Goldsmith assesses types of care offered by nursing homes, special patient needs, payment options, and hidden costs. (Prentice Hall, 1990. 267 pp. $9.95)

Staying Dry: A Practical Guide to Bladder Control, by Kathryn Burgio, K. Lynne Pearce, and Angelo J. Lucco. Three health experts describe a program developed by the National Institute on Aging and Johns Hopkins University in Maryland to help control incontinence, dispelling the myth that nothing can be done about this condition. (Johns Hopkins University Press, 1990. 169 pp. $12.95)

AIDS. *Surviving AIDS.* Michael Callen, who was diagnosed as having AIDS in 1982, explores the enigma of his own survival and that of a small but growing number of other long-term AIDS patients. The book draws on the author's experience, interviews with AIDS patients, researchers, and a review of the literature. (HarperCollins, 1990. 243 pp. $18.95)

Alzheimer's disease. *The 36-Hour Day: A Family Guide to Caring for Persons with Alzheimer's Disease, Related Dementing Illnesses and Memory Loss in Later Life* (2nd revised edition). Physician Peter V. Rabins and writer Nancy L. Mace explain the behavior of people with *dementia* (a breakdown of mental functions). This comprehensive guide to home care of such patients also addresses the medical, legal, financial, and emotional issues. (Johns Hopkins University Press, 1991. 329 pp. $9.95)

Arthritis. *Taking Control of Arthritis: A Noted Doctor Tells You Everything You Need to Triumph*, by physician Fred G. Kantrowitz. Kantrowitz answers common questions about many different types of arthritis, including age at onset, symptoms, physical examinations of patients, laboratory tests, treatments, sexual activity, and sports. (HarperCollins, 1990. 244 pp. $19.95)

Cancer. *The Race Is Run One Step at a Time: My Personal Struggle—and Every Woman's Guide to Taking Charge of Breast Cancer*, by Nancy

Brinker with writer Catherine McEvily Harris. This moving story of two sisters, by one who recovered from breast cancer (Brinker) but lost her sister to the disease, presents information about understanding breast cancer and making informed treatment decisions. (Simon & Schuster, 1990. 219 pp. $18.95)

Everyone's Guide to Cancer Therapy: How Cancer Is Diagnosed, Treated and Managed on a Day to Day Basis, by physicians Malin Dollinger and Ernest H. Rosenbaum, with writer Greg Cable. This guide is for people who want to be better informed and ask appropriate questions about cancer therapy and who want to act as partners with health professionals in dealing with their illness. (Somerville House, 1991. 624 pp. $19.95)

Diet and fitness. *The Vitamin and Mineral Encyclopedia.* Physician Sheldon Saul Hendler gives an overview of vitamin and mineral use. He describes the possible positive and negative effects of vitamins and minerals, and gives recommendations for intake and sources. (Simon & Schuster, 1990. 496 pp. $24.95)

The Duke University Medical Center Book of Diet and Fitness. Michael Hamilton, director of the Duke Diet and Fitness Center, along with three other medical experts at the center, describe its four-week program. (Ballantine Books, 1990. 417 pp. $19.95)

Health guides. *The American Medical Association Handbook of First Aid and Emergency Care* (revised edition), by Stanley Zydio, Jr., and James A. Hill, medical editors. This handbook, edited by two physicians, gives information on preparing for emergencies, preventing accidents, and giving first aid for a variety of conditions, including sports injuries. (Random House, 1990. 332 pp. $9.95)

Mayo Clinic Family Health Book: The Ultimate Home Medical Reference. Edited by physician David Larson, this easy-to-understand guide offers basic information about symptoms, diagnosis, treatment options, and self-help resources. It also covers emergencies, pregnancy, infant and child care, nutrition, stress, fitness, and disease prevention. (Morrow, 1990. 1,378 pp. $34.95)

Wellness Encyclopedia: The Comprehensive Family Resource for Safeguarding Health & Preventing Illness, by the editors of the University of California at Berkeley Wellness Letter. This guide includes a health risk assessment questionnaire and sections on longevity, nutrition, exercise, environment, and safety. (Houghton Mifflin, 1991. 541 pp. $29.95)

High blood pressure. *Controlling High Blood Pressure.* Physicians Frans H. Leenen and R. Brian Haynes explain what you should know about exercise, life style, diagnosis, drug

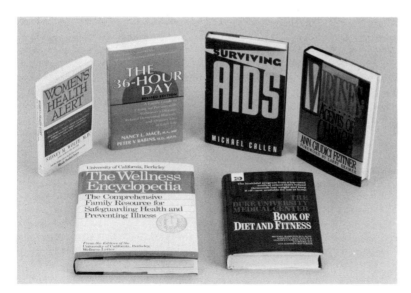

New books of note
New books on health and medicine include *Women's Health Alert,* a discussion of health risks involved in medical procedures for women; *The 36-Hour Day,* a guide to caring for patients with Alzheimer's disease; *Surviving AIDS,* an account of living with AIDS; *Viruses: Agents of Change,* an examination of the nature of viruses; *The Wellness Encyclopedia,* a family guide to health and preventing illness; and *The Duke University Medical Center Book of Diet and Fitness,* a description of the center's fitness program.

treatment, and diet in controlling blood pressure. (Prima Publishing, 1990. Reprint of 1989 ed.161 pp. $8.95)

Medical history. *Patenting the Sun: Polio, the Salk Vaccine, and the Children of the Baby Boom.* In this history of how the first polio vaccine was developed by Jonas Salk, writer Jane C. Smith claims that the supportive social and political environment in which Salk's groundbreaking research took place no longer exists. (Morrow, 1990. 413 pp. $22.95)

Strangers at the Bedside: A History of How Law and Bioethics Transformed Medical Decision Making. David J. Rothman, director of the Center for the Study of Society and Medicine at Columbia University in New York City, explores questions of legal and biological ethics involving doctors, patients, medicine, and society. (Basic Books, 1991. 303 pp. $24.95)

Mind and body. *The Healing Brain: A Scientific Reader.* Robert Ornstein and Charles Swencionis, editors. Medical researchers describe the brain's physiological and psychological roles in healing. (Guilford, 1990. 262 pp. $25.95)

Health and Optimism. Psychologist Christopher Peterson and writer Lisa M. Bossio use results from a 35-year study to examine whether optimism and pessimism can affect a person's health. (Free Press, 1991. 214 pp. $19.95)

Viruses. *Viruses: Agents of Change.* Medical writer Ann Giudici Fettner describes a wide variety of viruses, including those responsible for the flu, herpes, hepatitis, and AIDS. In layman's terms, she examines the complexity of viruses and their known and suspected roles in causing illness. Also discussed are the relationship between viruses and cancer, as well as between viruses and mental illness. (McGraw Hill, 1990. 287 pp. $19.95)

Women's health. *Women Talk About Gynecological Surgery from Diagnosis to Recovery.* Writers Amy Gross and Dee Ito draw on research and interviews with women patients and physicians to describe their experiences, to suggest what questions to ask, and to explain what steps to take to become better informed. (Crown, 1991. 353 pp. $22.95)

Women's Health Alert. Physician Sidney M. Wolfe with Rhoda Donkin Jones discuss risks associated with a variety of medical procedures and products, including birth control, Caesarean sections, weight-control products, hormone-replacement therapy, osteoporosis, breast implants, tranquilizers, and hysterectomies. (Public Citizens Health Research Group, 1991. 324 pp. $7.95)

☐ Margaret Moore

Brain and Nervous System

Work reported by British researchers in February 1991 brought neuroscientists a step closer to understanding the cause, or causes, of *Alzheimer's disease*, a severe form of mental deterioration that strikes many people over age 60. Neurologist Alison Goate and her colleagues at St. Mary's Hospital Medical School in London discovered a genetic *mutation* (a change in a gene) associated with the development of an inherited form of this devastating brain disorder.

Alzheimer's disease is one of the most common maladies of old age. Symptoms include confusion, forgetfulness, and, eventually, a complete loss of the ability to interact with other people or care for oneself.

Most cases of Alzheimer's seem to be *nonfamilial*—that is, they occur randomly, without any family history of the disorder. In about 10 per cent of cases, however, researchers have noted that the disease appears to be *familial*—having some hereditary basis and striking individuals in several generations.

Goate and her associates studied genetic material from members of families that have a high incidence of Alzheimer's disease. They focused on the gene coding for a protein called *amyloid precursor protein* (APP). This protein is converted in the brain into another protein, *beta amyloid*.

When researchers had previously examined brain tissue from deceased

Alzheimer's patients under the microscope, they noted extensive damage, including clumps of degenerated *neurons* (nerve cells) and large accumulations of beta amyloid. The protein collects in patches called *plaques*. The brains of deceased older people who never had Alzheimer's disease show similar changes, but to a much lesser degree.

Goate's research team found that in family members with Alzheimer's disease, the APP gene contained a mutation that was not present in healthy family members, in unrelated healthy individuals, or in persons who are suffering from the nonfamilial form of Alzheimer's disease. The mutation results in a slightly different form of the precursor protein—and thus of beta amyloid—being produced in brain cells.

Although the function of beta amyloid is not entirely clear, it appears to be necessary for the health of neurons. The presence of an abnormal form of beta amyloid, or the absence of the normal protein, may underlie familial Alzheimer's disease. The finding that those people with nonfamilial Alzheimer's disease do not have the APP mutation indicates that several genes may be involved in the disorder.

Animal "model" for Alzheimer's.
The creation of genetically engineered mice that have beta amyloid plaques in their brains was announced in July 1991 by scientists at two research institutions in the United States. The mice were expected to provide the first animal "model" of Alzheimer's disease, enabling investigators to observe the progression of the disease in the brain.

The scientists—working at California Biotechnology, Incorporated, in Mountain View and Miles Research Center in New Haven, Conn.—bred strains of mice that carry human genes coding for the increased production of beta amyloid in the brain. At the age of 2 years—equivalent to a human age of 50 years—the mice began to develop plaques. Besides serving as a model for studying the progression and possible causes of Alzheimer's disease, the mice will also make it possible for researchers to test new drugs against the disease.

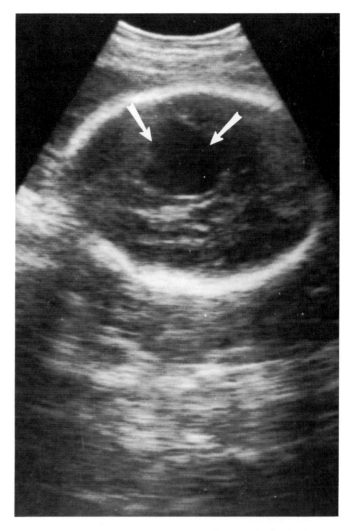

Prions and brain disease. Since the early 1980's, neuroscientists have debated the possible cause of *Gerstmann-Sträussler-Scheinker syndrome* (GSS), a rare degenerative brain disease with similarities to Alzheimer's. An important clue towards solving that puzzle came in December 1990 from neuroscientist Karen K. Hsiao and her colleagues at the University of California at San Francisco.

Like Alzheimer's disease, GSS causes a severe decline in mental abilities and is ultimately fatal. As with familial Alzheimer's, a tendency to develop GSS can be inherited. There is one characteristic, however, that sets GSS apart from all forms of Alzheimer's disease: It can be transmitted to laboratory animals by injecting them with

Prenatal brain damage
An ultrasound image (created with high-frequency sound waves) of a fetal brain shows a damaged area (indicated by arrows) that apparently caused the baby to be born with *cerebral palsy*, doctors from Magee-Women's Hospital in Pittsburgh, Pa., reported in November 1990. The researchers suggested that cerebral palsy, a disorder involving impaired movement, is often caused by brain damage incurred before birth.

brain material from deceased GSS patients.

The nature of the agent causing GSS has been the subject of intense investigation and controversy among brain scientists. The work of Hsiao and her associates indicates that the culprit is a tiny protein called a *prion*.

Prions were discovered in the early 1980's by neuroscientist Stanley B. Prusiner of the University of California at San Francisco, who was a coauthor of Hsiao's December 1990 research paper on GSS. In his earlier investigations, Prusiner studied a degenerative brain disease of sheep called *scrapie*, which is very similar to GSS. He found he could transmit scrapie to other animals by injecting them with pure protein extracts from scrapie-infected brain tissues.

The remarkable thing about this discovery was that the disease could apparently be transmitted through protein alone rather than by an infectious microorganism. The extracts contained no *nucleic acids*, the molecules that encode genetic information and carry out life functions, including reproduction. For example, *DNA* (deoxyribonucleic acid, the molecule genes are made of) is a nucleic acid. Because nucleic acids are so essential to living organisms, including infectious microorganisms, Prusiner's findings were greeted with skepticism by the scientific community in the 1980's.

Eventually, Prusiner was able to isolate and study the individual protein responsible for transmitting scrapie. He called this protein the *prion protein* (PrP). Soon afterward, Prusiner discovered the gene responsible for producing PrP, and subsequent studies revealed that PrP is a normal part of all animals' neurons. The cells of the human brain also produce PrP.

However, Prusiner later found that PrP in the brains of patients with GSS and animals with scrapie was different from the protein in healthy brains. And indeed, laboratory analysis revealed a difference of one *amino acid* between samples of PrP from a GSS-infected brain and from a normal brain. Amino acids are the building blocks of proteins, and just one wrong amino acid out of hundreds or even thousands can result in a malfunctioning protein.

Hsiao and her colleagues sought to prove that this tiny variation in the PrP protein was sufficient to produce disease. The scientists first made a synthetic gene fragment encoding the information for the production of the abnormal form of PrP. Next, they injected the gene fragments into fertilized mouse eggs. The eggs, with the gene fragments incorporated into the animals' genetic material, were then reimplanted into female mice and allowed to develop. Some of the baby mice that developed from the altered eggs produced abnormal PrP.

By the age of 6 months, those mice developed a brain disease almost identical to scrapie and GSS. Microscopic examinations of the mice's

Walking boots
Specially designed leather boots stabilize the ankles of a paraplegic patient, allowing him to walk with canes. According to an April 1991 report, some patients with completely paralyzed legs can learn to walk with the help of these custom-fitted boots, which are far less awkward and cumbersome than leg braces.

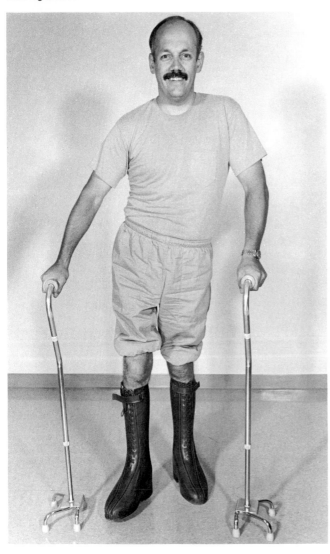

brains revealed abnormalities similar to those seen in scrapie and GSS brains. Thus, the investigators proved that the abnormal protein by itself is sufficient to cause spontaneous nerve cell degeneration and that a normal PrP protein is essential to maintaining the health of neurons.

Still to be learned is the function of normal PrP in neurons and whether the abnormal protein extracted from the brain tissue of the experimental mice can then transfer the disease to healthy mice. Showing that it can would confirm Prusiner's finding that a protein containing no genetic material can function as an infectious agent.

ALS gene found. The discovery of a genetic link to *amyotrophic lateral sclerosis* (ALS), a fatal neurological illness, was reported in May 1991 by researchers at several U.S. medical centers. The scientists, under the direction of neurologist Teepu Siddique of the Northwestern University Medical School in Chicago, found an association between ALS and a gene that is still unidentified.

ALS—better known as Lou Gehrig's disease, for the baseball player who died of it in 1941—is a disorder in which neurons that transmit electrical impulses to muscles die for reasons unknown. ALS patients become progressively weaker and usually die within five years.

Although most cases of the disease occur randomly, 5 to 10 per cent of ALS cases occur in families that have been stricken through several generations. In those instances, the disease is clearly hereditary, indicating that a faulty gene is involved.

In search of that gene, Siddique and his colleagues studied the chromosomes—the structures that carry the genes—of 23 families with multiple cases of ALS. Human beings have 23 paired chromosomes, one copy of each pair from the mother, the other copy from the father. The researchers concentrated on the two copies of chromosome 21, which preliminary studies had indicated were the probable location of the ALS gene.

The scientists examined about 100 identifiable sequences of DNA. These sequences, known as *markers*, serve as reference points for researchers

Hot lines for headaches
Two national organizations operate toll-free telephone numbers to offer free literature and other information about headaches and lists of physicians in the caller's area who might be of help:

The National Headache Foundation in Chicago, 1-800-843-2256.

American Council for Headache Education in West Deptford, N.J., 1-800-255-2243.

trying to locate specific genes. In this case, the scientists were looking for an association between particular markers and the occurrence of ALS.

Although they were unable to link any single marker with ALS, the investigators found that four markers in one part of the chromosome were often present in the ALS patients. The scientists said their research indicated that the sought-for gene was located close to the markers.

In some of the ALS families, however, no linkage could be found between the chromosome-21 markers and the disease. That finding indicates that familial ALS may not be one disease, but may be several similar disorders

Magnetic field imaging
Magnetic fields detected by high-tech sensors called SQUIDs produce an image of nerve activity in the brain. Researchers in the United States and Europe in 1990 and 1991 were exploring the use of SQUIDs, which someday may be used to diagnose and treat brain disorders such as Alzheimer's disease and epilepsy.

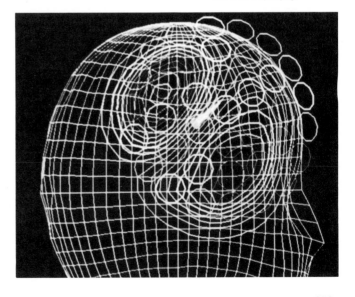

which are caused by different abnormal genes.

Center of attention. "Pay attention!" is an order almost everyone receives at least once. But what part of the brain is involved in obeying that command? In January 1991, neuroscientist José V. Pardo and his associates at Washington University in St. Louis, Mo., reported that "paying attention" occurs in the right half of the brain.

Using a scanning technique called *positron emission tomography* (PET), Pardo and his colleagues studied blood flow through different regions of the brain in normal individuals whom they asked to "pay attention." The sci-

entists asked the volunteers to look at objects shown to them or to note touches to one of their big toes and to concentrate on the pattern and frequency of those stimuli.

The researchers noted increased blood flow through the right half of the brain regardless of which side of the body was touched or from which side an object was presented. The increases occurred in addition to greater blood flow in the right side of the brain in areas dealing with vision or sensation. ☐ Gary Birnbaum

In the Special Reports section, see CLOSING IN ON PARKINSON'S DISEASE. In WORLD BOOK, see BRAIN; NERVOUS SYSTEM.

Cancer

Scientists gained important insights during 1990 and 1991 into the genetic changes that occur when a normal cell becomes cancerous. One series of research studies reported during that period pointed to a mutation in a specific gene called *p53* as a critical factor in the occurrence of a wide variety of cancers. The gene is particularly interesting to researchers because it is one of a number of genes, called *suppressor genes,* whose normal function is to suppress cell growth.

Bladder cancer. In May 1991, scientists reported new findings linking the

mutated p53 gene to cancer of the bladder. A team headed by geneticist Bert Vogelstein of the Johns Hopkins School of Medicine in Baltimore found defects in the p53 gene in 11 of 18 bladder cancers that were removed surgically from patients.

The scientists then developed a test that identified bladder cancer cells in the patients' urine by detecting cells with the same genetic defect among the large number of normal cells. This raised the possibility of developing a routine urine test to screen people at high risk for bladder cancer. The study was reported by scientists from the M. D. Anderson Hospital in Houston,

Tests for cancer

Early detection of cancer can often save lives. The American Cancer Society has developed some general guidelines for tests available for various types of cancers that indicate who should have those tests and when.

Type of cancer	Type of test	Who should be screened and when
Cervical	Pap smear	Women 18 years and older, each year Girls under 18 who are sexually active, each year
Prostate	Rectal examination Ultrasound and blood test	Men aged 40 and older, each year Not recommended for general screening
Breast	Examination by physician Mammogram	Women aged 20 to 40, every three years Women over 40, each year Women 35 to 39, once in four years Women 40 to 49, every one or two years Women over 50, each year
Ovarian	Ultrasound and blood test	Not recommended for general screening
Colon	Rectal examination Stool blood test Sigmoidoscopy	Men and women 40 and older, each year Men and women 50 and older, each year Men and women 50 and older, every 3 to 5 years
Lung	X ray	Not recommended for general screening

Source: The American Cancer Society.

the University of Southern California in Los Angeles, and Harvard University Medical School in Boston.

The scientists noted that the still-experimental urine test could be used for early identification of a recurrence of bladder cancer among patients who had previously undergone treatment. The scientists stressed, however, that much work remains to be done before their test will be ready for routine clinical use.

Liver cancer. Studies reported in April 1991 also implicated p53 in liver cancer. Two scientific groups found genetic mutations at the same location in the p53 gene in liver cancer patients who were exposed to a known liver carcinogen (cancer-causing agent) called *aflatoxin B1.*

The first group, led by oncologist (cancer specialist) Curtis Harris of the National Cancer Institute (NCI) in Bethesda, Md., found the mutation in liver cancer patients from a region of China near Shanghai. The second group, led by oncologist Mehmet Ozturk of the Massachusetts General Hospital's Cancer Center in Charlestown, Mass., looked at patients from southern Africa.

Liver cancer is one of the leading cancer killers in these regions of China and Africa, and aflatoxin B1 exposure is also common in both places. Aflatoxin B1 is produced by fungi that form on moldy food crops, such as rice and wheat. Such molds tend to develop in hot humid regions and can also result when crops are improperly harvested or stored. Although scientists note that aflatoxin's role in mutating the p53 gene is unproven, they do know from laboratory tests that aflatoxin B1 can cause mutations in other genes.

Another known risk factor for liver cancer in these regions is infection by the hepatitis B virus. With the new information on the p53 mutation, scientists can now focus more closely on the sequence of events or exposures to carcinogens that result in high rates of liver cancer in these areas. It is possible, for example, that a hepatitis B virus infection makes liver cells divide more rapidly, increasing the possibility of errors during cell replication. This, in turn, might increase the possi-

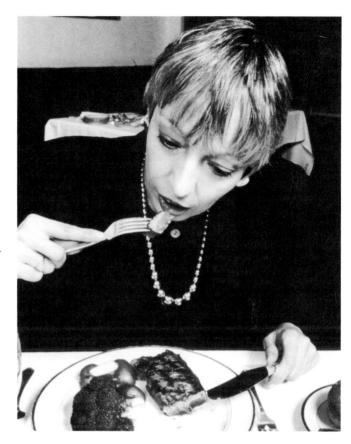

bility of a mutation in the p53 gene due to exposure to aflatoxin.

Li-Fraumeni syndrome. A p53 mutation has also been found in families with a genetic susceptibility to a spectrum of common cancers, according to a study reported in November 1990. Geneticists reported finding an inherited p53 mutation in patients with a condition known as the Li-Fraumeni syndrome.

By age 30, people who have inherited this extremely rare syndrome begin to develop one or more of several different cancers, including brain tumors, osteosarcoma (a bone cancer), leukemia (a blood cancer), and breast cancer. More than 90 per cent of patients with Li-Fraumeni syndrome have cancer by the time they are 70 years of age.

The finding suggests that the p53 gene defect is a high-risk factor for cancer development in these families. The research was reported by geneticist Stephen Friend and colleagues at

Red meat and cancer
A daily diet of red meat, such as beef, pork or lamb, may be hazardous to your health. A study in December 1990 by researchers at Harvard University's School of Public Health in Boston showed that women who ate red meat daily had a 2.5 times greater risk of developing colon cancer than those who ate red meat less than once a month.

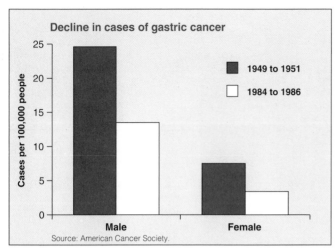

Decline in cases of gastric cancer

Cases per 100,000 people

■ 1949 to 1951
□ 1984 to 1986

Male   Female

Source: American Cancer Society.

The number of cases of gastric cancer among men and women in the United States has significantly declined since the early 1950's. Some scientists believe the decline may be due to a lessening of gastric infections caused by a bacterium known as *Helicobacter pylori,* which has been linked, along with other factors, to gastric cancer.

Massachusetts General Hospital's Cancer Center; Frederick Li and Joseph Fraumeni of the NCI, who discovered the syndrome that bears their name; and geneticist Louise Strong of the M. D. Anderson Cancer Center.

Colon cancer gene. In August 1991, Vogelstein and colleagues at the Cancer Institute in Tokyo and the Howard Hughes Medical Institute at the University of Utah in Salt Lake City reported isolating a gene in patients who have an inherited form of colon cancer called familial adenomatous polyposis (FAP). The FAP gene contains instructions that the cell uses to make a particular protein product, and

evidence suggests that this protein has the ability to tap into the mechanism by which a cell signals growth. The scientists believe that the FAP gene's normal counterpart acts as a suppressor of cell growth, and that a mutated FAP gene could interfere with this function. If this hypothesis is true, it would explain why people who inherit the mutated FAP gene have such a high risk of colon cancer. See DIGESTIVE SYSTEM.

Gene therapy. Scientists at the National Institutes of Health (NIH) in Bethesda, Md., began the first federally approved attempt to treat a human being using gene therapy in September 1990. Gene therapy involves inserting new genes into cells to treat or cure certain diseases. See GENETICS (Close-Up). In January 1991, the first cancer patients were treated using this approach.

The NIH team was led by surgeon and immunologist Steven A. Rosenberg; R. Michael Blaese, an NCI expert on childhood immune diseases; and gene therapy research pioneer W. French Anderson of the National Heart, Lung, and Blood Institute. They gave two patients with advanced melanoma, a life-threatening form of skin cancer, transfusions of special cancer-killing cells. To create these cells, the researchers first removed cells called *tumor-infiltrating lymphocytes* (TIL's) from the patients' own tu-

Although women with a family history of breast cancer face an increased risk of developing the disease themselves, that risk declines with age, according to a study reported in 1990 by physicians at Chicago's Rush-Presbyterian-St. Luke's Medical Center. The study of 9,000 women compared women with a family history of breast cancer and those without a family history. By age 64, the risk of developing breast cancer was the same for both groups.

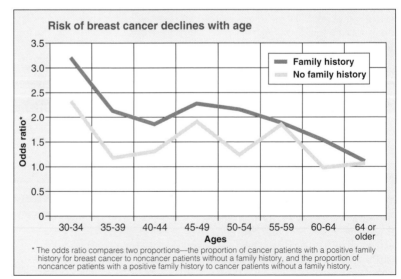

Risk of breast cancer declines with age

Odds ratio*

— Family history
— No family history

Ages: 30-34 35-39 40-44 45-49 50-54 55-59 60-64 64 or older

* The odds ratio compares two proportions—the proportion of cancer patients with a positive family history for breast cancer to noncancer patients without a family history, and the proportion of noncancer patients with a positive family history to cancer patients without a family history.

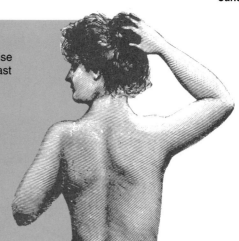

mors. TIL's are cancer-fighting cells that migrate from other parts of the body to the cancer site and invade the tumor.

The researchers then inserted into the TIL's a gene capable of producing a potent antitumor toxin called *tumor necrosis factor* (TNF). The modified cells were then transfused back into the patients. Researchers believe that TIL's may have the ability to recognize and destroy tumor cells that have spread to distant parts of the body. They hope that the modified TIL's will be particularly effective at finding and killing tumor cells.

In July 1991, Rosenberg issued his first report on the preliminary results of the treatment and noted that the first two patients were still alive. Before the treatment began, they were not expected to live beyond March. Rosenberg said the early results indicate the treatment is not dangerous, as some feared, but he cautioned that it was too soon to say that the therapy was working. Rosenberg said that two more patients with advanced melanoma have been added to the treatment program.

Rectal cancer treatment. Findings published in March 1991 demonstrated that a combination of radiation therapy and cancer drugs following surgery decreases the high risk of tumor recurrence in rectal cancer patients and improves their chances for survival. The NCI considered the findings so significant that it mailed information on the study to 150,000 physicians in the United States. The NCI's announcement also included newer, unpublished data from a second study about rectal cancer treatment.

The published study was led by oncologist James E. Krook of the Duluth Clinic in Duluth, Minn., and involved a number of community-based oncologists in the Midwest. The physicians treated patients after surgery with radiation and the cancer drug *5-fluorouracil,* which is available by prescription, and the drug *methyl-CCNU,* which is still being tested for its effectiveness in humans.

The unpublished data from a second study suggested that postsurgical radiation treatment with 5-fluorouracil alone (without methyl-CCNU) provided nearly equivalent results. This means that oncologists who might not have access to methyl-CCNU can still use a treatment regimen that is widely available to reduce recurrence of tumors in rectal cancer patients and improve chances for survival.

News for barbecue lovers. Scientists reported in March 1991 the discovery of a new class of highly carcinogenic chemicals that form in meats grilled over a hot fire. These chemicals, called *heterocyclic aromatic amines,* are formed from amino acids (building blocks of protein) and from *creatinine,* which is found in muscle fiber in meats. The discovery was made by scientists at NCI; the Lawrence Livermore National Laboratory in Livermore, Calif.; and the National Cancer Center in Japan.

For the carcinogens to form, the meat must be cooked at a very high temperature—above 212 °F (100 °C). This generally is achieved when grilling, frying, and broiling.

Fortunately, according to the scientists, precooking meats by microwaving them for two to three minutes and pouring off the resulting liquid will remove about 90 per cent of the substances that help form the carcinogens. The meat then can be grilled more safely, though it should not be well-done.

Never too late to quit. The health benefits of quitting cigarette smoking extend well into later life, according to a study reported in June 1991. Epidemiologists from the National Institute on Aging in Bethesda, Md.; Harvard Medical School; Yale University School of Medicine in New Haven, Conn.; and the University of Iowa in Iowa City studied the cigarette-smoking habits of 7,178 people aged 65 and older.

Overall risk of death doubled in current smokers. But people who had quit smoking, regardless of when they quit, experienced virtually no excess risk of death due to heart disease compared with people who had never smoked. The risk of death due to cancer, however, remained high for former smokers compared with nonsmokers. The highest death rates from cancer occurred among those who had smoked for 40 years or more, according to the study.

The findings are consistent with what is known of the biologic effects of cigarette smoking. Most scientists believe that the effects of cigarette smoking on heart disease are due to current tobacco use, whereas cancer occurs as a result of cumulative exposure to the carcinogenic agents in cigarette smoke.

□ Patricia A. Newman-Horm
In the Special Reports section, see COMBATING PROSTATE CANCER. In WORLD BOOK, see CANCER.

Child Development

Deaf babies of deaf parents babble with their hands in the same repetitive way as hearing babies babble with their voices, according to research reported in March 1991 by psychologists Laura Ann Petitto and Paula F. Marentette of McGill University in Montreal, Canada. According to the researchers, this finding suggests that the brain possesses an inborn capacity to learn language in a sequential way, regardless of whether communication relies on spoken words or hand signs.

Previous studies of language development have revealed that during the first year of life, the babbling of hearing babies, though meaningless, includes increasingly complex sounds.

This development occurs, apparently, in preparation for saying the first words. Thus, many researchers assumed that normal hearing and the maturation of the nerves and muscles controlling the mouth and vocal cords were necessary for the development of language among infants.

Petitto and Marentette examined the hand movements and sounds made by two deaf babies and three babies with normal hearing. Both deaf babies had deaf parents who communicated by American Sign Language, a common form of sign language. The parents of the hearing babies spoke either French or English at home. When the babies reached 10, 12, and 14 months of age, the researchers videotaped the babies alone and with their parents.

An analysis of the babies' hand movements and vocal expressions provided the first evidence that deaf babies babble and that their language development follows the same pattern as that of hearing babies. Hearing infants produce repetitive but meaningless sounds. From these sounds, infants learn the basic units of vocal language and the combinations of sounds that can be used to make words. At about 10 or 11 months, many hearing infants begin to string sounds together to form their first words.

The researchers found that the deaf babies also began to babble by repeatedly making hand gestures that were essentially meaningless but similar to the signs for letters and numbers that they saw their parents use. Their hand movements grew more complex with time, and they began to sign their first words at the age of 10 or 11 months.

Part-time work hazards. Many parents see part-time work by their teen-aged children as a means of building character and developing responsibility. But psychologists reported in March 1991 that high school students who work at outside jobs for more than 10 hours per week are more likely to have serious academic, psychological, and social problems than students who do not hold jobs or who work fewer hours. Working students were less interested in school, received lower grades, experienced more psychological distress, reported more physical problems, had higher rates of drug and alcohol use and delinquency, and relied less on their parents for guidance.

Laurence Steinberg of Temple University in Philadelphia and Sanford M. Dornbusch of Stanford University in Stanford, Calif., surveyed 3,989 students aged 15 to 18 at nine high schools in California and Wisconsin. The students, who represented a variety of economic and ethnic backgrounds, responded to survey questions in the fall of 1987 and again about six months later.

Compared with nonworking students, students with outside jobs

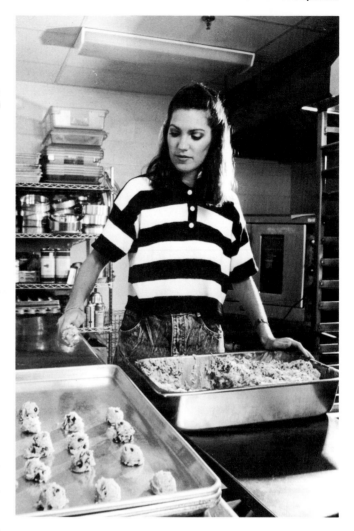

were as self-reliant, expressed as much self-confidence, and had equally positive attitudes about work. As the number of hours of part-time work increased, however, working students reported exerting less effort in school and resorting more often than nonworking students to such actions as cheating on schoolwork, copying assignments from others, and cutting classes.

According to the researchers, the study did not indicate that extensive teen-age employment causes serious problems. Students may work long hours because they already dislike school and have other family or social problems, they suggested. The researchers also theorized that student workers may, for unknown reasons,

The hazards of working
Part-time jobs may not benefit high school students. According to a March 1991 study, teenagers who worked more than 10 hours per week were more likely to have lower grades, have higher rates of alcohol and drug use, and have more psychological distress than students who did not work or worked fewer hours.

be more willing to report bad grades, drug use, and other problems.

Teen self-esteem. Children of both sexes tend to lose some of their self-confidence as they approach and go through adolescence. But from ages 9 to 16, girls lose confidence in themselves to a much greater extent than do boys, according to the results of a survey released in January 1991.

The survey also revealed that preteen and teen-aged girls have much less enthusiasm for mathematics and science, less confidence in their academic abilities, and fewer aspirations to professional careers than do boys. The survey of 2,400 girls and 600 boys in public schools throughout the United States was commissioned by the American Association of University Women in Washington, D.C.

According to the survey, both girls and boys lost some self-confidence between elementary school and high school. But the decline for girls was much steeper. The percentage of boys who said they always "feel happy the way I am" dropped from 67 per cent in elementary school to 46 per cent in high school. But with girls, the numbers fell from 60 per cent to 29 per cent.

According to the psychologists who designed the survey, the results raise questions about the role schools play in undermining girls' self-esteem. Interestingly, the survey found that black

girls were much more likely to have a positive self-image in high school than were white girls. The psychologists theorized that one reason for this finding was that black children were more likely than white children to draw their confidence from their families and communities rather than from school. The psychologists called for intensive studies of how girls and boys are treated in the classroom and how teaching styles and techniques may erode girls' self-confidence.

A different view of adolescent self-esteem was presented in a study published in February 1991. The two-year investigation of 128 boys and girls progressing through junior high school found no striking sex differences in self-esteem.

About one-third of the youngsters surveyed consistently reported feeling strongly self-confident, achieving good grades, and maintaining rewarding friendships throughout junior high school, reported psychologist Barton J. Hirsch of Northwestern University in Evanston, Ill., and his colleagues. Another third of the students in the study experienced small increases in self-esteem.

About 13 per cent of the students had persistently low self-esteem and school achievement. And the rest—about one in five youngsters—started out with good grades, high self-esteem, and numerous friends, only to

Perils of rejection
Children who have problems getting along with others are more likely to experience difficulties in school or with the law than their more popular classmates, according to studies reported in 1990. Researchers found that children rejected by classmates because they were insensitive or too aggressive performed badly in school and were more likely to have been arrested or to have dropped out of school by age 18.

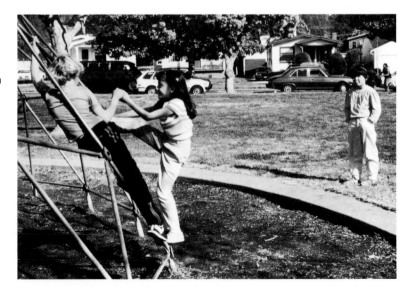

report dramatic drops in all these areas during junior high school. So far, the reasons for these plunges in self-esteem remain unclear, Hirsch said.

Sweet soothing for babies. A few drops of sugar-sweetened water eases the crying of newborn babies more effectively than does a pacifier. Sugar water also markedly reduces crying and, apparently, pain among infants undergoing medical procedures, such as blood collection and circumcision, according to a report published in September 1990.

Psychologist Elliott M. Blass of Cornell University in Ithaca, N.Y., and his colleagues studied 16 healthy babies, who were 1 to 3 days old, in a quiet hospital nursery. After monitoring each baby's crying for five minutes, the researchers squirted a tiny drop of sugar water (0.1 milliliter) on each infant's tongue once a minute for five minutes.

Crying virtually stopped while the sugar solution was being administered and for five minutes afterward. A second study revealed that newborns given a drop of sugar water once per minute for up to 10 minutes cried much less than those sucking on a pacifier for that amount of time.

Moreover, infants given 2 milliliters of sugar water just before having a sample of blood collected or undergoing circumcision cried about half as much as infants given unsweetened water prior to the same procedures, Blass noted. Sugar's sweet taste may be calming because it somehow activates natural pleasure-inducing chemicals in the brain known as *opioids*, the researchers suggested. They were unable to say whether a few drops of sugar water might calm an irritable baby, but they planned to conduct further studies.

Effects of divorce. A study published in June 1991 challenged the common belief that children of divorced parents have emotional, behavioral, and academic problems purely because of the stress of the divorce and its aftermath. According to sociologist Andrew J. Cherlin of Johns Hopkins University in Baltimore and his colleagues, many of these childhood problems appear before parents divorce. Moreover, growing up in a family continually disrupted by marital conflict may cause serious problems for children, regardless of whether the parents eventually divorce, the researchers said.

Previous studies of divorce's effects on children focused on the months or years after parents separated. Cherlin's group looked at children both before and after their parents split up.

The investigators conducted a statistical analysis of long-term surveys of more than 11,600 unrelated children in Great Britain from 1965 to 1969 and of 822 unrelated children in the United States from 1976 to 1981. In Great Britain, each child was studied twice—at ages 7 and 11. In the United States, the children were also studied twice, between ages 7 and 11 and between 11 and 16. The researchers compared information about youngsters whose parents divorced after the survey began with information about those whose parents stayed together. The data came from parent and teacher ratings of the children's behavioral and emotional problems as well as from the children's scores on academic achievement tests.

The researchers found that about half the behavioral, psychological, and achievement problems observed among boys following the divorce had existed before the parents separated. Parental conflict before divorce accounted for about 25 per cent of the girls' academic problems but none of their behavioral problems.

The findings of the study suggest that conflict between parents affects boys more than it does girls. The researchers noted, however, that girls may get just as upset as boys, but their distress may be manifested in other ways, such as feelings of depression and anxiety. If this is the case, they may be less likely than boys to exhibit behavioral or academic problems.

Although the study found that divorce itself is not as traumatic as researchers had believed, the findings also suggest that parental conflict may harm children even if the parents stay together. □ Bruce Bower

In the Special Reports section, see WHAT'S BEHIND SHYNESS?; MEASLES ON THE RISE. In WORLD BOOK, see CHILD.

Childbirth
See Pregnancy and Childbirth

Contraception
See Birth Control

Dentistry

Safety of "silver" fillings

Mercury amalgam fillings, which dentists use to fill about 80 per cent of all cavities, came under fire in 1990. A study reported in August raised concern that the fillings might release harmful mercury vapors into the body. But experts reviewing research on amalgam said the fillings seemed to pose no direct health threat.

Concern about the possible hazards posed by mercury in dental fillings arose in August 1990 when researchers at the University of Calgary in Canada reported that 6 sheep given 12 mercury amalgam fillings showed a serious decline in kidney function. The study seemed to support critics of the use of mercury amalgam fillings, who have charged that the fillings release vapors that can cause health problems.

About 80 per cent of all fillings used by dentists in the United States have been made of mercury amalgam, which is composed of 50 per cent mercury and a 50 per cent mixture of silver, copper, tin, and zinc. Many experts dismissed the Canadian study as inappropriate for determining the health effects of such fillings in human beings. The American Dental Association (ADA) issued a statement saying that amalgam fillings are safe and that no practical substitute exists for the material.

Nevertheless, the National Institutes of Health asked a group of experts to review the research on mercury amalgam and determine what risks, if any, the substance posed. The panel reported in August 1991 that the small amounts of mercury released by amalgam fillings did not seem to present a direct threat to human health, but that further research was needed to fully determine their safety.

The safety of fluoridated water. Fluoride in drinking water does not cause cancer in human beings, and cities should continue to fluoridate water to prevent tooth decay, according to a February 1991 report from the United States Public Health Service (PHS). These conclusions were based on a PHS study designed to resolve questions raised about the safety of fluoridation.

In the study, scientists reviewed about 50 other studies of fluoride's effects in human beings. They determined that if water fluoridation poses any risk to the public, it is too small to be detected. The study also confirmed that water fluoridation is highly effective in reducing tooth decay.

Before fluoride was added to water, the average child had developed 10 cavities by his or her 12th birthday. Today, children drinking fluoridated water develop an average of only 3 cavities.

The report noted that in addition to fluoridated water, more than 90 per cent of all toothpastes and some types of mouthwash contain fluoride. Swallowing or regularly using large amounts of toothpaste containing fluoride could substantially increase exposure to fluoride, according to the report. Thus, the report advised parents to instruct their children to use only small amounts of toothpaste and then to have them rinse thoroughly after brushing.

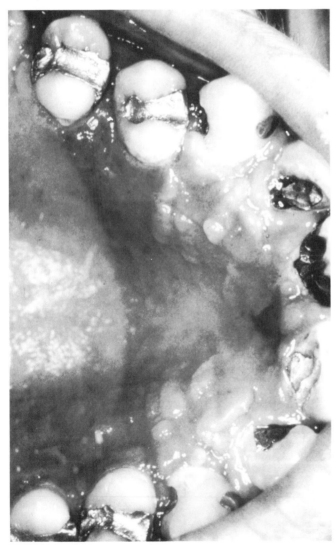

Smokers and periodontal disease. People who smoke cigarettes face a high risk of developing *periodontal disease,* a disease of the gums and other tissues surrounding the teeth. A study reported in April 1991 found that smokers were five times more likely than nonsmokers to have periodontal disease, which is the leading cause of adult tooth loss.

Periodontal disease damages the tissues that hold teeth firmly in the jaw. It is caused by *plaque,* a sticky deposit that accumulates on the surface of teeth and is formed from food debris and bacteria.

In 800 healthy adults aged 28 to 75 years, the researchers measured the depth of "pockets" that had developed between the teeth and gums. These pockets enlarge, trap plaque, and become infected as periodontal disease progresses. Cigarette smokers were five times more likely than nonsmokers with comparable oral hygiene habits to have pockets deep enough to fit the definition of periodontal disease.

AIDS and dentists. Confirmation that a dentist had transmitted the AIDS virus to five patients prompted the ADA to issue new recommendations for dentists. See also HEALTH POLICY; AIDS.   □ Michael Woods

In WORLD BOOK, see DENTISTRY.

Researchers reported closing in on the location of a gene believed responsible for one form of the type of diabetes called *non-insulin-dependent diabetes*. This finding was published in February 1991 by scientists at the universities of Chicago, Michigan, and Pennsylvania.

Diabetes is a disease in which the body fails to produce or efficiently use the hormone insulin to maintain normal levels of *glucose* (sugar) in the blood. It affects more than 12 million people in the United States. There are two basic types. The more severe kind, Type I diabetes, also known as *insulin-dependent* or *juvenile-onset diabetes*, requires daily injections of insulin. The more common kind, Type II diabetes, also known as non-insulin-dependent or *adult-onset diabetes*, sometimes requires oral medication that induces the body to produce more insulin.

Researchers believe several genes are involved in the regulation and secretion of insulin in the body. In the new study, the researchers homed in on a gene associated with a form of Type II diabetes known as *mature-onset diabetes of the young*. The researchers studied five generations of a 275-member family in which the disease occurred commonly. The re-

Diabetes

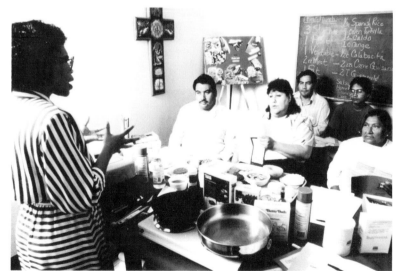

Combating diabetes through nutrition
A dietitian provides classes in cooking low-sugar, low-fat meals to help Hispanic residents of San Antonio battle the obesity and high blood-sugar levels that accompany diabetes. In some of the city's Hispanic neighborhoods, as many as 1 person in 5 has diabetes.

searchers traced the gene to a particular region of chromosome 20. (Chromosomes are the tiny threadlike structures in a cell nucleus that carry the
genes. Most human cells contain 23
pairs of chromosomes.)

Experts called the finding a "historic"
advance in understanding the genetics of diabetes. One of the researchers cautioned that much work remains
before the exact location of the diabetes gene is found, but he acknowledged "we now know where to look."

Off that couch. Regular exercise
may help prevent Type II diabetes, researchers reported in July 1991. A
study done at the University of California in Berkeley found that inactive
men were twice as likely to develop
the disease as physically active men.

The researchers also found that the
risk of developing Type II diabetes was
even higher for sedentary men who
had other risk factors, such as a family history of diabetes. Previous studies
had indicated that exercise can improve the body's ability to use sugar.

Bloodless blood-glucose tests. A
device now being tested may enable
people to measure the level of glucose in their blood without the pain of
drawing blood. The new device, announced at the International Diabetes
Federation Congress held in June
1991 in Washington, D.C., shines a
beam of *infrared* light—an invisible
form of light—through the skin. Within
five seconds, it provides a blood-glucose reading based on how much
light the body has absorbed. The device was developed by Futrex, Incorporated, of Gaithersburg, Md.

To maintain blood glucose levels as
close to normal as possible, people
with diabetes need to test their blood
several times a day. Since the early
1980's, the standard technique has
been to prick a finger with a needle,
draw a small amount of blood, and
test it using a handheld machine. If
proven effective, the painless infrared
monitor could prompt people with diabetes to monitor their blood sugar
more often, independent experts said.

Early onset of retinopathy. A complication known as *diabetic retinopathy* often begins several years before

diabetes is diagnosed, researchers reported at the international diabetes
congress in June. Retinopathy, a condition in which small blood vessels in
the eye become damaged, can lead
to blindness.

The finding indicates that many
adults who are likely to develop diabetes are not regularly screened for
the disease, according to the American Diabetes Association. The association recommends a screening test
every three years for people who are
over 40, overweight, and have diabetes in their family.

More than 2,000 people with Type II
diabetes were tested for retinopathy
by researchers at the U.S. National Institutes of Health; the University of
Wisconsin in Madison; and Sir Charles
Gairdner Hospital in Perth, Australia.
About one-fifth of the Americans and
one-tenth of the Australians tested
had developed retinopathy by the time
their diabetes was diagnosed.

The study indicated that Type II diabetes usually begins 9 to 12 years before it is diagnosed and that retinopathy may start from 4 to 7 years before
the diabetes diagnosis. That time lag
is critical, the researchers said, because people with diabetes may go
without treatment during several years
when high blood glucose levels could
cause severe damage not only to the
eyes, but to the heart, blood vessels,
kidneys, and nerves as well.

Diabetes-enzyme link. Scientists reported the discovery of an *enzyme* (a
protein that speeds up or causes
chemical reactions) linked to the development of Type I diabetes. The discovery, reported in September 1990,
led scientists to speculate about a
possible screening test for the enzyme
that could identify people likely to develop Type I diabetes up to eight years
before symptoms first appear. Type I
symptoms include excessive thirst
and urination, fatigue, weight loss,
and blurred vision.

The enzyme-diabetes link was reported in the journal *Nature* by researchers at Yale University in New
Haven, Conn., and the University of
California at San Francisco. The researchers found that the enzyme
stimulates the production of *antibodies* that somehow play a role in de-

stroying special insulin-producing cells, called *beta cells*, in the pancreas. (Antibodies are proteins produced by the body's disease-fighting immune system in response to what it perceives to be an invader.) Scientists believe that many cases of Type I diabetes develop when the immune system malfunctions.

The enzyme, *glutamic acid decarboxylase* (GAD), was found in 80 per cent of those tested—people newly diagnosed with diabetes or who later developed it. Sufficiently early detection of GAD might enable physicians to save the remaining beta cells and halt the onset of the disease, the researchers said.

Stopping beta-cell destruction.
Researchers reported at the June diabetes congress on initial success in interfering with the destruction of the body's beta cells. University of Florida researchers, in Gainesville, found that *azathioprine*, a drug used to suppress the immune system, helped children with newly diagnosed diabetes maintain better blood sugar levels and natural insulin production.

The university is coordinating a nationwide study of azathioprine in people with certain prediabetic conditions who are likely to develop Type I diabetes over the next three to seven years.   ☐ William H. Allen
In WORLD BOOK, see DIABETES.

Cancer researchers reported in August 1991 that they had discovered the gene responsible for an inherited form of colon cancer. Researchers from the Johns Hopkins School of Medicine in Baltimore, the Cancer Institute In Tokyo, and the Howard Hughes Medical Institute at the University of Utah reported that *mutations* (alterations) in a gene called *adenomatous polyposis coli* (APC) is the first in a series of mutations in colon and rectal cells that lead to colon cancer.

People who inherit the defective gene develop a rare condition called *familial adenomatous polyposis* (FAP).

This results in the unrestrained growth of thousands of *polyps* (tiny mushroom-shaped growths) in the rectum or colon. Some of these polyps can become cancerous and, if not removed, develop into invasive tumors. Although only about 1 in 5,000 people suffer from FAP, the researchers said flaws in the APC gene, whether inherited or acquired later in life, may also play a crucial role in triggering most cases of colon cancer. This disease kills approximately 60,000 Americans a year, according to the American Cancer Society.

The researchers said the APC gene is on chromosome 5. Each human cell

Digestive System

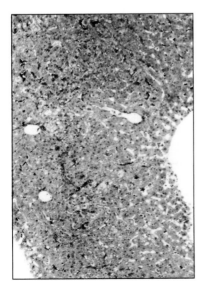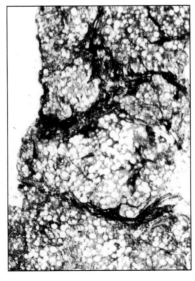

Combating cirrhosis
Liver tissue from a baboon fed *lecithin* (a soybean extract) along with an alcohol-laden diet, *far left,* shows little sign of *cirrhosis* (scarring of the liver). By contrast, tissue from a baboon fed the same diet without lecithin, *left*, has dark bands that indicate heavy scarring. Researchers at two New York City medical centers reported in December 1990 that their study of cirrhosis in baboons indicated lecithin may prevent or halt the disease in human beings.

has 23 pairs of chromosomes, which contain the genes that determine an individual's physical characteristics. Evidence suggests that a defect in the APC gene is the first of several genes to be mutated in a multistep process that leads to colon cancer.

The researchers noted that discovery of the APC gene will allow doctors to identify people with an inborn predisposition to colon cancer. The discovery could also lead to tests to detect colon cancer in its early stages.

Detecting intestinal bleeding. Researchers in May 1991 described the use of a recently developed instrument for locating the source of bleeding within the small intestine. The new instrument, a thin, very flexible tube called a *Sonde enteroscope*, allows physicians to examine previously inaccessible parts of the small intestine for sources of chronic or severe bleeding that traditional diagnostic methods such as X rays fail to uncover. An enteroscope is a type of *endoscope* (a tube for viewing internal organs and body cavities) used for viewing the small intestine.

Until the development of the Sonde enteroscope, doctors were unable to directly view all of the small intestine's 16 feet (4.9 meters) except through surgery. This was due to the construction of most endoscopes, which have rigid steering cables that prevent the instrument from passing through the many twists and turns of the small intestine. A pediatric colonoscope, a relatively flexible endoscope used for the examination of children's colons, can be pushed about 4 feet (1.2 meters) into the upper small intestine, but this still leaves some 12 feet (3.7 meters) hidden from view.

Unlike other endoscopes, the new Sonde instrument has no rigid steering cables. Its outer sheathing is also made of more flexible plastic than other endoscopes. It is nearly 9 feet (3 meters) long and slightly more than 1/4 inch (about 0.5 centimeter) in diameter. It has a lens at the tip and a thin, flexible bundle of fiber-optic strands that transmit light and images along its entire length.

The device, which is inserted down the throat, moves through the small bowel as a result of *peristalsis* (wave-like muscular contractions of the small bowel), a process that takes about eight hours. A doctor then slowly withdraws the instrument while viewing the inside of the small intestine.

Doctors can currently identify sources of bleeding in the *gastrointestinal tract* (esophagus, stomach, and small and large intestine) in about 95 per cent of patients. The remaining 5 per cent are more difficult to diagnose, because most of the bleeding in this group occurs in the small intestine.

Stopping bleeding. Findings presented in May 1991 show that a new

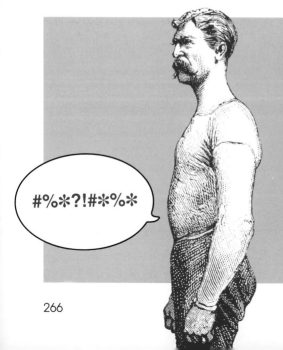

Stomach statements
Do your stomach rumblings make you look around to see if anyone else could hear them? According to doctors, those abdominal growls are probably nothing to worry about, especially if you're on a high-fiber diet. Rhythmic contractions called *peristalsis* move food down the digestive tract. If there is no food present, peristalsis moves whatever gas or liquid remains, which can produce those embarrassing growls and gurgles. A high-fiber diet can also contribute to the hullabaloo. Although high-fiber foods may offer health benefits, such as lowering the level of cholesterol in the blood, their digestion also creates gas, which makes the process more audible. However, intestinal noises accompanied by pain may be a sign of bowel obstruction, an ulcer, or other problems. If this is the case, consult a doctor.

#%✳?!#✳%✳

technique for controlling bleeding of veins and arteries in the esophagus is as effective as conventional methods and reduces the severity of *ulcers* (breaks in the skin or membrane) that often result from conventional treatment called *sclerotherapy*. With sclerotherapy, a physician injects a *sclerosing* (hardening) agent into the ruptured blood vessel. This substance creates thick deposits that clog the vessel, thus controlling bleeding. But sclerosing agents can kill surrounding esophageal tissue and cause deep, bleeding ulcers.

With the new treatment, developed by researchers at the University of Colorado Health Science Center in Denver, the physician stops the flow of blood to an affected artery or vein by tying the blood vessel off with a small rubber ring similar to a rubber band. This technique is called *ligation*. Doctors perform ligation with a special tube that fits over a fiber-optic endoscope.

Greg Van Steigman, a gastrointestinal surgeon and one of the developers of the technique, reported that ligation stops bleeding of veins and arteries in the esophagus as effectively as sclerotherapy. He reported that in 120 patients, 60 of whom received ligation and 60 sclerotherapy, 20 per cent of sclerotherapy patients developed serious, bleeding ulcers compared with 3 per cent of the ligation patients.

Liver disease such as cirrhosis or hepatitis is the most common cause of bleeding esophageal blood vessels. When the liver is damaged, blood flow through the organ can be disrupted, which increases pressure in the vein that drains the intestines, spleen, and liver. The body tries to relieve this pressure by diverting blood to veins and arteries around the esophagus and chest. The increased pressure can rupture these veins and arteries, causing serious bleeding.

Small intestine transplant. The first successful small intestine transplant was reported by medical researchers at the University of Pittsburgh School of Medicine in May 1991. The procedure will aid people who suffer from underdeveloped or missing sections of the small intestine. These people cannot digest food properly and must receive all nourishment intravenously.

Researchers said that a new anti-rejection drug, FK506, aided their success. The small intestine contains a high number of *lymphocytes*, white blood cells that play a major part in the body's rejection of transplanted organs. Previous attempts at small intestine transplants using other anti-rejection drugs had all failed.

□ James Franklin

In the Special Reports section, see New Options for Treating Gallstones. In World Book, see Cancer; Colon; Digestive system.

Drug Abuse
See Alcohol and Drug Abuse

Drugs

In July 1991, the commissioner of the United States Food and Drug Administration (FDA) ordered a major review of regulations that the FDA had proposed for food and drug manufacturers over the past 30 years. David Kessler, appointed commissioner in September 1990, said that about 400 regulations had been proposed but never implemented. They ranged from stipulating the size of print on prescription drug warnings, proposed in 1961, to the listing of ingredients by percentage on baby food labels, proposed in 1976. Kessler said the FDA will act on the regulations it considers important and drop the rest.

The commissioner's review was termed the second phase of his plan to reform the FDA, which increasingly had been criticized by members of Congress and the food and drug industries for losing credibility because of allegations that it had not done enough to protect the public health. During Kessler's first reform phase, which began shortly after he took office, the FDA hired about 100 criminal investigators. Their tasks include investigating possible fraud, such as in the generic drug scandal of 1989, when several companies falsified test data presented to get FDA approval of their generic versions of established drugs. Also under the first reform phase, the agency banned food and drug manufacturers from using misleading words on their product labels, such as "fresh" on products that actually were processed.

New cancer drugs. Idarubicin, marketed as Idamycin, was approved on Sept. 27, 1990, to treat *acute myeloid leukemia* (a type of blood cancer) in adults. Several studies had shown significantly greater rates of remission and longer survival with treatment that included idarubicin than in treatments without this drug.

In December 1990, altretamine, formerly known as hexamethylmelamine and sold under the name Hexalen, received FDA approval for the treatment of cancer of the ovaries. Altretamine caused tumor regression and reduced tumor-related symptoms in some women who did not respond to other drugs.

In addition to approving drugs to fight cancer, the FDA approved a medication aimed at easing the side effects of some cancer drugs. Nausea and vomiting are among the adverse reactions commonly associated with drugs used to treat cancer. On Jan. 4, 1991, the FDA approved odansetron, marketed as Zofran, to combat nausea and vomiting. Ondansetron is the first of a new class of drugs called *serotonin type 3 receptor antagonists.* In clinical studies, ondansetron was proven more effective in human beings than other drugs used to combat nausea, including in people taking high-dose *cisplatin*, an anticancer

drug that is particularly troublesome due to the nausea it causes. Ondansetron is marketed in an *intravenous* (administered directly into the veins) form, but researchers are evaluating a form that can be taken orally.

Preventing infection in cancer patients who are receiving *chemotherapy* (drug therapy) is a critical problem because the treatment suppresses the production of white blood cells in the body's bone marrow. White cells fight infection in the body. In early 1991, the FDA licensed two *colony stimulating factors*, substances that regulate the production of blood cells in the bone marrow.

Studies showed that the first drug, *filgrastim*, licensed on Feb. 20, 1991, reduced the occurrence of infection in cancer patients on chemotherapy. Experts suggested that this new drug, also known as *granulocyte-colony stimulating factor* and marketed as Neupogen, could benefit an estimated 225,000 patients with cancer in the United States.

Licensed on March 5, the second drug, sargramostim (also known as *granulocyte macrophage-colony stimulating factor* and marketed under the names Leukine and Prokine) speeds bone marrow recovery in patients who have undergone *autologous bone marrow transplantation*. In this procedure, doctors remove marrow from the patient, destroy the diseased cells

Drug recall
A clerk removes Sudafed 12-hour decongestant capsules from a Seattle store in March 1991 as part of a nationwide recall after a product-tampering scare. In February, two people died and a third became ill after taking Sudafed capsules that had been laced with cyanide. Authorities discovered that at least six packages of the capsules, all bought in stores in the Tacoma-Seattle region, had been tampered with.

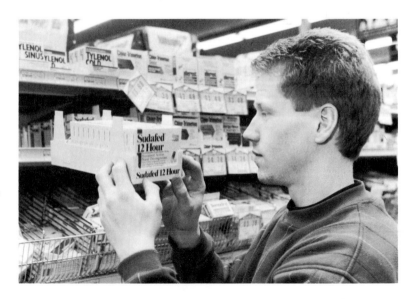

in the sample, and return the healthy marrow cells to the patient's body. Immune system cells come from the bone marrow. Because doctors destroy the patient's marrow after the marrow sample is taken, the patient is vulnerable to infection for a period of several weeks, until the cleansed marrow is able to rebuild the body's immune system. As many as 5,000 people undergo these transplants each year in the United States, including some with *Hodgkin's disease*, a type of cancer of the lymph system.

Lung surfactant. Exosurf Neonatal, licensed on Aug. 2, 1990, is the first lung surfactant product for premature infants with *respiratory distress syndrome* (RDS). As many as 50,000 premature infants in the United States develop RDS every year. Approximately 5,000 of them die from the disorder. Premature infants frequently lack natural surfactant, a substance that coats the inside of the lungs so that the lungs will not collapse during breathing. When the amount or quality of surfactant is inadequate, the work of breathing increases, and the infant tires, causing progressive respiratory failure. Exosurf Neonatal, which is used to treat RDS in infants, is administered through the *trachea* (windpipe).

Lead poisoning treatment. On Jan. 30, 1991, the FDA approved the first oral treatment for severe lead poisoning in children, a drug called *succimer*, available as Chemet. Lead poisoning is the number-one environmental disease of young children, say health experts. They estimate that 3 million to 4 million children in the United States may have blood lead levels that are high enough to cause behavioral and health problems. The major source of lead poisoning in children is the lead-based paint on surfaces such as window and door frames in some houses and apartment buildings.

Researchers have found that succimer is well tolerated by young patients. And unlike other lead-poisoning therapies, it does not significantly deplete essential minerals from the body.

Many faces of interferon. Alpha interferon, marketed as Intron A, became the first drug approved for the

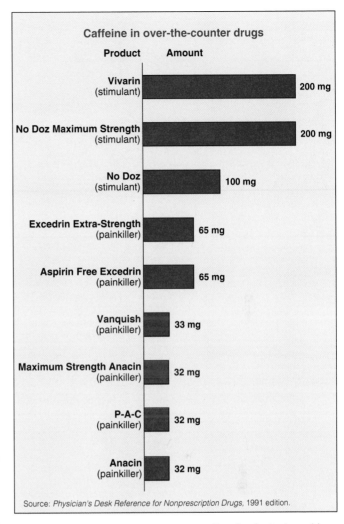

Caffeine in over-the-counter drugs

Product	Amount
Vivarin (stimulant)	200 mg
No Doz Maximum Strength (stimulant)	200 mg
No Doz (stimulant)	100 mg
Excedrin Extra-Strength (painkiller)	65 mg
Aspirin Free Excedrin (painkiller)	65 mg
Vanquish (painkiller)	33 mg
Maximum Strength Anacin (painkiller)	32 mg
P-A-C (painkiller)	32 mg
Anacin (painkiller)	32 mg

Source: *Physician's Desk Reference for Nonprescription Drugs*, 1991 edition.

treatment of chronic hepatitis C in February 1991. (This disease was formerly included in a group of hepatitis infections called non-A, non-B hepatitis.) There are an estimated 150,000 new cases of this liver disorder in the United States each year. Alpha interferon had already been approved for the treatment of *hairy-cell leukemia* (a blood cancer), AIDS-related *Kaposi's sarcoma* (a skin cancer that develops in some people with AIDS), and genital warts. Alpha interferon is also being evaluated in patients with hepatitis B and other forms of hepatitis.

Contraceptive implants. The FDA approved a unique new contraceptive formulation on Dec. 10, 1990. Marketed as Norplant, *levonorgestrel* is a

People who try to avoid caffeine may be surprised to learn that the drug is an ingredient in many over-the-counter medications. Caffeine acts as a stimulant by making people more alert and increasing their heartbeat and breathing rate. In some nonprescription pain relievers, caffeine is added to speed the effect of acetaminophen and aspirin.

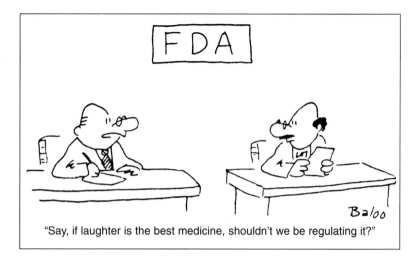

"Say, if laughter is the best medicine, shouldn't we be regulating it?"

synthetic hormone that is implanted into a woman's body. The implants consist of six flexible rods, each about the size of a matchstick. The rods, which are inserted under the skin of the upper arm through a small incision, continuously release the synthetic hormone and provide contraceptive effectiveness for up to five years. The hormone blocks ovulation and thickens mucus in the *cervix* (the opening to the uterus) so that sperm cannot enter the uterus. The implants must be removed after five years and, if desired, new ones can be inserted.

Drug for yeast infections. The FDA approved the first over-the-counter drug for vaginal yeast infections in November 1990. Clotrimazole, sold as Gyne-Lotrimin, had been available only through a doctor's prescription since the late 1970's. During that time, it proved to be a highly effective treatment with little risk, according to the FDA's Center for Drug Evaluation and Research.

Vaginal yeast infections are caused by the fungus *Candida*, which normally exist in relatively small numbers in the vagina. Experts estimate that 75 per cent of all women get at least one yeast infection during their lifetime. The fungus can multiply when the body's natural balance is upset. For example, the taking of birth control pills or antibiotics can trigger a yeast infection, as can warm weather. Also, women with diabetes seem to have a greater risk of getting this infection

than others, according to some health experts.

The nonprescription yeast-infection treatment is intended for use by women who have had vaginal yeast infections previously diagnosed by a physician and who are experiencing the same symptoms. These symptoms include itching and irritation of the vaginal area and sometimes a thick, white discharge. Women who experience these symptoms for the first time should consult a physician because symptoms of yeast infections can be the same as for other conditions, such as for some sexually transmitted diseases.

Drugs "normalize" cancer cells. A new class of drugs, which may be effective against a wide range of cancers, causes cancer cells to revert to normal behavior, according to a report given at the American Chemical Society's annual meeting in August 1991. The experimental drugs are now tested on a very limited number of people, but the first clinical trials may begin by the end of 1991. Researchers had thought that once a cell starts to become cancerous, the process could not be reversed. But the new studies indicate that at least in some cancer cells, the new drugs can reverse the progression, triggering the cells to mature almost normally.

☐ Daniel A. Hussar

In the Health Studies section, see PRESCRIPTION DRUGS AND HUMAN HEALTH. In WORLD BOOK, see DRUGS.

A combination of two drugs may be the most effective way to treat persistent middle-ear infections, physicians at Bnai Zion Medical Center in Haifa, Israel, reported in December 1990. These infections, which cause a build-up of fluid and pus that can damage the eardrum and cause hearing loss, are among the most common childhood ailments.

The researchers studied 136 children, ages 4 to 10, with stubborn infections in the middle ear and slight hearing loss. The physicians divided the children into three groups and pre-scribed a different drug treatment for each group. Forty-nine children received *amoxicillin*, an antibiotic, in combination with a *placebo* (an inactive substance). Fifty children received amoxicillin and *prednisone*, a *corticosteroid* (a drug used to reduce inflammation). Two placebos were given to the remaining 37 children.

After two months, the doctors examined the children and tested their hearing. In the group that had taken both drugs, 20 children had completely recovered from the infection and regained normal hearing, and 25 children had improved. Twenty children had also recovered in the group that had received amoxicillin and a placebo, but of the other 29 children in that group only 9 showed improvement. Of the 37 children receiving two placebos, 21 had improved due to

their bodies' own natural defenses, but none had recovered completely.

The researchers speculated that the two-drug combination proved most effective because it works in complementary ways: Amoxicillin destroys the bacteria responsible for the infection, while prednisone works to reduce swelling in the inner ear, allowing fluid to drain out.

Ear damage from aerobics. The repetitive jumping in some aerobic exercise programs may cause hearing and balance problems. That finding was reported in December 1990 by neurologist Michael Weintraub at New York Medical College in Valhalla.

Weintraub treated five women who either worked as aerobics instructors or regularly did high-impact aerobic workouts. All the women had developed *vertigo* (dizziness) or *tinnitus* (ringing in the ears). Weintraub also surveyed 37 aerobics instructors. Five had frequently suffered vertigo, and eight said they had tinnitus.

Weintraub noted that the symptoms affecting the women are similar to symptoms sometimes experienced by runners. The jarring impacts of long-distance running can damage delicate structures in the inner ear, and apparently the more energetic forms of aerobics can have the same effect. Weintraub recommended that people engaging in high-impact aerobics who

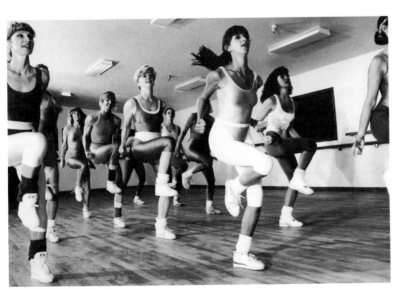

Inner-ear hazard?
The jarring motions of a high-impact aerobic work-out may damage structures in the inner ear, causing hearing and balance disorders, a New York researcher reported in December 1990. The scientist found that people who worked out hard and often—particularly aerobics instructors—frequently developed persistent inner-ear problems.

develop tinnitus or vertigo take up another form of exercise.

Laser surgery for the inner ear.

The use of a *laser* (a device emitting an intense beam of light) to treat *otosclerosis*, an inner-ear condition that leads to hearing loss, was reported in December 1990 by a team of surgeons from hospitals affiliated with the University of California at Irvine and at Sacramento.

Otosclerosis is an abnormal growth of spongy bone around the *stirrup*, a tiny bone that conducts sound waves into the inner ear. As the disease progresses, the growth prevents the stirrup from transmitting sound, which results in a gradual loss of hearing.

The conventional treatment for severe otosclerosis is to fold back the eardrum and remove the bone deposits with a drilling instrument. However, the drilling often causes excessive bleeding, and it can damage surrounding nerves.

The California surgeons used a laser to treat 10 patients with advanced otosclerosis. As well as vaporizing the abnormal bone growths, the laser's concentrated light energy sealed off blood vessels, preventing bleeding. Also, because the laser was free of vibrations, it caused no damage to nerves. ☐ Beverly Merz

In WORLD BOOK, see DEAFNESS; EAR.

Emergency Medicine

Motorcycle riders who wear a safety helmet are less likely to die or suffer severe injuries in an accident than riders who are not helmeted. In addition, according to two recent studies, helmeted riders who are injured spend less time in the hospital, recover more quickly from their injuries, and have lower medical bills than do their helmetless counterparts.

Laws requiring motorcycle riders to wear safety helmets have aroused much debate. Some critics of helmet laws have argued that helmets limit the driver's vision and hearing. Critics have also contended that the added weight of a helmet on the head aggravates the severity of neck injuries. Since 1975, a number of states have repealed their helmet laws.

The first study, reported in autumn 1990, investigated the effects of helmet use in Kansas before and after the repeal of that state's helmet law in 1975 and in Louisiana before and after the passage of that state's helmet law in 1981. Researchers from several institutions in Texas and Louisiana found that while the laws were in effect, the death rate and severity of injuries from motorcycle accidents decreased. The length of time injured cyclists were hospitalized or disabled, and their medical costs, also fell.

Zeroing in on arteries

A tiny ultrasound transmitter in the tip of a "smart needle," developed at the University of California in San Francisco, enables physicians to locate arteries quickly and so eliminates the need for repeated needle sticks. High frequency sound waves emitted by the transmitter are reflected by blood moving through an artery. The return signal, amplified and emitted by an attached monitor, guides physicians directly to the artery.

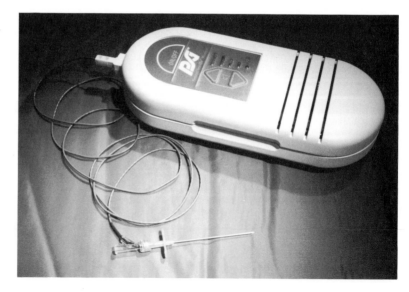

The second study, reported in May 1991, was conducted at the University of Nebraska Medical Center in Omaha. Researchers found that medical costs for injured motorcyclists who had been wearing helmets were 38 per cent lower than those for injured cyclists who were not helmeted.

New CPR technique. A new form of *cardiopulmonary resuscitation* (CPR) is more effective than standard CPR in reviving a patient who has stopped breathing or whose heart has stopped beating. Patients resuscitated with the new technique also suffered less brain damage, according to research reported in November 1990 by physicians from St. Joseph's Hospital in Paterson, N.J.

In standard CPR, one or two rescuers alternate blowing oxygen into the victim's lungs by mouth-to-mouth breathing and compressing the victim's chest to squeeze the heart and circulate blood through the body. In the modified form of CPR, called *interposed abdominal compressions CPR* (IAC-CPR), one person compresses the upper abdomen at the same time a second person releases pressure on the chest. The pressure on the abdomen squeezes the large blood vessels that run through this area, forcing more blood into the brain. The pressure also helps to fill the heart before the next chest compression. Although IAC-CPR requires further testing, ex-perts believe the technique has the potential to improve the odds of survival for many patients whose breathing or heart action has stopped.

Stopping bleeding. The development of a nonsurgical technique that can stop serious bleeding from small, hard-to-reach blood vessels was reported by researchers at the University of Southern California at Los Angeles in November 1990. According to the researchers, the technique may be especially useful in cases in which bleeding vessels are deeply buried in delicate organs or when injuries are so severe that surgeons cannot locate the bleeding vessel.

In this technique, called *microcatheter embolization*, a *catheter* (tubing) about the diameter of a strand of spaghetti is threaded into a large blood vessel near the injury site. A dye that shows up on an X ray is injected into the large vessel and smaller blood vessels branching from it. Once the source of the bleeding has been identified by X rays, a microcatheter about the diameter of a human hair is inserted into the larger catheter and pushed into the bleeding blood vessel. Finally, tiny platinum coils are pushed through the microcatheter and deposited at the bleeding point. By slowing the flow of blood, the coils cause a blood clot to form, effectively halting the bleeding. ☐ Robert D. Powers

In WORLD BOOK, see HOSPITAL.

Testimony from witnesses opposed to the granting of a license for a low-level radioactive waste dump in southeastern California was presented at three simultaneous public hearings in July 1991. If approved, the license would be the first granted under a 1985 federal law that made each state responsible for disposing of its own radioactive wastes.

The proposed dump site is located in Ward Valley, near the border with Arizona. Foes of the proposed site note its close proximity—13 miles (21 kilometers)—to the Colorado River, which supplies water to about 15 million people in southern California, Arizona, and parts of Mexico. The proposed dump site also lies above a vast underground water basin used as a water supply.

Among those who testified against the granting of the license was Hugh Kaufman, special assistant to the director of the Environmental Protection Agency's (EPA's) Hazardous Site Control Division. Kaufman warned that the proposed dump could threaten southern California's water supply with low-level radioactive contamination. The hazardous life of low-level waste ranges from hours to hundreds of thousands of years.

Leukemia and electromagnetic fields. In December 1990, the EPA reported that a review of scientific studies "suggests a causal link" be-

Environmental Health

tween extremely low-frequency electromagnetic fields and *leukemia* (a blood cancer). The EPA report noted, however, that electromagnetic fields are only "a possible, but not proven, cause of cancer in humans." The report called for further research.

Electromagnetic fields are produced wherever there are electric currents. Such fields are found around high voltage power lines and all household appliances. The fields are part of the *electromagnetic spectrum*, which also includes radio waves, microwaves, infrared light, visible light, ultraviolet light, X rays, and gamma rays. However, electromagnetic fields give off so little energy that many scientists have difficulty understanding how the fields could be biologically harmful.

For example, electric currents in the United States and Canada operate at an extremely low *frequency* (the rate at which the electromagnetic waves vibrate, or *cycle*, per second) of 60 cycles per second. By comparison, ultraviolet light, which is known to be biologically harmful, has an extremely high frequency that starts at 1,000,000,000,000,000 cycles per second. Radiation at such a high frequency has enough energy to break apart the chemical bonds that hold atoms together and so could damage genes that control cell growth.

Some scientists speculate that although low-frequency electromagnetic radiation is not energetic enough to break chemical bonds, it may interfere with electrical signals at cell membranes. Such signals are involved in communications between cells that govern cell growth.

Air pollution and lung damage.
Air pollution caused by automobiles or industrial plants can permanently damage lung tissue, according to the results of an 11-year study reported in March 1991 by epidemiologist Roger Detels of the School of Public Health at the University of California at Los Angeles. Detels observed that "damage from air pollution may begin at a very young age, years before any symptoms of respiratory problems appear." Those breathing problems increase with age, he noted, indicating that air pollution may cause permanent impairment to lung function.

Three southern California cities—Long Beach, Glendora, and Lancaster—were selected for the study. Long Beach and Glendora have particularly high levels of sulfur, nitrogen oxides, and hydrocarbon gases as well as sulfates in solid granular form given off by automobile and industrial emissions. Lancaster, however, is a rural community relatively free of air pollution and was selected for the study for purposes of comparison.

The researchers gave breathing tests to adults and children in the three communities in 1972 and then again in 1983. The subjects ranged in

Radiation train
Frenchmen demonstrate radiation-testing equipment in a "hospital train" designed to speed to the scene of any nuclear accident that might occur in France. The new train is equipped to monitor the radiation exposure of as many as 5,000 people each day.

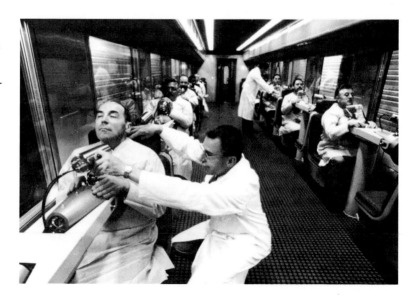

Plants that fight pollution

Indoor plants can remove air pollutants from homes and offices, according to the Foliage for Clean Air Council, based in Falls Church, Va. The council said its findings were based on studies conducted by retired scientist Bill Wolverton, formerly with the National Aeronautics and Space Administration. A single house plant, according to the scientist's findings, can remove about 87 per cent of some pollutants in a 100 square-foot (9.3 square-meter) area. Tropical plants and flowering plants reportedly were especially effective. The chart below lists many common indoor pollutants and the plants that were found to most effectively remove them.

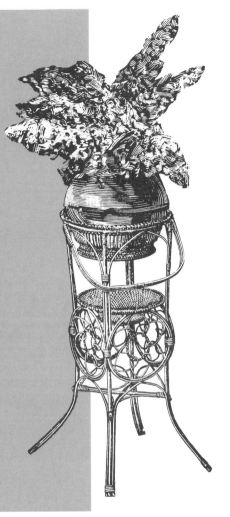

Pollutant	Solutions
Formaldehyde	Philodendron
	Spider plant
(Found in foam insulation,	Golden pothos
plywood, clothes, carpeting,	Bamboo palm
furniture, household cleaners)	Corn plant
	Chrysanthemum
Benzene	English ivy
	Marginata
(Found in tobacco smoke,	Janet Craig
gasoline, synthetic fibers,	Chrysanthemum
plastics, inks, oils, detergents)	Gerbera daisy
	Warneckei
	Peace lily
Trichloroethylene	Gerbera daisy
	Chrysanthemum
(Found in dry cleaning, paints,	Warneckei
varnishes, lacquers, adhesives)	Marginata

age from 7 to 59 years old. The study found that high levels of pollution in Long Beach and Glendora were linked with chronic bronchitis and *emphysema* (lung disease involving destructive changes in tiny air sacs) and/or impaired lung function. In Lancaster, however, lung function decline was related to normal aging processes.

Lead poisoning. Health officials issued a call for annual blood tests for lead poisoning in young children following a March 1991 report from the U.S. Centers for Disease Control (CDC) in Atlanta, Ga. The report documented the death of a 28-month-old Wisconsin boy who ingested lead from paint chips that littered the floor of his family's living quarters. The fed-

eral government banned most uses of lead-based paint in 1977, but a 1988 report by the U.S. Public Health Service revealed that 52 per cent, or 42 million, of the nation's households still have lead-based paint on walls and woodwork.

The symptoms of lead poisoning depend largely on the amount of lead in the body and on how long lead has been accumulating in the body. Some of the symptoms include abdominal pains, muscular weakness, and fatigue. Severe exposure can cause nervous-system disorders, high blood pressure, and death.

Epidemiologist Tom Matte of the CDC called for yearly testing of blood lead levels because prompt treatment can prevent brain damage. Most pa-

Lead poisoning victim
A Maryland child poses with her parents two years after she suffered lead poisoning while her home's exterior was sanded and repainted. In 1991, United States health officials recommended that young children be given annual blood tests for lead. Children who ingest paint or drinking water that contains lead may suffer serious health effects, including brain damage.

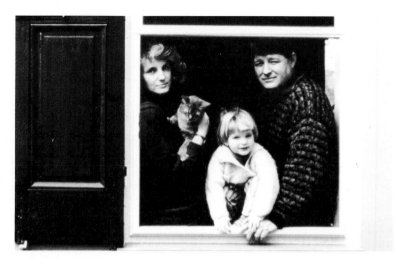

tients are given drugs called *chelating agents*, which bind to the metal in the bloodstream and are then excreted.

Matte noted that an estimated 3 million children in the United States may have excessive levels of lead in their blood. Lead in the bloodstream inhibits the production of *hemoglobin*, which is used by red blood cells to carry oxygen to tissues throughout the body. Lead also blocks essential enzymes in the brain and nervous system. These two factors lead to the destruction of brain tissue.

In addition to lead-based paint, another source of exposure to lead is tap water contaminated by lead pipes or the lead solder in copper plumbing.

In May 1991, the EPA mandated virtually all of the nation's water suppliers—about 79,000 utilities—to begin testing households for lead levels in drinking water.

The EPA also approved new regulations that reduce the current permissible level of 50 parts of lead per 1 billion parts of water to 15 parts per billion. The testing program, which was due to begin on Jan. 1, 1992, in the nation's 800 largest cities, will involve hundreds of thousands of households, and the new standards will affect about 230 million people.

☐ Laura M. Lake

In WORLD BOOK, see ENVIRONMENTAL POLLUTION.

Exercise and Fitness

Evidence continued to accumulate during 1990 and 1991 that physically active men have a reduced risk of coronary heart disease, the leading cause of death in Western nations. A long-term follow-up study of the association between physical activity and coronary heart disease found in 1990 that men who engage in regular vigorous exercise significantly reduce their risk of coronary heart disease, compared with men who engage in nonvigorous exercise. The study defined as vigorous exercise that which improves *aerobic fitness* (makes the heart and lungs work harder and so improves their ability to meet the muscles' need for oxygen).

Epidemiologist Jeremy Morris of the

London School of Hygiene and Tropical Medicine in England, who has been studying the relationship between exercise and coronary heart disease since 1953, began this latest study in 1976. The study involved 9,376 middle-aged males—British civil servants who engaged in sedentary office work and were free of clinical heart disease. Because prior research had raised questions regarding the kind of exercise that protects against heart disease, Morris sought to determine whether the intensity, type, frequency, or duration of exercise influenced the cardiac benefits associated with being physically active. Morris reported his initial findings from this ongoing research program in June 1990.

At the study's onset, the participants described in detail the type of leisure-time physical activity they engaged in over the prior month. The researchers then identified those men who experienced a heart attack or death due to coronary heart disease over the next 10 years.

Among men who engaged in vigorous sports at least twice a week, such as jogging, swimming, and singles tennis, the risk of coronary attack during the follow-up period was reduced by 60 per cent, compared with men who did not participate in vigorous sports. However, participation in non-vigorous sports, such as golf and bowling, was not associated with a reduction in the risk of a heart attack.

Similarly, civil servants who walked regularly at a "brisk" pace—greater than 4 miles (6 kilometers) per hour—reduced their risk of heart attack by 75 per cent. Those men who walked at a "fairly brisk" pace—3 to 4 miles (5 to 6 kilometers) per hour—for more than 30 minutes a day had a 50 per cent lower risk, compared with men who walked at a leisurely pace.

Other forms of regular vigorous exercise, such as cycling and calisthenics, also were associated with reduced coronary attack rates among men 55 to 64 years of age. In contrast, "recreational work," such as gardening and do-it-yourself jobs around

Increasing the risk of heart disease
In 1990, the federal Centers for Disease Control in Atlanta, Ga., issued a report comparing physical conditions and life style practices associated with an increased risk for coronary heart disease. Based on data gathered during the mid-1980's, the report noted that about 58.6 per cent of American adults either do not exercise or have fewer than three 20-minute workouts per week. Such a sedentary life style results in a twofold increase in the risk of death due to coronary heart disease, compared with physically active people.

The most common risks for heart disease

Per cent of adults with risk factors

Source: Centers for Disease Control.

the house, was not associated with a lower risk of coronary attacks, whatever the quantity or intensity of the work. In addition, total energy expended in leisure-time nonvigorous activity was not related to the coronary attack rate. In short, only activity that was vigorous and habitual afforded a degree of protection from coronary attacks.

Exercise and blood pressure. Exercise—even moderate exercise—may help lower blood pressure in elderly women, according to the results of a study reported by researchers at the University of California at San Diego in February 1991. This study is one of only a few that have examined the relationship between physical activity and cardiovascular risk factors in older people or women. Because high blood pressure is an important risk factor for coronary heart disease and stroke in older women, the researchers were particularly interested in a possible association between physical activity and lower blood pressure.

More than 600 women aged 50 to 89 years who resided in a predominantly white, upper middle-class community in southern California were examined from 1985 to 1987. The researchers measured blood pressure and heart rate and interviewed the women about their medical history and their use of cigarettes, alcohol, and medications. The women also

were asked about their participation in each of 17 different leisure-time physical activities during the previous two weeks.

The researchers classified the activities on the basis of their relative intensity. For example, light-intensity activities included walking, gardening, bowling, and golfing; moderate-intensity activities included swimming, hiking, and biking; and heavy-intensity activities included jogging, running, and aerobic exercise.

The study showed that the higher the intensity of reported activity, the lower the level of the measured blood pressure. This was true for both *systolic blood pressure* (SBP)—the pressure blood exerts against the walls of the arteries when the heart is contracting—and *diastolic blood pressure* (DBP)—the pressure blood exerts when the heart is relaxed. (The pressure exerted by blood in the arteries is expressed as the height in millimeters that it will move a column of mercury.)

For example, the age-adjusted mean SBP was 142 millimeters of mercury (mmHg) among sedentary women and 130 mmHg among women who engaged in heavy-intensity activity. Similarly, the age-adjusted mean DBP was 77 mmHg among sedentary women and 72 mmHg among heavy-intensity exercisers. Older women who participated in moderate activity or only light activity also had lower SBP and DBP than

Exercise and the heart

Aerobic exercise raises the heart rate and helps strengthen the circulatory and respiratory systems. Several health organizations have calculated target heart rates individuals of various ages should aim for while exercising, *below*. This can help determine whether a workout is providing aerobic benefits. But some experts say that exercising regularly is more important to health than tracking heart rate.

Heart rate (beats per minute)				
Age	American Heart Association	American College of Sports Medicine	Institute for Aerobics Research Men	Women
25	117 to 146	117 to 176	125 to 154	127 to 156
30	114 to 143	114 to 171	124 to 152	124 to 152
35	111 to 139	111 to 167	122 to 150	120 to 148
40	108 to 135	108 to 162	120 to 148	117 to 144
45	105 to 131	105 to 158	119 to 146	114 to 140
50	102 to 128	102 to 153	117 to 144	111 to 136
55	99 to 124	99 to 149	115 to 142	107 to 132
60	96 to 120	96 to 144	114 to 140	104 to 128
65	93 to 116	93 to 140	112 to 138	101 to 124

sedentary women, though the magnitude of the difference was less.

Screening tests for exercisers.
Treadmill tests do not improve the ability of physicians to predict whether men free of symptoms of heart disease but with high levels of *cholesterol* (a fatlike substance) in the blood can safely begin an exercise program, according to research reported in February 1991. Investigators at the University of Washington in Seattle conducted the research.

A treadmill test, also called *exercise electrocardiography,* involves measuring the electrical currents given off by the heart with an electrocardiograph

while the patient is exercising on a treadmill. Some physicians have recommended that men aged 40 years and older with risk factors for coronary heart disease, such as high blood cholesterol, undergo exercise electrocardiography before beginning an exercise program. However, this recommendation was controversial because no research studies had been done to directly assess the ability of such treadmill tests to identify people at risk for sudden exercise-related "cardiac events," such as fatal and nonfatal heart attacks.

☐ David S. Siscovick
In WORLD BOOK, see ELECTROCARDIOGRAPH; PHYSICAL FITNESS.

Eye and Vision

In January 1991, a team of eye surgeons at Barnes Hospital in St. Louis, Mo., reported that they had used a new technique to restore normal vision in an eye that had been declared legally blind. Ophthalmologists Henry J. Kaplan and Matthew Thomas developed the procedure to treat *macular degeneration,* a principal cause of blindness in older people. The condition affects the *macula,* the central area of the *retina,* the structure that transmits visual signals to the optic nerve, which carries them to the brain.

The aging process, an infection, or a blow to the eye can produce cracks in retinal tissue, including the macula. When blood vessels or scar tissue grow through cracks in the macula, the retina loses its capacity to transmit visual signals. Vision loss begins with the development of a black spot in the center of the visual field. As more of the retina is overrun with blood vessels, the spot expands until the entire visual field is blotted out.

The Barnes ophthalmologists treated a woman who had rapidly lost the vision in her left eye following an infection called *histoplasmosis*, which is caused by a soil-dwelling fungus. They began by making a series of tiny incisions in the side of the eye and inserting tiny forceps no larger in diameter than a human hair. Using a microscope to monitor their progress, the doctors lifted a small section of the retina and plucked away a sliver of scar tissue. Within two hours, they

had repeated the process several hundred times and had removed all of the scar tissue obstructing the retina. Although the vision in the woman's eye did not begin to improve until six weeks after the operation, her vision had returned to normal within six months. The Barnes ophthalmologists planned to use the procedure to treat other patients with vision loss due to histoplasmosis, and, eventually, in patients with macular degeneration.

Glaucoma treatment. In November 1990, researchers released the results of the first large study to test whether glaucoma is more effectively controlled with drugs or laser surgery. (A laser is an instrument that uses a narrow, intense beam of light.) The results of the study indicated that the two forms of therapy were equally effective, though laser surgery was somewhat more convenient.

Glaucoma is a condition in which pressure inside the eye increases due to a build-up of *aqueous humor*—the fluid that nourishes the cornea and the lens. Excess fluids accumulate when a meshlike tissue surrounding the eye becomes constricted, curtailing the drainage of fluids from the eye. As fluid pressure increases, the blood vessels supplying the optic nerve are also constricted. Deprived of nutrients, optic-nerve cells begin to die, and the visual field narrows.

Standard treatment for glaucoma begins with eye drops containing

Monitoring
eye disease

Scientists at the University of Texas in San Antonio, *right,* demonstrate the use of a device they invented to detect early signs of *diabetic retinopathy,* a leading cause of blindness. The device, called a *vascular entoptoscope,* enables diabetics to see small blood vessels in their own eyes, *below left,* and so monitor changes in their eyes between regular eye checkups. Patients can be taught to detect abnormal changes in the eye's blood vessels, *below right,* which can become a serious threat to their vision if not treated promptly. The scientists hope to develop a version of the vascular entoptoscope for home use.

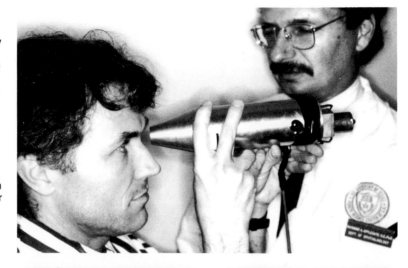

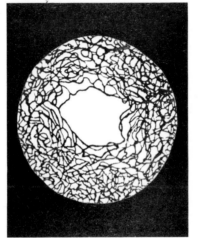

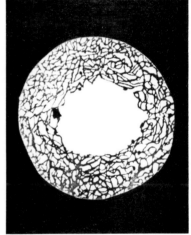

timolol, a pressure-lowering drug. Additional drugs are used if timolol does not lower pressure in the eyeball sufficiently. If all drugs fail, ophthalmologists may then try to lower pressure within the eye by using a laser to burn microscopic holes in the tissue to increase its drainage capacity.

Because laser surgery had been so successful in correcting early glaucoma, ophthalmologists wondered if it should replace drug treatment as the first line of therapy for the disorder. The National Eye Institute in Bethesda, Md., had sponsored the Glaucoma Laser Trial in part to answer that question.

The study, which was conducted at eight eye treatment centers in the United States, involved 271 patients with newly diagnosed, untreated glaucoma. Each patient had one eye treated with laser surgery and the other with eye drops. If either treatment failed to sufficiently reduce pressure in the eye, additional drugs were added.

After the two-year study ended in 1989, the researchers determined that 44 per cent of the eyes that first underwent laser surgery needed no pressure-lowering drugs, 26 per cent needed timolol, and 19 per cent required two or more drugs. Eleven per cent still had pressures that were considered high enough to cause damage or loss of sight.

In comparison, 30 per cent of the eyes treated with drops needed only timolol, while 66 per cent needed two or more drugs. Four per cent still had excessive pressure. However, the average pressure of the laser-treated eyes was significantly lower than that of the eyes treated with drops alone.

The researchers concluded that laser surgery was at least as good as treatment with eye drops. They added that, if used first, laser treatment might delay or eliminate the inconvenience of using eye drops several times a day.

Lasers remove corneal scars. In April 1991, researchers from four eye treatment centers reported the successful use of a laser to erase scars on the *cornea,* the transparent front part of the eye. Ophthalmologists at centers in Minneapolis, Minn.; Oklahoma City, Okla.; Ft. Myers, Fla.; and Louisville, Ky., treated 33 patients who had corneal scars from a variety of causes, including eye injuries, birth defects, genetic diseases, and infections. The researchers used *excimer lasers*, which produce ultraviolet light beams, to smooth the surface of the cornea by burning away tiny bits of corneal tissue.

Because the patients' symptoms varied considerably, the researchers did not compare results among patients. However, they noted that many patients had improvements in vision and that none suffered any additional scarring or other serious side effects from the procedure. Most of the patients experienced mild to severe pain following treatment, but the pain was relieved by taking medication, applying ice packs, or bandaging the eye.

What causes cataracts? Dietary supplements of certain vitamins and minerals may play a role in reducing the risk of *cataracts,* an age-related condition that causes a clouding of the lens, according to a study reported in February 1991. Because cataracts are the main cause of blindness in human beings and because the total cost of cataract surgery has surpassed $2.5 billion a year in the United States alone, ophthalmologists have begun to focus on preventing cataract formation. To better determine what causes cataracts, several research groups have begun studies to determine if life-style factors influence their development.

The Lens Opacities Case-Control Study, conducted by researchers at the State University of New York at Stony Brook and Harvard Medical School in Boston, looked at the habits of 945 people who had cataracts and 435 people who did not. They found that people who regularly took dietary supplements containing certain vitamins and minerals—such as vitamins C and E, carotene, riboflavin, niacin, thiamine, and iron—had a reduced risk of cataracts. Those who smoked, were overweight, and had jobs that required working outside in sunlight for long periods, increased their risk.

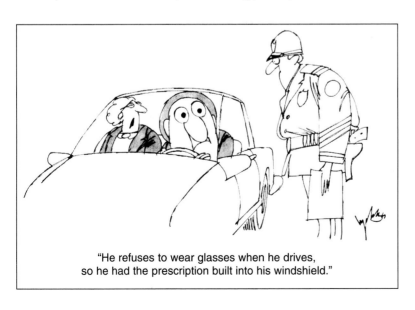

"He refuses to wear glasses when he drives,
so he had the prescription built into his windshield."

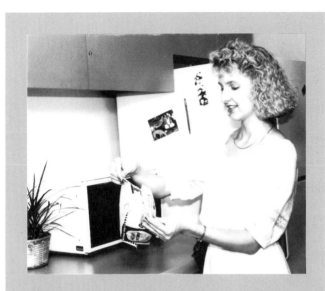

Popcorn lovers beware!
A hasty peek into a microwave popcorn bag may hasten an injury to the eyes, according to a letter published in the Oct. 25, 1990, issue of *The New England Journal of Medicine.* Two New Jersey physicians described three patients who suffered burns to the *cornea,* the transparent outer covering of the eye, caused by steam escaping from microwave popcorn bags as the bags were opened. Two of the patients temporarily experienced blurred vision as a result of the burns, though normal vision was restored after they were treated with antibiotics and/or wore an eye patch for several days. The two physicians called for manufacturers of microwave popcorn bags to place warnings on their packages, noting the possible danger to eyes due to escaping steam.

Massachusetts Eye and Ear Infirmary in Boston, according to an October 1990 report by researchers at Harvard Medical School. Although an estimated 33,000 sports-related eye injuries occur in the United States each year, little information exists concerning the risk of injury for particular sports.

The 202 patients who were treated injured their eyes playing basketball (58 patients), baseball or softball (40 patients), racquetball (23 patients), tennis or soccer (15 patients each), and football or hockey (9 patients each). The remainder were injured while skiing, surfing, or playing golf, lacrosse, field hockey, or volleyball.

Most of the basketball players were jabbed by fingers or elbows. Most of the baseball, softball, tennis, and racquetball players were struck by balls. The soccer injuries were proportionately the most severe; 5 of the 15 players had bleeding inside the eye.

The researchers noted that protective headgear was responsible for minimizing eye injuries in such sports as hockey and football. They also reported that while only 5 per cent of the injured players said they usually wore protective eye gear before they were injured, 31 per cent said they were using eye protection a year later. The researchers recommended wearing protective goggles or glasses during most sports activities.

Dining room danger. The dining room may pose less frequent but possibly greater danger to the eye than the athletic field, according to a study reported in January 1991. Researchers from the University of Illinois in Chicago, the University of Miami (Fla.), and the Medical College of Wisconsin in Milwaukee reported that they had treated six patients whose eyes were punctured by eating utensils.

Because the patients, who ranged in age from 11 months to 52 years, were eating at the time of the accidents, the utensils were coated with as many as 42 different species of bacteria found in human saliva. As a result, even though all were treated with antibiotics, five of the six patients developed severe eye infections that resulted in vision losses.

In a second study, researchers at the Harvard School of Public Health in Boston followed up on a few earlier reports linking cataract formation with the use of tranquilizers. The scientists analyzed medical records of 45,301 people who were treated at a health maintenance organization in Seattle. They found that those who had taken antipsychotic drugs or tranquilizers containing phenothiazine had 3.5 times the average risk of developing cataracts. There was also a greater, but less pronounced risk, for patients who had taken tranquilizers containing benzodiazapines.

Eye injuries. Basketball was the leading cause of sports-related eye injuries among 202 patients at the

Beverly Merz

In WORLD BOOK, see EYE.

Health-care spending in the United States continued to rise, prompting concern during 1990 and 1991 in both the public and private sectors. Final figures for 1989 (the last year for which final data were available) revealed that overall U.S. health-care spending rose to $604.1 billion, an increase of 11.1 per cent over spending for 1988. The 1989 amount represented 11.6 per cent of the nation's *gross national product* (GNP), the total value of all goods and services produced—the highest percentage in U.S. history.

Despite efforts to control spending, the federal government's share of the bill increased slightly to 28.9 per cent of total expenditures. The share of state and local expenditures declined by 0.1 per cent from 1988 to 17.1 per cent of total expenditures in 1989. Private health insurance accounted for 33 per cent of the total, and personal out-of-pocket spending by patients accounted for 21 per cent.

Federal health-care spending increased to $174.4 billion. State and local government spending rose by $7.3 billion from 1988 to $78.8 billion in 1989.

Most of the money went for hospital care, which represented 39 per cent of total costs. Other personal health services, such as dental care and home health care, accounted for 22 per cent of costs. This was followed by physicians' services at 19 per cent, other spending, such as private health insurance costs, at 12 per cent, and nursing home care at 8 per cent.

The U.S. Department of Commerce has predicted that total health-care spending for 1990 would climb to $675.7 billion, or 11.9 per cent of GNP. That would represent an average of $2,660 for every person living in the United States, the highest per capita rate in the world. The report also predicted that without effective cost controls, health-care spending would continue to rise by 12 to 15 per cent each year for the next five years.

Medicare's future. Despite the gloomy news about soaring medical costs, the Health Care Financing Administration (HCFA) predicted in January 1991 that higher Medicare payroll taxes and efforts at cost control could keep the Medicare trust funds solvent until the year 2008. HCFA is the agency that oversees Medicare (a program that pays for the health-care expenses of people over the age of 65 and certain other groups) and Medicaid (a federal and state program for low-income patients).

This optimistic forecast, however, was not shared by Medicare's trustees, who estimated in May 1991 that the trust funds might be solvent until 2005 but could be depleted as early as 2001. Even under optimal condi-

Financing Medical Care

The prognosis for Medicare looks bleak, according to 1990 estimates by the Health Care Financing Administration, the federal agency that administers the health-insurance program. In January 1991, the agency estimated that Medicare's trust fund for hospitals will go broke by 2005 unless there are higher payroll taxes and efforts at cost control.

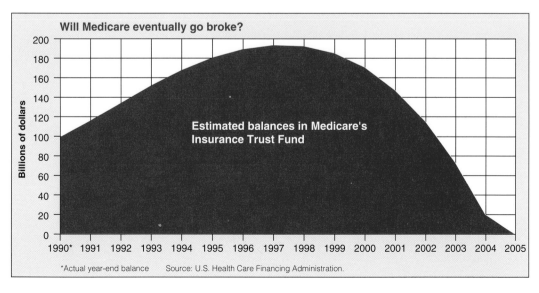

Will Medicare eventually go broke?

Billions of dollars

Estimated balances in Medicare's Insurance Trust Fund

1990* 1991 1992 1993 1994 1995 1996 1997 1998 1999 2000 2001 2002 2003 2004 2005

*Actual year-end balance   Source: U.S. Health Care Financing Administration.

tions, the trustees warned, the fund might be bankrupt by the year 2018.

Government officials made some controversial efforts to contain the red ink. The Administration of President George Bush, as part of a five-year budget agreement worked out with Congress in 1990, had said it would limit Medicare cuts. However, the Administration's 1992 budget proposal included deeper reductions than had been expected.

Medicare fee changes. Even more controversial was a plan proposed in June 1991 by HCFA to change the way Medicare pays physicians. Congress had mandated in 1989 that as of 1992, doctors be paid on the basis of the "relative value" of each procedure. The relative value scale was expected to increase payments for primary care providers, such as family and general practitioners, and reduce pay for medical specialists, such as surgeons and cardiologists, who perform surgery and other procedures that involve the use of more sophisticated, technological tools.

Accompanying that change was a provision for "volume performance standards," which set limits on the total amount Medicare could pay doctors in the course of a year. If those limits are exceeded, payments to doctors would be cut back the following year. HCFA's proposed fee schedule for 1992 would have reduced physi-

cian payments substantially. In August 1991, however, under pressure from Congress, the HCFA dropped the planned reductions.

Medicaid's woes. The Medicaid program underwent expansion and came under criticism. In October 1990, as part of the five-year budget agreement, states were required to phase in Medicaid coverage for all children from age 6 to 18 years in families with incomes below the federal poverty level (defined as an annual income of $12,675 or less for a family of four). Previously, the Medicaid program did not require that children in this age group be covered. Nevertheless, some states did provide some coverage for children aged 6 to 18 years.

Because Medicaid is partially funded by states, and because most states faced budget deficits in 1990 and 1991, the mandates brought outcries from all 50 governors. They complained that federal responsibilities for health care were being shifted to states without adequate federal funding being provided.

In April 1991, Health and Human Services Secretary Louis W. Sullivan and Richard G. Darman, director of the Office of Management and Budget, announced that estimates of federal spending on Medicaid were far too low. The two men estimated that the federal share of the program was likely to increase by $15 billion, or 30

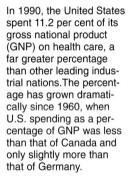

In 1990, the United States spent 11.2 per cent of its gross national product (GNP) on health care, a far greater percentage than other leading industrial nations. The percentage has grown dramatically since 1960, when U.S. spending as a percentage of GNP was less than that of Canada and only slightly more than that of Germany.

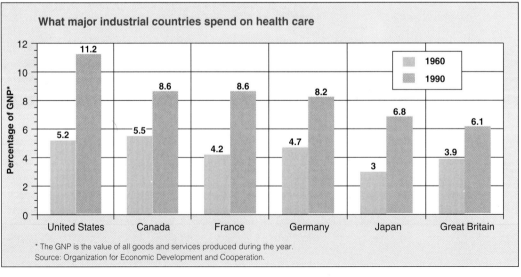

What major industrial countries spend on health care

Percentage of GNP*

Legend: 1960, 1990

United States — 5.2 (1960), 11.2 (1990)
Canada — 5.5 (1960), 8.6 (1990)
France — 4.2 (1960), 8.6 (1990)
Germany — 4.7 (1960), 8.2 (1990)
Japan — 3 (1960), 6.8 (1990)
Great Britain — 3.9 (1960), 6.1 (1990)

* The GNP is the value of all goods and services produced during the year.
Source: Organization for Economic Development and Cooperation.

per cent, from 1990 to 1992. Darman and Sullivan launched a federal investigation of Medicaid expenditures, which resulted in plans to increase monitoring of state Medicaid programs and to use better techniques for estimating costs.

Private coverage. In 1988 (the last year for which final data were available), 188.4 million Americans had private health insurance coverage, according to the Health Insurance Association of America. Of that total, 153.3 million had workplace-related coverage.

Commercial insurers covered the largest number—93.3 million. The single biggest insurer remained the non-profit Blue Cross and Blue Shield plans, with 74 million members. About 71.3 million people were covered by other plans, including self-insured employer programs and health maintenance organizations.

Private health insurers collected $98.2 billion in premiums in 1988 and paid out $171.1 billion in claims. Although commercial firms reported underwriting losses of $3.8 billion, Blue Cross and Blue Shield plans earned $1.1 billion, a turnaround from a 1987 loss of $1.9 billion.

☐ Emily Ann Friedman

In WORLD BOOK, see MEDICAID; MEDICARE.

Food

See Nutrition and Food

Genetics

In mid-1991, about nine months after their first attempts to use *gene therapy* to repair a human genetic disorder, researchers at the National Institutes of Health (NIH) in Bethesda, Md., reported promising, though still inconclusive, results. Gene therapy involves the insertion of new genes into cells to repair a disease-causing defect.

In this case, the NIH physicians gave genetically altered white blood cells to two girls with a rare immune disorder. The cells contained a new gene coding for an *enzyme* (a type of protein) that the girls' bodies were unable to produce. The girls' immune systems were reportedly functioning properly in late 1991, but the long-term effects were still uncertain.

The researchers also used gene therapy to treat two patients with a deadly form of skin cancer. Although the patients tolerated the therapy well, the physicians said it was too soon to tell whether their cancers had been significantly affected. See Close-Up.

Fragile X syndrome. The identity of a mutated gene responsible for a disorder called *fragile X syndrome* was reported in May 1991 by researchers in the United States and the Netherlands. The syndrome is the most common inherited form of mental retardation. The faulty gene may also be involved in several behavioral disorders, such as hyperactivity, and in many cases of learning disability.

Fragile X is named for the characteristic appearance of the *X chromosome.* Chromosomes, of which human beings have 23 pairs in each cell, are the structures that carry genes. The X chromosome is one of the two chromosomes that determine an individual's sex. With fragile X syndrome, a portion of the X chromosome carrying the abnormal gene is attached to the rest of the chromosome by just a sliver of genetic material, creating a fragile, or easily broken, site. The faulty gene, as researchers had expected, was pinpointed very near the fragile site.

Human females have two X chromosomes; males have one X and a smaller sex chromosome called the Y chromosome. According to genetic theory, all males carrying a *mutant* (changed) gene on the X chromosome should be affected by that gene. The reason is that there is no corresponding normal form of the gene on the Y chromosome to counteract the effects of the mutation. If the mutant form of the gene is *recessive* (requires two copies of the gene in each cell for the gene to produce its trait in the body), females with only one mutant gene should be unaffected because a normal version of the gene resides on the other X chromosome.

That is not how it works with fragile X syndrome, however. About 20 per cent of males who have the gene somehow escape the syndrome. Those males can pass the gene to their daughters—who are also unaf-

Gene Therapy: A New Era in Medicine

Since the early 1970's, when researchers first learned to isolate genes and transplant them from one organism to another, scientists have held out hope for a new era in medicine. In that era of gene therapy, diseases would be prevented or cured by altering the genetic machinery inside our cells.

Prediction became reality on Sept. 14, 1990, when a 4-year-old girl with a rare immune-system disorder received the first of several infusions of white blood cells carrying copies of a gene her body lacked. The experimental treatment, done at the National Institutes of Health (NIH) in Bethesda, Md., was the first federally approved foray into gene therapy.

By January 1991, the NIH's gene therapy trials had expanded on two fronts. Physicians there began treating a second patient, a 9-year-old girl, with the same immune disorder, called *adenosine deaminase* (ADA) *deficiency*. That same month, NIH physicians started administering genetically engineered cancer-fighting cells to two patients suffering from advanced *melanoma*, a deadly form of skin cancer.

Gene therapy is the latest episode in a medical revolution that began early in the 1900's. That revolution has included the development of vaccines and antibiotics, which protect against many disease-causing viruses and bacteria. A number of illnesses are caused, however, not by infectious microorganisms but by flaws in our own molecular makeup. Those conditions are targeted by gene therapy.

Human beings have an esti-mated 50,000 to 100,000 genes inside each cell of the body. A gene carries a coded "recipe" for making a protein. The tens of thousands of proteins produced by cells shape our bodies and regulate all the chemical processes of life.

This genetic "symphony" is incredibly fine-tuned. Just one tiny glitch in a single gene can cause cells to produce a malformed version of an essential protein. Deprived of the normal protein, the body or mind may be severely impaired. More than 4,000 inherited diseases, including cystic fibrosis, muscular dystrophy, and sickle cell anemia, have been tracked to defects in a solitary gene.

ADA deficiency, too, has been traced to a single abnormal gene. The gene causes cells to manufacture faulty ADA, a protein required by the immune system. Without properly functioning ADA, the body cannot rid itself of certain *toxins* (poisons). As the toxins build up, they destroy white blood cells, which are crucial in defending against disease.

Most victims of ADA deficiency die of infection in early childhood. Fortunately, the disorder is quite rare, affecting fewer than 10 children born in the United States each year.

In the experimental treatment at the NIH, teams of researchers led by molecular biologists W. French Anderson and R. Michael Blaese inserted a normal copy of the human ADA gene into a virus that usually infects mice. The virus had been genetically engineered to make it incapable of causing disease. The scientists then mixed the virus with batches of white blood cells taken from the two young patients. The virus entered the cells and inserted its genes, including the spliced-in ADA gene, into the cells' own genes.

In each treatment, the girls received about a billion altered white blood cells apiece, infused into the blood through a vein. The therapy appeared

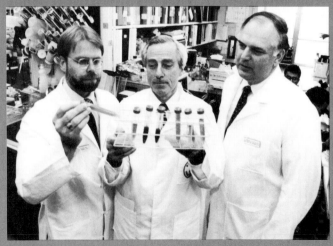

Medical researchers discuss a new gene-therapy treatment.

successful, though the girls will need further treatments every few months. In late 1990, the researchers reported that both girls' immune systems seemed to be working normally.

NIH cancer researcher Steven A. Rosenberg, aided by Anderson and Blaese, took a similar approach with the melanoma therapy. But in this case, foreign genes were used not to compensate for an inborn defect but to enhance the natural tumor-killing powers of certain of the patients' own cells.

Rosenberg extracted those cells—cancer-fighting white blood cells called *tumor-infiltrating lymphocytes*—from the tumors of two melanoma patients. He inserted into the cells copies of a gene coding for a potent anticancer protein called *tumor necrosis factor* (TNF).

The cells were then returned to the patients' bodies. The researchers hoped the lymphocytes would home in on clusters of tumor cells that had spread throughout the body and kill them by flooding them with large amounts of TNF.

Although there had been some concerns about the safety of the therapy, Rosenberg later reported that the patients had not been harmed. He said it was still too early to tell if they had been helped.

The NIH scientists hope the gene-therapy trials will prove successful enough to smooth the way for further tests. Even optimistic experts expect gene therapy to advance slowly, with disappointments along the way. Yet the era of genetic medicine is here, and many researchers believe it will transform health care. ☐ Yvonne Baskin

fected, as one would expect. But both the male and female children of those daughters can inherit the syndrome.

A clue to the unusual inheritance pattern of fragile X syndrome was provided earlier in May by researchers in France and Australia. They found that the DNA fragment that is prone to breaking away from the X chromosome is longer in people with the syndrome than in those without it.

How the larger fragment size results in mental impairment is a question that geneticists must now try to answer. While that research proceeds, medical scientists will work on developing a prenatal diagnostic test for fragile X syndrome.

Genes and cancer. New insights into the genetic basis of cancer emerged from several studies published in late 1990 and early 1991. The research centered on *tumor suppressor genes,* one of two broad categories of genes involved in the development of cancer.

The other gene category consists of *oncogenes.* When these genes are either mutated or functioning inappropriately, they transform normal cells into cancerous cells. By contrast, tumor suppressor genes normally control cell growth, preventing the wild cell division that characterizes cancer. When suppressor genes are mutated or absent, however, their regulatory action is missing and cells multiply unchecked.

One recent study shedding new light on the cancer process focused on the role of tumor suppressor genes in a rare hereditary disorder known as *Li-Fraumeni syndrome.* The syndrome afflicts about 100 families worldwide and makes its victims prone to developing cancer relatively early in life—often before age 30. Another study researched colon cancer, one of the leading causes of cancer deaths in the United States.

The Li-Fraumeni research, reported in November 1990, was conducted by a team of scientists at the Massachusetts General Hospital Cancer Center in Boston. The team, led by cancer researcher Stephen Friend, was probing the relationship between tumor suppressor genes and the development of cancer in adults. Li-Fraumeni families are good subjects for such re-

A "protective" gene that causes cancer

Researchers reported in November 1990 that a gene called *p53* is involved in many cases of cancer. Ordinarily, p53 is a type of gene that prevents uncontrolled cell growth. But if p53 becomes *mutated* (changed), cancer can develop.

Most human cells have two copies of p53 in their *chromosomes,* the structures that carry the genes. Some people inherit a mutated p53 on one chromosome, but it causes no harm as long as the other copy of p53 is normal.

If the normal copy of p53 mutates, perhaps from a cancer-causing substance circulating in the body, the gene ceases to carry out its protective function and instead allows cell growth to run wild—the start of cancer.

Scientists have linked p53 with a number of cancers, including cancer of the brain, breast, soft tissues, blood, adrenal glands, and bones. A screening test for the p53 defect would identify people at high risk of developing those cancers.

search because they are susceptible to a variety of cancers.

Friend and his colleagues focused on an important tumor suppressor gene called *p53,* which has been implicated in breast cancer, brain cancer, and several other malignancies. Analyzing the DNA (deoxyribonucleic acid, the molecule that composes genes) of five Li-Fraumeni families, the scientists discovered four specific mutations in the p53 gene. Each cancer patient in those families had one of the p53 mutations in his or her cells.

The mutations were found in normal as well as cancerous cells and were apparently present in every cell of the patients' bodies. That finding indicated that the mutations were inherited instead of occurring in cells after birth.

A genetic mutation that is inherited is present in cells throughout the body, whereas a mutation that is acquired in life affects only a limited number of cells.

The researchers also found at least two cancer-free individuals in the Li-Fraumeni families who had p53 mutations in their cells. Those people were considered to be at high risk for developing cancer.

The investigators said many people in Li-Fraumeni families apparently inherit one copy of the mutated gene along with a normal copy of the gene. (With certain exceptions, each body cell contains two copies of any given gene.) If the normal copy of the p53 gene in just one body cell is somehow knocked out of commission during a person's life—a highly probable occurrence—cancer results.

People in families that are not afflicted with high rates of cancer inherit two normal p53 genes. But they, too, can develop p53-related cancers if both copies of the gene in a cell become mutated. Cancer researchers now suspect that a mutated p53 gene may be the most common genetic defect involved in human cancers. See also CANCER.

Colon cancer. Researchers reported in March and August 1991 the discovery of two apparent tumor suppressor genes, which, when mutated, seem to trigger the development of *colorectal cancer* (cancer of the colon and rectum). The research groups—which included investigators from the Molecular Genetics Center at Johns Hopkins University in Baltimore, the University of Utah in Salt Lake City, and the Cancer Institute in Tokyo, Japan—named the genes MCC, for *mutated in colorectal cancer,* and APC, for *adenomatous polyposis coli.*

Doctors hope a screening test can be devised to detect mutations in the MCC gene. Such a test could identify individuals who have colorectal cancer while the disease is still in an early stage. Meanwhile, biologists are trying to determine the function of the proteins that the MCC and APC genes code for. Once the proteins' roles are understood, colorectal cancer might

be prevented with drugs that replace missing protein products. See also CANCER and DIGESTIVE SYSTEM.

Continued work on the genetics of cancer is leading specialists toward an understanding of the disease that recognizes the importance of both oncogenes and tumor suppressor genes in the development of malignancies. Research indicates that the process of transforming a normal cell into a cancer cell always involves a complex series of steps in which both kinds of genes play important roles.

Lou Gehrig's disease. The location of a gene associated with an inherited form of *amyotrophic lateral sclerosis* (ALS), a fatal nervous-system disorder, was reported in May 1991 by a team of scientists at several medical centers in the United States. ALS is commonly known as Lou Gehrig's disease, for the famous baseball player who died of the illness in 1941.

ALS usually strikes after age 50. The disorder causes nerve cells controlling the skeletal muscles to deteriorate and die. There is no effective treatment, and the disease is usually fatal within five years of onset. Although the underlying cause of ALS is not known, 5 to 10 per cent of cases run in families, indicating that those cases have a genetic basis.

To find the gene involved in hereditary ALS, the researchers—led by neurologist Teepu Siddique of North-

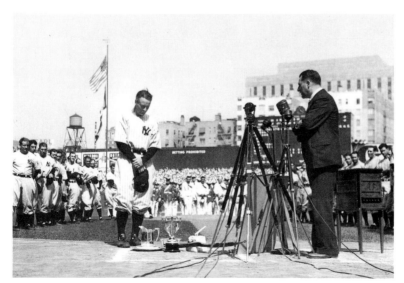

Lou Gehrig's disease
Researchers in May 1991 reported finding the approximate location of a gene associated with an inherited form of *amyotrophic lateral sclerosis* (ALS), a fatal disorder of the nervous system. ALS is commonly known as *Lou Gehrig's disease* for the New York Yankees first baseman who died of ALS in 1941. Gehrig, *left,* head bowed, was honored at Yankee Stadium in July 1939, shortly after the disease ended his career.

western University Medical School in Chicago—studied the DNA of 23 families in which the disease has afflicted individuals in several generations. The scientists used a technique called *genetic linkage analysis,* which enabled them to trace a particular gene to a segment of a chromosome.

The investigators narrowed the location of the ALS gene to a region of chromosome 21. Finding the approximate location of the gene is the first step toward isolating the gene and learning its function. That, in turn, could lead to an understanding of ALS and perhaps to ways of treating or preventing the disease.

Because the inherited form of the disease is indistinguishable from the nonhereditary form, geneticists think that the same biochemical abnormality may underlie all cases of ALS. People who contract nonhereditary ALS may acquire a genetic defect, perhaps caused by an environmental factor. That same defect is present at birth in those who develop the inherited form of the disease. More than one gene may be involved in the disease, however, and Siddique's group concluded from their research that other genes on other chromosomes may also cause ALS.   □ Joseph D. McInerney

See also BRAIN AND NERVOUS SYSTEM. In WORLD BOOK, see CELL; GENETICS; CANCER.

Glands and Hormones

Contrary to common belief, vigorous exercise does not disrupt a woman's menstrual cycle nor does it cause a weakening of the bones. Those conclusions were reported in November 1990 by a team of researchers from the University of British Columbia in Vancouver, Canada. According to the researchers, bone loss in female athletes as well as female nonathletes may result from subtle abnormalities in the menstrual cycle.

In the past, some studies have found reduced levels of sex hormones in women who exercise vigorously. As a result, many researchers hypothesized that strenuous exercise causes women to stop *ovulating* (releasing an egg). The cessation of ovulation, in turn, leads to a reduction in the production of the female hormone *estrogen.* Estrogen slows the destruction of bone tissue, which is replenished constantly. But when the body fails to make enough new bone, a significant loss of bone mass may lead to *osteoporosis,* a crippling bone disorder.

The researchers charted the menstrual cycles of 21 female marathon runners and a similar group of less active women for one year. The medical researchers also estimated the loss of bone mass in the women's spines using an X-ray technique. They reported that the athletes were no more likely to have irregular menstrual cycles than were the less active women. In addition, the researchers reported no difference in the loss of bone mass between the women in the two groups.

The researchers did, however, find a significant bone loss in women with two subtle menstrual irregularities, regardless of how strenuously they exercised. These irregularities were a failure to ovulate and a shortened *luteal phase* of the menstrual cycle. The luteal phase of the cycle is the interval between ovulation and the beginning of menstrual bleeding. During this second phase of the menstrual cycle, the level of the hormone *progesterone* rises. The irregularities are difficult to detect because they do not affect the length of the menstrual cycle or the heaviness of the flow.

The researchers reported that women with either of the irregularities lost an average of 4 per cent of their spinal bone mass during the year of the study. In contrast, the women with normal menstrual cycles either lost no spinal bone mass or gained a small amount during the study.

The researchers theorized that the bone loss in women with the irregularities resulted from deficiencies in progesterone, which may stimulate the development of new bone tissue. They reported that women with the greatest amount of bone loss had the lowest levels of progesterone.

Benefits of estrogen. The benefits of taking estrogen supplements after menopause outweigh the risk of developing cancer. That conclusion was reported in January 1991 by medical

A Health & Medical Annual Close-Up

A Medical Mystery at the White House

When President George Bush set off on his daily run on May 4, 1991, he stepped into a medical mystery. After jogging for only a few hundred yards, Bush became winded.

Doctors found that the President had developed *atrial fibrillation*. In this condition, the contractions of the heart's upper chamber are more rapid and weaker than normal, and so less oxygen-rich blood is pumped into the body. Bush's shortness of breath occurred because his heart could not meet his body's oxygen demands. Doctors soon determined that his erratic heartbeat was caused by Graves' disease, a condition that had also been diagnosed in his wife, Barbara, 18 months earlier.

Graves' disease is an *autoimmune disorder*—a condition in which blood cells that normally fight disease-producing organisms attack the body's own tissue. In Graves' disease, the targets are mainly the thyroid and eye sockets.

The thyroid, a gland located in the front of the throat, produces *thyroxine*, a hormone that helps regulate the activity of several organs, including the heart, and the nervous system. Thyroxine also regulates the body's *metabolic rate*, the rate at which the cells consume food energy.

In Graves' disease, the body's disease-fighting cells cause the thyroid to produce excess amounts of thyroxine. As a result, people with the disease may develop an irregular heartbeat, feel fidgety, and lose weight even though they are eating normally. The disease may also weaken the muscles holding the eye in place and cause the tissues behind the eyes to swell.

The cause of Graves' disease is unknown. Many scientists suspect that it may be triggered when a virus or other microorganism whose surface resembles that of the cells of the thyroid and eyes infects the body. When the immune system attacks the invader, it also attacks those body cells.

Although both Bushes had sudden, unexplained weight losses, other symptoms of the disorder varied. Mrs. Bush developed blurred vision and dry eyes rather than an irregular heart rate.

When treating patients with Graves' disease, doctors first reduce the thyroid's production of thyroxine to normal levels. Because thyroxine levels may fluctuate, some physicians prefer to give Graves' patients drugs to regulate the hormone only when its level rises. Other doctors prefer to correct the problem by surgically removing part of the thyroid. Doctors sometimes have patients drink solutions containing a small amount of radioactive iodine, which selectively kills cells in the thyroid gland. President Bush underwent this treatment.

Patients with mild inflammation of the eyes may find relief by sleeping with their head elevated to reduce swelling or by using medicated drops to keep the eyes moist. Those with severe inflammation may require stronger medication. Some patients, such as Mrs. Bush, also undergo radiation treatments to destroy swollen tissue behind the eyes.

In addition to the Bushes, Millie, the Bushes' dog, was diagnosed as having an autoimmune disease—a condition related to rheumatoid arthritis. Because such an occurrence was so unusual, White House physicians ordered tests of the Bushes' water supply. But these analyses failed to reveal any clues to the puzzle. Researchers hoped, however, that the first family's problems would lead to an increased effort to find the cause of Graves' disease. ☐ Beverly Merz

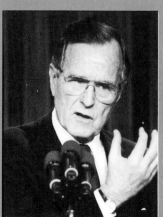
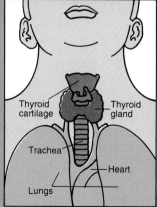

Thyroid cartilage

Thyroid gland

Trachea

Heart

Lungs

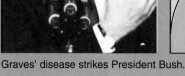
Graves' disease strikes President Bush.

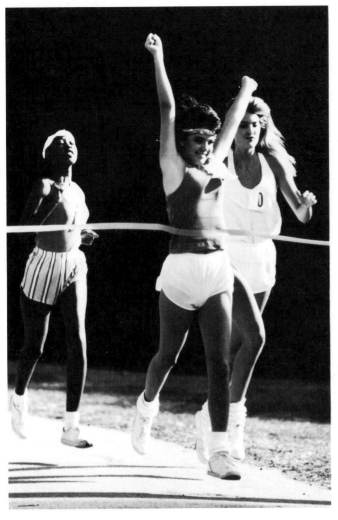

A win for exercise
Vigorous exercise does not disrupt a woman's menstrual cycle or weaken her bones, according to a November 1990 study. Canadian researchers compared female athletes with less active women and found menstrual irregularities and bone loss equally common in both groups. The scientists theorized that bone loss in some women resulted from abnormalities in the menstrual cycle unrelated to exercise.

researchers at the University of Southern California (USC) in Los Angeles.

Estrogen, which is produced in smaller amounts after *menopause* (the time in a woman's life when menstruation ceases), is often prescribed to prevent hot flashes, osteoporosis, stroke, and heart disease in postmenopausal women. Previous studies, however, had found that women who take the hormone are more likely than nonusers to develop cancer of the uterus. Some studies have also found an increased risk of breast cancer, though other studies have failed to confirm these findings.

The USC researchers followed the medical history of 8,853 post-menopausal women for 7½ years. They found that the death rate for women

who took estrogen supplements at some time after menopause was 20 per cent lower than the rate for the women who did not take estrogen. Moreover, the death rate for women who took the supplements for at least the last 15 years of their life was 40 per cent lower than it was for non-users. In practical terms, the findings indicate that women who have taken estrogen supplements at some time after menopause may live 1.2 years longer, while long-term users may live 2.5 years longer than nonusers.

The researchers also reported that women who took estrogen supplements were three times more likely to develop uterine cancer than nonusers. There was no difference, however, in the rate of breast cancer between the two groups, and the overall death rate from cancer among estrogen users was no higher than that of nonusers.

High blood pressure. A plant substance used as a heart drug may also be produced naturally by the human body, scientists reported in September 1990. Furthermore, the hormone-like substance, called *ouabain*, may play an important role in the development of many cases of high blood pressure. Ouabain is a member of the digitalis family of drugs, which have long been used to treat some types of heart disease.

Scientists from the University of Maryland in Baltimore and the Upjohn Company in Kalamazoo, Mich., reported that they had found higher-than-normal levels of ouabain in the blood of 60 per cent of the patients in their study. The cause of the patients' high blood pressure, like that of the majority of people with the condition, was unknown.

The researchers theorized that ouabain causes high blood pressure by interfering with the action of a protein that regulates the movement of sodium out of body cells. Scientists believe that excessive levels of sodium in cells lead to a build-up of calcium. Calcium, in turn, stimulates muscle contractions in the walls of blood vessels, triggering an increase in blood pressure. ☐ William Jubiz

In the Special Reports section, see THE PUZZLE OF PMS. In WORLD BOOK, see GLAND; HORMONE.

Hospitals and other health-care facilities were at the center of major political and legal disputes in the United States in 1990 and 1991. One controversy concerned whether nonprofit hospitals should retain their state and federal tax exemptions. The Internal Revenue Service in 1969 had eliminated a requirement that nonprofit hospitals provide some charity care to the uninsured poor in order to retain tax exemptions. In 1990, federal and state officials questioned whether hospitals continued to offer enough charity care to merit their $8.5-billion tax break.

Hospitals were challenged, and also sometimes taxed, in Utah, Pennsylvania, and Texas, and by mid-1991, at least 17 other states were considering similar actions. Although hospitals claimed that they were providing sufficient "community benefit" to merit their exemptions, representatives submitted legislation to Congress in 1991 that would force hospitals to provide a minimum amount of charity care to retain their tax breaks.

Patient "dumping." The long-standing legal controversy over patient "dumping" flared again during 1991. Dumping is the practice of transferring a patient from one hospital to another because the patient is uninsured and unable to pay for care. In July 1991, the U.S. Department of Health and Human Services won its case against a Texas physician who in 1986 had become the first doctor charged under federal law with dumping. The physician had transferred an uninsured woman in labor to a hospital 170 miles (274 kilometers) away.

Patient rights. Hospitals became more involved in the ongoing issue of patients' rights and termination of treatment in 1990 and 1991. A provision in the 1990 Omnibus Budget Reconciliation Act called for each patient admitted to a hospital to be informed of his or her rights, under state law, to refuse care and to draw up living wills or other advance directives concerning medical care.

A living will is a document written by a mentally competent adult that states the person does or does not wish certain medical procedures to be taken on his or her behalf to prolong life should that person become terminally ill. The Patient Self-Determination Act was scheduled to go into effect on Dec. 1, 1991.

Public hospitals (those owned by cities, counties, or states) in 1991 were serving a rising number of medically indigent people—individuals who are too poor to pay for hospital insurance but who do not qualify for government assistance. AIDS patients and emergency cases arising from violent crime added to overcrowding of public hospitals in 1990 and 1991.

Health-Care Facilities

Sensored for safety
An infant born in Malden Hospital in Malden, Mass., wears an ankle bracelet containing an electronic sensor as part of the hospital's program to deter kidnapping. In February 1991, the hospital began issuing the devices, which set off alarms at specially wired exits.

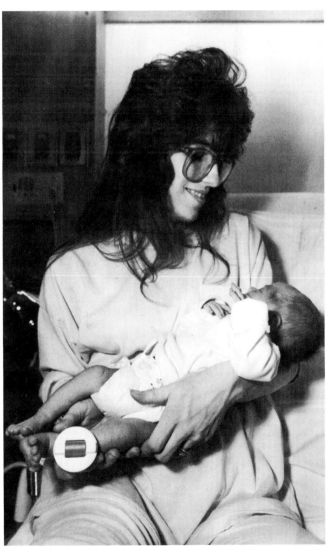

In January 1991, the National Association of Public Hospitals reported results of a 1988 survey of 57 large public hospitals in major cities that illustrated the strains on these institutions. Despite local and state financial assistance, the hospitals surveyed averaged a loss of $9.4 billion in 1988. These hospitals also averaged 19,000 drug-related emergency room visits, accounting for nearly 30 per cent of total emergency cases. The survey also found that the wait for admission to these hospitals averaged 5.5 hours, but could be as long as 10 days.

Hospital finances. The overall *margins* (income that exceeds expenses) of U.S. hospitals were down in 1990, averaging 4.8 per cent as opposed to 5.0 per cent in 1989. It cost hospitals more to care for patients in 1990 than they received through billing for patient care, according to the American Hospital Association (AHA). Charitable donations, investments, and other revenues not involving direct care to patients paid the difference between expenses for and revenues from patient care, the AHA said.

The levels of reimbursement from the two largest public programs, Medicare and Medicaid, contributed to hospitals' shaky finances. The AHA reported that neither program paid all of the costs for treating patients it covered. In 1991, the AHA released the results of a 1989 survey that had

found on average, Medicaid paid only 78.3 per cent of the cost incurred by covered patients. Illinois paid the least—only 53 per cent of the cost. New Jersey paid the most, 106 per cent, or slightly more than the hospitals' costs. Total losses to hospitals due to insufficient Medicaid payments and the unpaid medical bills of uninsured patients were $13.2 billion in 1989, nearly four times the $3.5 billion reported in 1980.

Financial troubles contributed to the closing of 63 hospitals in 1990, down from 80 in 1989. Texas had the most closings, with 13 hospitals. More rural hospitals closed in 1990 than urban facilities—28 versus 22. Although 43 hospitals opened, 37 of these were facilities specializing in psychiatric or substance-abuse care.

The trend of declining patient admissions continued, although at a relatively moderate pace, with admissions for 1990 down 0.5 per cent from those in 1989. In contrast, from 1980 through 1990, total admissions dropped by 12 per cent. However, outpatient visits continued to rise, reaching 243.4 million in 1990, a 6 per cent increase over the 1989 total.

Although hospitals continued to face staff shortages in 1990 and 1991, the national nursing shortage did ease somewhat. As of April 1990, 11 per cent of positions for registered nurses were unfilled, down from 12.7 per cent in 1989. However, the rate varied

The emergency room is the largest drain on a hospital's finances, according to a 1990 survey of hospital executives. But only 10 per cent of these executives said they would reduce emergency room services if under financial pressure to keep their hospitals open. Obstetrics is considered the next most unprofitable hospital service, and 22 per cent of the executives surveyed said they would cut back in this area if financially pressured.

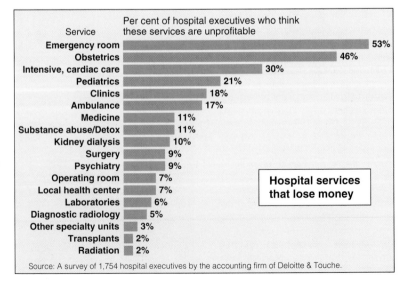

Service	Per cent of hospital executives who think these services are unprofitable
Emergency room	53%
Obstetrics	46%
Intensive, cardiac care	30%
Pediatrics	21%
Clinics	18%
Ambulance	17%
Medicine	11%
Substance abuse/Detox	11%
Kidney dialysis	10%
Surgery	9%
Psychiatry	9%
Operating room	7%
Local health center	7%
Laboratories	6%
Diagnostic radiology	5%
Other specialty units	3%
Transplants	2%
Radiation	2%

Hospital services that lose money

Source: A survey of 1,754 hospital executives by the accounting firm of Deloitte & Touche.

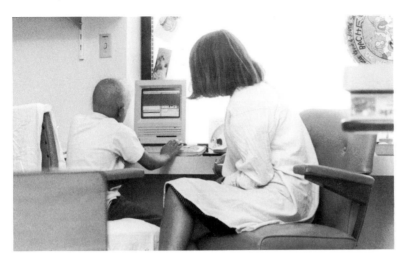

according to region, with New England having the fewest vacancies and southern and southwestern states having the most.

Nursing homes. There were an estimated 18,900 nursing homes in the United States in 1990, according to the American Health Care Association. They had 1.6 million beds and were caring for 1.5 million residents, 1.3 million of whom were 65 years old or older.

The increasing use of nursing home care by older Americans was documented in a federal study published in February 1991. The study predicted that 43 per cent of Americans who turned 65 in 1991 would eventually require at least some nursing home care during the rest of their lives.

Beginning Oct. 1, 1990, new federal rules for nursing home care required patient care plans that involved the patient and the family. The rules also limited the use of restraints and drugs on patients when done for the sole purpose of helping the staff control undesirable behavior. Some states were reluctant to accept the rules.

□ Emily Ann Friedman

See also FINANCING MEDICAL CARE; HEALTH POLICY. In the People in Health Care section, see CARING FOR THE TERMINALLY ILL. In WORLD BOOK, see HOSPITAL.

Health Policy

Health insurance for the uninsured, questions about the risk of infection with the virus that causes AIDS, and the ongoing debate over abortion dominated health policy discussions in 1990 and 1991.

Health insurance. The effort to find a means of providing health coverage for the growing number of Americans without health insurance gained momentum in 1990 and 1991 as several powerful interests entered the fray. An estimated 31 million to 37 million Americans lack any form of health insurance.

The Democratic Party leadership in the United States Congress in June 1991 announced a broad health-care reform strategy called *HealthAmerica*. If enacted, the program would require all employers to either provide subsidized health insurance to their workers, or pay a 5 to 8 per cent payroll tax. HealthAmerica would use the tax funds to provide insurance for those employees not covered by a subsidized plan. The plan also called for a new public program called *AmeriCare* to supersede the financially beleaguered Medicaid program and to cover the unemployed Americans who would not be covered under HealthAmerica. (Medicaid is a joint state-federal program that provides health coverage to some low-income and disabled people.)

The bill had strong political support

A Health & Medical Annual Close-Up

The Legacy of Nancy Cruzan

More than seven years after the 1983 auto accident that rendered her permanently unconscious, Nancy Beth Cruzan, age 33, died in a Missouri nursing home on Dec. 26, 1990. Her plight and its resolution brought to national attention issues regarding the right of patients and their families to refuse or terminate treatment.

Because Cruzan's condition left her unable to swallow, she was kept alive by a feeding tube that provided fluid and nutrition. In January 1984, her parents were appointed her legal guardians. Convinced that their daughter would not wish to continue in what doctors described as a "persistent vegetative state" with no possibility of returning to consciousness, they sued in 1988 for the right to end the artificial sustenance.

Missouri Circuit Court Judge Charles E. Teel, Jr., granted their petition, based on reports that she had told friends she would not wish to live a life that was not "at least halfway normal." However, the attorney general of Missouri appealed the decision to the state supreme court, which denied the Cruzans' request, saying the state had a compelling interest in preserving life.

The Cruzans appealed to the Supreme Court of the United States, which upheld Missouri in a 5 to 4 decision on June 25, 1990. The court based its decision on the lack of "clear and convincing evidence" of Nancy Cruzan's wishes. However, the Supreme Court's ruling accepted the argument put forward by attorneys for the Cruzans that a competent adult has the right to refuse treatment.

In her concurring opinion, Justice Sandra Day O'Connor stated that if Cruzan had designated a surrogate to make health decisions for her in the event of her being unable to do so, Justice O'Connor may well have supported a surrogate's decision to end life support.

In December 1990, the Cruzans again appeared before Judge Teel, asking that the tube be disconnected, based on new testimony. Three of Nancy Cruzan's friends testified that she had explicitly stated her opposition to living in a comatose state, thus offering "clear and convincing evidence" of her wishes. Judge Teel again decided in favor of the Cruzans, and on Dec. 14, 1990, the tube was removed.

What was Nancy Cruzan's legacy? Her case was the first instance in which the U.S. Supreme Court recognized a person's right to refuse treatment. In addition, the opinion of Justice O'Connor that designating surrogates could prevent similar situations from occurring set off a sudden round

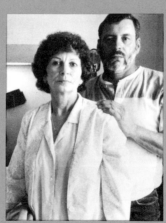

Nancy Cruzan's parents.

of interest in health-care surrogates and *living wills.* (A living will is a legal document stating a person's wishes regarding the circumstances under which he or she would refuse further treatment.) At least 45 states have enacted living-will statutes, and 29 states allow individuals to give power of attorney to another person in case the individual becomes legally incompetent.

The Cruzan case also helped spur the U.S. Congress to pass the Patient Self-Determination Act in 1990. The new law requires that every patient being admitted to a hospital or nursing home be informed of state law regarding his or her rights to refuse treatment. The new law, which goes into effect on Dec. 1, 1991, also stipulates that health-care providers must inform patients of state law regarding the patient's right to execute advance directives, such as designating a surrogate or stipulating whether he or she would want extraordinary measures to be taken in order to be kept alive.

It remains to be seen whether the Supreme Court's decision or the Patient Self-Determination Act will help establish sufficient guidelines for judging the often-difficult ethical issues posed by the so-called right-to-die. The legal wrangling is over for Nancy Cruzan's parents, but not for many others. It seems likely that state laws will continue to vary. Thus, legal experts believe, the fate of patients and families may depend primarily on where they live, a situation that is sure to lead to more litigation.

□ Emily Ann Friedman

among Democrats, but Republicans were less enthusiastic. Louis W. Sullivan, secretary of the U.S. Department of Health and Human Services, in February 1991 said he opposed a federally funded and controlled insurance system but supported expansion and reform of Medicaid. Other key officials of the Administration of President George Bush, including Richard G. Darman, head of the Office of Management and Budget, predicted that the Administration would unveil a health-care reform proposal before the 1992 presidential election.

Health-care reform activity continued at the state government level as well. Some states have been at the forefront of health-care reform, enacting plans to provide coverage for the uninsured without waiting for the federal government to act. But some of those early programs encountered problems during the year.

Faced with a massive budget deficit, Republican Governor William F. Weld of Massachusetts in February 1991 sought repeal of the state's universal coverage statute. The legislature did not comply but in its spring session failed to appropriate funds for the program, thus making its full implementation in 1992 highly unlikely. The Minnesota legislature passed a modified universal access statute, but Republican Governor Arne H. Carlson vetoed it in June 1991, citing lack of funds.

The Oregon legislature in June 1991 adopted a plan for "rationing" Medicaid services by limiting what types of care would be provided but increasing enrollment in the program for women and children by raising income eligibility to the federal poverty line. Of some 700 services that could be covered, 122 were eliminated, including treatment for patients with Alzheimer's disease and patients with end-stage AIDS who were unlikely to survive for five years.

However, the cutbacks cannot be implemented without permission from either Congress or the Health Care Financing Administration (HCFA). Oregon was likely to seek such permission from HCFA Administrator Gail Wilensky, who appeared receptive to the state's plan.

AIDS testing and disclosure. Legal and political battles loomed over legislative proposals that would require physicians and dentists who have AIDS to disclose their disease to patients. The controversy was sparked by the revelation in January 1991 that David J. Acer, a Florida dentist, had apparently infected at least five of his patients with human immunodeficiency virus (HIV), the cause of AIDS. One of those patients, Kimberly Bergalis, waged a highly visible and emotional campaign for required HIV testing of health-care providers before she became too ill to continue.

Higher death rates among blacks	
Disease	Death rate
Tuberculosis	8.9 times higher
Hypertensive heart disease	6.5 times higher
Asthma	4.4 times higher
Pneumonia and bronchitis	3.8 times higher
Appendicitis	3.2 times higher
Rheumatic heart disease	2.8 times higher
Cervical cancer	2.6 times higher
Hernias	2.4 times higher
Acute respiratory disease	2 times higher
Gallbladder infection	1.6 times higher
Influenza	1.3 times higher

Source: International Journal of Epidemiology.

American blacks are more likely than whites to die of 11 preventable or easily controlled diseases, health officials in Washington, D.C., reported in a September 1990 study. Of the nearly 122,000 Americans who died of these diseases from 1980 to 1986, more than 80 per cent were black, though blacks account for only 12 per cent of the total United States population.

In March 1991, the U.S. government identified 19 cities that were eligible for $171 million in federal grants to combat their very high infant mortality rates. Based on data for a five-year period, the figures show that Washington, D.C., had the highest rate of the 19 cities, with an average of 21.1 deaths in the first year of life per 1,000 live births. Each year in the United States, about 40,000 infants die before their first birthday.

Infant mortality in the United States (1984-1988)

(Average annual number of deaths in the first year of life per 1,000 live births)

Washington, D.C.	21.10	St. Louis, Mo.	15.13
Detroit	20.38	Kansas City, Mo.	13.85
Newark, N.J.	18.61	Indianapolis	13.63
Baltimore	17.43	Boston	13.41
Memphis	17.00	New York City	12.83
Philadelphia	16.68	Milwaukee	12.79
Atlanta	16.50	Jacksonville, Fla.	12.67
Chicago	16.26	Houston	11.43
Cleveland	16.11	Los Angeles	10.54
New Orleans	15.31		

Source: U.S. Health & Human Services.

The American Dental Association on Jan. 17, 1991, recommended that dentists infected with HIV inform their patients or stop performing procedures that could infect patients. And after much debate at its summer meeting in July 1991, the American Medical Association (AMA) voted to oppose mandatory testing of patients or health-care providers as too unwieldy and expensive. But the AMA encouraged voluntary testing of those who might be at higher risk of carrying the virus.

On July 18, in a surprise vote, the U.S. Senate passed a bill providing for jail terms of up to 10 years for HIV-positive health-care providers who "knowingly" fail to disclose their status to patients. Sponsored by Senator Jesse Helms (R., N.C.), the bill was not expected to survive in the U.S. House of Representatives. However, a second bill, also passed by the Senate in July 1991, asking states to enact tougher guidelines for testing and protective practices involving health-care providers, was thought to have a better chance of passage.

Abortion counseling. On May 23, 1991, the Supreme Court of the United States dealt another blow to abortion rights advocates. In *Rust v. Sullivan*, the court ruled that federal regulations banning the counseling or even mention of abortion by staff at family planning clinics receiving federal funds were constitutional. Several groups, including the AMA and the

American College of Obstetricians and Gynecologists, protested the decision as interference in the private relationship between a doctor and a patient. By September, the House and Senate had passed legislation overturning the ban.

In 1990, the Louisiana legislature passed a stringent abortion law that prohibited the procedure except in cases of rape, incest, or risk of the mother's life. Democratic Governor Charles E. (Buddy) Roemer III vetoed the measure, but on June 18, 1991, the legislature voted to override the veto. The law, which provides for fines and jail sentences for physicians who perform abortions that do not meet these conditions, faced its first legal challenge in August when a federal district court judge ruled the new law unconstitutional.

Right to die. Nancy Beth Cruzan died on Dec. 26, 1990, ending an emotional case that pitted the state of Missouri against the comatose woman's parents, who had sought to end artificial nutrition and hydration for their daughter (see Close-Up). In July 1991, a county probate judge in Minnesota ruled that a local hospital could not remove life support from Helga Wanglie, a comatose 87-year-old woman, as the hospital had wanted to do. Her husband had sued to prevent the removal. Helga Wanglie died three days after the court decision. □ Emily Ann Friedman

In WORLD BOOK, see HEALTH CARE.

Hearing
See Ear and Hearing

A new battery-powered device that helps a failing heart pump blood was first implanted into a patient on May 9, 1991, by surgeons at the Texas Heart Institute at St. Luke's Episcopal Hospital in Houston. The implant was designed to support the heart's functioning until doctors could perform a heart transplant.

The pump, called a *left ventricular assist device*, does not replace the entire heart, as did a type of artificial heart that was implanted in several patients in the 1980's. Instead, the new device helps the heart's main pumping chamber, the *left ventricle*, pump blood into the *aorta*, the body's main artery.

Surgeons place the pump in the abdomen and use tubing to attach it to the left ventricle and to the aorta. Blood drains from the left ventricle through the tubing and into the pump, where it is then pushed through another tube and into the aorta. A wire runs from the pump to an external battery pack that the patient wears like a holster slung over the shoulder. This design allows the patient to leave the hospital and move about freely.

Women and heart disease. Women fare worse than men after a heart attack and are more likely than men to die during surgery to bypass clogged arteries, according to two independent studies reported in 1990 and in 1991. Cardiology researchers in Israel reported in February 1991 an evaluation of the death rates of women and men who had experienced a heart attack. The rates were adjusted for age because women with heart disease are older, and older people have higher overall death rates compared with younger people.

The researchers found that among 1,524 women who were hospitalized for a heart attack, the age-adjusted death rate was 23 per cent. The age-adjusted rate for 4,315 men studied was 16 per cent. When the researchers considered all the factors known to influence survival after a heart attack, female gender alone appeared to account for an increased death rate during hospitalization and one year after a heart attack.

Cardiac surgeon Thierry Follinguet

of Downstate Medical Center in New York City reported at a November 1990 American Heart Association (AHA) meeting in Dallas that women are more likely than men to die during *coronary artery bypass surgery*, an operation that uses part of a vein or artery taken from the patient's leg or chest to detour around clogged portions of an artery. In a study of 1,297 patients, Follinguet found that 12 per cent of women undergoing bypass surgery died within two months of the operation, contrasted with a death rate of 7 per cent for men.

An evaluation of 15 factors—including age—that may affect survival dur-

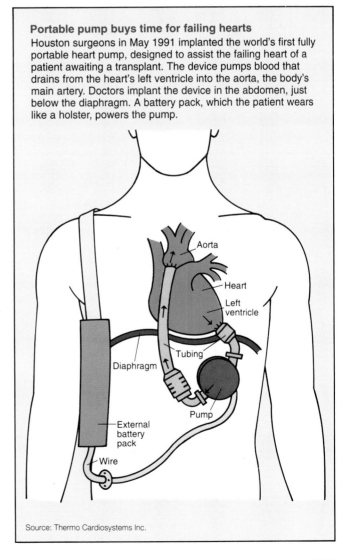

Portable pump buys time for failing hearts
Houston surgeons in May 1991 implanted the world's first fully portable heart pump, designed to assist the failing heart of a patient awaiting a transplant. The device pumps blood that drains from the heart's left ventricle into the aorta, the body's main artery. Doctors implant the device in the abdomen, just below the diaphragm. A battery pack, which the patient wears like a holster, powers the pump.

Aorta

Heart

Left ventricle

Tubing

Diaphragm

Pump

External battery pack

Wire

Source: Thermo Cardiosystems Inc.

ing bypass surgery did not explain the difference in death rates. Follinguet concluded that women's anatomy and physiology differs from that of men in some way that affects the results of surgery. For example, he noted that women's typically smaller blood vessels may be harder to sew together and may clog more quickly than men's vessels.

These studies and others raised concern in Congress that not enough federally funded research is directed at heart and *vascular* (blood vessel) disease in women. Cardiologist Bernardine Healy, director of the National Institutes of Health in Bethesda, Md., announced that she would form a special research group to study women's diseases.

Although *coronary artery disease* (CAD)—a progressive narrowing or blockage of blood vessels leading to the heart—is the number one cause of death for both men and women, most research has targeted men. Scientists have generally assumed that conclusions they based on studies of men would also pertain to women. These recent studies contradict this assumption and challenge the medical community to study women more thoroughly in the future.

Cholesterol and heart disease. The first scientific evidence showing that reducing cholesterol in the blood decreases the risk of dying from coronary heart disease was published in October 1990. Although physicians have thought that high levels of blood cholesterol increased the risk of developing coronary artery disease, previous studies showed no improvement in overall death rates when cholesterol levels were lowered.

The new, 10-year study evaluated 838 patients at six U.S. medical centers who had suffered one heart attack and had high cholesterol levels. About half of the patients were delegated as the control group. They received standard medical treatment, which included instructions to eat a diet that limited fat and cholesterol. Many patients in this group also took cholesterol-lowering drugs at some time during the study. More than 30 per cent were taking one or more such drugs at the end of the study.

The other group of patients underwent surgery in which doctors detached a section of the small intestine that passes cholesterol into the blood and reattached it to the large intestine. The large intestine excretes cholesterol in feces rather than routing it to the bloodstream. These patients also received dietary instructions. Only a small proportion of surgical patients took cholesterol-lowering drugs, and less than 4 per cent were taking such drugs at the end of the study.

Total cholesterol levels (a combination of two kinds of cholesterol: one that clogs the arteries and one that helps clear arteries) in the intestinal bypass patients were about 23 per cent lower than levels in the control group of patients who did not have the intestinal bypass. The type of cholesterol that can build up in the arteries and lead to heart disease was nearly 38 per cent lower in the surgical patients than in the control group. This decline in cholesterol levels was much greater than decreases noted in previous studies that used other cholesterol-lowering techniques.

The overall death rate among the intestinal bypass patients was not significantly lower than that of the control group, primarily because intestinal bypass patients whose hearts were badly damaged at the beginning of the study did not appear to benefit from lowered cholesterol levels. However, bypass patients whose hearts were not damaged when the study began had a 36 per cent lower death rate than the control patients. They also had fewer heart attacks after surgery and needed fewer invasive procedures to correct clogged arteries. Tests of the intestinal bypass patients confirmed that their coronary arteries had less build-up of fatty deposits.

Although the bypass surgery dramatically lowered blood cholesterol, the researchers did not advocate it as a means of achieving that goal. More studies are required to determine surgery's role in managing coronary heart disease, they said.

Aspirin studies inconclusive. Aspirin can prevent heart attacks in certain individuals but may not decrease the risk of stroke, according to a report presented at an AHA meeting in

Common heart disorder affects President Bush

A common heart abnormality, *atrial fibrillation,* became news when President George Bush was hospitalized in May 1991. Doctors treated Bush with drugs to slow the abnormally fast heartbeat that characterizes the disorder and determined that the problem was caused by an overactive thyroid gland. Atrial fibrillation, which affects about 1 million Americans, can have other causes but is not usually life-threatening.

When the heart beats normally, its upper chambers (the left atrium and the right atrium) and its lower chambers (the left and right ventricles) work in a coordinated fashion to receive and pump blood. The atria contract to force blood into the ventricles, which, in turn, contract to push the blood into the aorta and the pulmonary artery, the chief arteries of the heart. In atrial fibrillation, the atria's contractions are too rapid and weak. As a result, blood may collect in the atria or back up into the lungs and cause shortness of breath. If the atrial fibrillation is untreated, blood clots may form, enter the bloodstream, and cause a stroke or a heart attack.

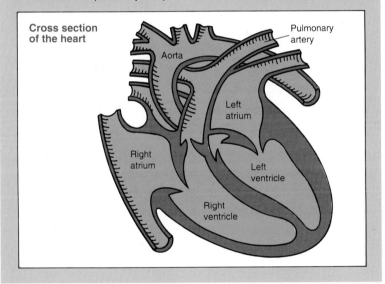

Cross section of the heart

Pulmonary artery

Aorta

Left atrium

Right atrium

Left ventricle

Right ventricle

Dallas in November 1990. The finding resulted from the Physicians Health Study, an ongoing project sponsored by the National Heart, Lung, and Blood Institute, which is researching the health of 20,000 U.S. physicians.

Heart attacks occur when *platelets*, small disklike structures in the blood, stick to fatty deposits in the arteries leading to the heart. This causes a blood clot to form, which narrows the artery and prevents a normal flow of oxygen-rich blood to the heart. Without adequate blood and oxygen, part of the heart stops functioning.

Scientific evidence has shown that aspirin can prevent heart attacks by stopping a build-up of platelets on fatty deposits. This knowledge has led physicians to prescribe an aspirin a day for some people who are at increased risk for a heart attack.

This study, presented at the AHA meeting, focused on 333 physician-patients who had coronary artery disease. About half of the physicians were randomly assigned to take one aspirin every other day. The others were given *placebos* (pills containing an inactive substance). The physicians who took aspirin had one-third fewer heart attacks than the physicians who took placebos. However, the physicians who used aspirin were five times more likely to have a stroke than were those who used no aspirin. Consequently, the overall death rate was the same for both groups.

A British study reported in 1988 had also showed an increased rate of

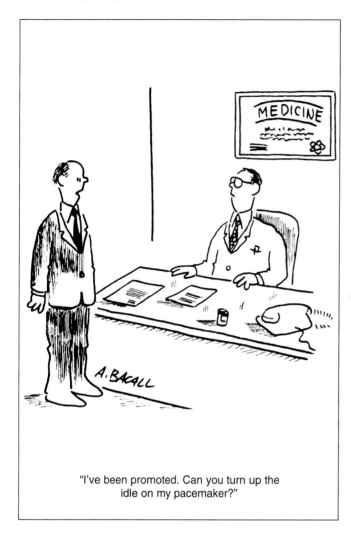

"I've been promoted. Can you turn up the idle on my pacemaker?"

If heart-attack victims obtain medical attention within a few hours after they start to feel chest pain, doctors can give them a drug that may dissolve the blood clot plugging their coronary artery and prevent severe heart damage. In this study, physicians compared the effectiveness of three clot-dissolving drugs. Streptokinase, the standard drug, costs about $200 per dose, while newer drugs, tissue plasminogen activator (tPA) and anisoylated plasminogen-streptokinase activator complex (APSAC), cost about $2,000 per dose.

All three drugs showed the same rate of success in treating a heart attack and restoring normal heart function. However, in patients who took the newer drugs, the incidence of strokes caused by bleeding in the brain was twice as high as in those who received streptokinase.

Heart valve replacement. In a study published in February 1991, cardiologists in Scotland reported that two types of artificial heart valves caused problems in patients. When one of the valves that controls the flow of blood in the heart becomes severely diseased, surgeons can often replace it with an artificial valve. Physicians use two major types of prosthetic valves: those made of animal tissue and those made of metal or plastic (mechanical valves).

In the study, the researchers compared 533 patients who had been randomly assigned to receive one of the two types of valves. After 12 years, four times as many patients with animal-tissue valves required further surgery to correct valve failure, compared with patients who had mechanical valves. But significant bleeding occurred three times as often in the patients with mechanical valves as in those with animal-tissue valves.

Bleeding occurred more often with mechanical valve users because these patients usually require lifelong drugs to prevent blood clots from forming on the valve. Because these drugs inhibit clot formation throughout the body, patients who take them may require hospitalization to control episodes of bleeding. ☐ Michael H. Crawford

In WORLD BOOK see HEART; HEART ATTACK; CHOLESTEROL.

Hospitals
See Health-Care Facilities

stroke among physicians who took aspirin. In that study, however, no evidence existed to show that aspirin significantly reduced heart attacks.

Clot-dissolving drugs. Standard, less expensive drugs for heart-attack victims work just as well as—and may be safer than—newer, more costly drugs. Cardiologist Peter Sleight of Oxford University in England reported this conclusion at a meeting of the American College of Cardiology in Atlanta, Ga., in March 1991. Sleight reported the finding as part of the results of the Third International Study of Infarct Survival, which involves more than 40,000 patients treated at medical centers in North America, Europe, and New Zealand.

Scientists in February 1991 reported that an experimental drug is more effective than conventional antibiotics in combating *gram-negative bacteremia* (blood poisoning). This serious blood infection strikes about 300,000 Americans each year, killing as many as 100,000 of them.

The infection results when normally harmless bacteria in the stomach and intestines enter the blood as a result of an injury or surgery. Once in the blood, the bacteria can release toxic chemicals called *endotoxins* that can trigger kidney failure and other life-threatening reactions.

The new drug, made with genetic engineering techniques, contains an engineered protein called HA-1A that is similar to *antibodies* (disease-fighting proteins) produced by the immune system. HA-1A attaches to bacterial endotoxin and inactivates it.

Medical researchers from more than 30 American and European medical centers tested HA-1A on 200 patients with gram-negative bacteremia and found that it reduced the death rate from blood poisoning by 39 per cent. The new drug is designed to be administered along with conventional antibiotics.

Childhood vaccinations. In October 1990, the American Academy of Pediatrics (AAP) in Chicago recommended vaccinating children beginning at age 2 months rather than at 15 months against *Hemophilus influenzae type b* (Hib), an infection that can cause bacterial meningitis in young children. Bacterial meningitis is an inflammation of membranes around the brain and spinal cord that can cause permanent hearing loss and even death. Children are most at risk from the infection between the ages of 2 months and 18 months. Meningitis strikes approximately 10,000 children a year under the age of 18 months, according to the AAP.

The AAP recommendation followed the October 1990 Food and Drug Administration approval of a new vaccine against Hib for children under 15 months old. The new drug is called HbOC and will be marketed under the brand name Hibtiter. Although there are other vaccines against the dis-

ease, it was the first time one had been licensed for children under the age of 15 months. The new drug may be given in three doses, two months apart, and in combination with other vaccines, such as those for measles and polio, as well as for diphtheria, tetanus, and pertussis (DTP).

Hepatitis vaccination. In March 1991 an advisory committee of the United States Centers for Disease Control (CDC) in Atlanta, Ga., said that the vaccine for hepatitis B should be added to the list of vaccines administered to American children. The list, *the standard pediatric immuniza-*

New immunization schedule
The Centers for Disease Control (CDC) recommended in March 1991 that the hepatitis B vaccine be added to the childhood immunization schedule, starting at age 2 months. Children should now be immunized against nine diseases. Protection against diphtheria, tetanus, and pertussis (whooping cough) is included in one vaccine. The American Academy of Pediatrics lowered the recommended age for receiving *Hemophilus influenzae* type b (Hib-conjugate) vaccine to 2 months from 15 months in October 1990. The CDC has concurred.

Vaccine	2 mos.	4 mos.	6 mos.	12-15 mos.	15 mos.	15-18 mos.	4-6 yrs.	11-12 yrs.	14-16 yrs.
Diphtheria/tetanus/ pertussis (DTP)	x	x	x				x	x	x
Polio	x	x					x	x	
Measles					x		x		
Mumps					x		x		
Rubella					x		x		
Hemophilus influenzae type b (Hib-conjugate)*	x	x	x	x	x				
Hepatitis B	x								

Source: Centers for Disease Control.
*Dose schedule varies according to vaccine type used.

Cholera Strikes a Continent

Cholera began to spread in early 1991 through the crowded shantytowns that ring cities in Peru. The infection soon erupted into a full-blown epidemic, spreading to neighboring Ecuador, Colombia, Chile, and Brazil. It was South America's first major cholera epidemic this century. By August, the disease had afflicted nearly 300,000 people, killing more than 3,000, according to the World Health Organization.

Cholera, an infection of the intestinal tract, thrives in areas with unclean drinking water and inadequate sewage systems—the unsanitary conditions often found in developing nations. The microscopic culprit that causes the disease is the bacterium *Vibrio cholerae*. The bacteria are transmitted primarily in water and in food, especially shellfish and unwashed fruits and vegetables, that have become contaminated by an infected person's *feces* (solid body wastes).

The cholera bacteria produce a *toxin* (poison) that attacks the victim's small intestine, triggering the secretion of large amounts of fluid. This, in turn, produces severe, watery diarrhea and vomiting. If these symptoms go untreated, a cholera victim can die of *dehydration* (the loss of vital body fluids), sometimes within hours.

Most cholera deaths can be prevented through early treatment, which consists of replacing lost body fluids with a solution of water, salts, and sugar. Antibiotics can help curtail the diarrhea.

Many people who swallow *V. cholerae* never become ill. But when these so-called "healthy carriers" live in unhygienic conditions, they can infect others through bacteria in their feces.

The 1991 outbreak began in three cities along Peru's northern coast—Chancay, Piura, and Chimbote. The disease quickly reached Lima, Peru's capital, where more than half of the city's 7 million people live in shantytowns without running water or enclosed sewers. The Rímac River, which flows through Lima, was soon contaminated with *V. cholerae*. The bacteria also contaminated the fish that are eaten raw in *seviche*, a popular Latin-American dish.

As the disease spread to other South American countries, health officials launched public education campaigns. They encouraged people to boil drinking water and cook food well, avoid raw seafood and food purchased from street vendors, and wash their hands before eating. The epidemic was expected to continue, however, largely because of poor sanitation and the scarcity of medical resources.

Travelers to affected regions were also advised to watch what they ate and drank. Vaccinations were not generally recommended, because they provide only short-term protection and are not effective for everyone. People who developed diarrhea or began vomiting during or right after a trip to a cholera-stricken area were told to seek medical help at once.

By mid-1991, health officials had reported 14 cases of cholera in the United States and 1 in Canada. The illness had afflicted only individuals who had traveled to South America or eaten illegally imported South American crab meat.

A widespread cholera outbreak in the United States was unlikely because of the excellent sanitation system, the U.S. Centers for Disease Control in Atlanta reported in spring 1991. But a surge of cholera cases in Mexico led U.S. public health officials to issue a cholera alert in August. Officials worried especially about an outbreak near rivers along the Mexican border into which untreated sewage was dumped.

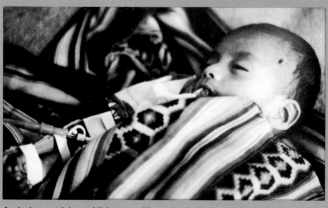

A cholera-stricken child gets a lifesaving infusion of fluids.

☐ Richard Trubo

tion schedule, now includes vaccinations against diphtheria, tetanus, pertussis, rubella, measles, mumps, and polio.

Hepatitis B is a viral disease of the liver that has been increasing in recent years, with most cases among adults. About 200,000 to 300,000 cases of hepatitis B occur each year, according to the CDC.

Although an effective vaccine for the disease has existed since 1982, prevention focused mostly on identifying people at risk—such as intravenous drug users—and vaccinating them. Despite this preventive method, the number of cases increased about 30 per cent between 1979 and 1989, according to the CDC.

The CDC concluded that vaccination of children offered the best prospect of controlling hepatitis B, eventually resulting in generations of adults immune to the disease. Thus, health officials put the vaccine on the standard pediatric immunization schedule. The vaccine would be given in three or four doses, with the first given about two months after birth.

Bacteria and stomach cancer. A type of bacteria suspected of causing many cases of stomach ulcers may also play a role in the development of stomach cancer, according to a May 1991 report. The bacteria, *Helicobacter pylori* (previously called *Campylobacter pylori*), can thrive in the highly acidic environment of the stomach, where they may cause inflammation of the stomach lining. Many experts believe that the inflammation plays an important role in the development of peptic ulcers. (A peptic ulcer is an open sore in the lining of the stomach or upper part of the small intestine.)

A team of researchers at Stanford University in Stanford, Calif., detected *H. pylori* in the stomachs of about 90 per cent of patients with the most common form of stomach cancer. The researchers also found *H. pylori* in the stomachs of 32 per cent of other patients with a similar but less common form of stomach cancer.

Researchers concluded that infection with *H. pylori* may be a risk factor for stomach cancer, which causes an estimated 13,400 deaths in the United States each year, according to the American Cancer Society. Although incidence of the disease has declined in the United States, stomach cancer is a leading cause of death worldwide, according to medical experts.

Lyme disease vaccine research. In October 1990, researchers at Yale University in New Haven, Conn., announced an advance toward a vaccine that would protect people, pets, and other animals from Lyme disease, a bacterial infection spread by deer ticks. It can cause chronic arthritis, heart abnormalities, nerve damage, and other disorders.

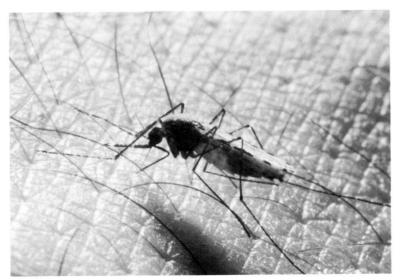

Malaria on the rise
The *Anopheles* mosquito transmits a parasite that causes malaria, which kills as many as 2 million people worldwide each year. World health officials reported that cases of malaria continued to increase in 1990 and 1991 as drug-resistant strains of the disease spread. Researchers searched for new weapons to use in the battle against the disease, such as stronger drugs and ways to lessen the parasite's drug resistance.

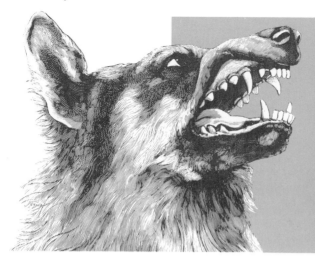

Hot line for rabies and tick bites
The Centers for Disease Control in Atlanta has established a 24-hour hot line (404-332-4555) that provides recorded information on rabies, a deadly infection that people most often contract from the bite of an infected animal. Callers can receive information on animal bites, rabies-prevention recommendations for international travelers, and information on how to report rabies vaccine reactions. The hot line also provides information about Lyme disease and Rocky Mountain spotted fever (illnesses contracted through tick bites) and other infectious diseases. Callers can also request written information.

Using genetic engineering techniques, the researchers produced large quantities of a key protein found on the surface of *Borrelia burgdorferi*, the bacterium that causes Lyme disease. This protein causes the human immune system to produce antibodies that fight *B. burgdorferi*.

Tests of the experimental vaccine showed that it was effective in protecting laboratory mice from infection. Scientists predicted that a human vaccine could be available by 1999.

In addition to the research at Yale on a new vaccine, researchers at the National Institutes of Health in Bethesda, Md., reported in May 1991 the development of a new test to detect infection with the Lyme disease bacterium. Current tests used to diagnose the disease are "indirect" tests. They identify antibodies made by the body in response to Lyme disease bacteria. These tests may fail to diagnose infection in people who produce low levels of such antibodies. But the new test determines the direct presence of *B. burgdorferi* in the body by detecting certain proteins produced by the disease-causing bacterium.

☐ Michael Woods

In the Special Reports section, see THE SPECTER OF AIDS; MEASLES ON THE RISE; SEXUALLY TRANSMITTED DANGER. In WORLD BOOK, see HEPATITIS; LYME DISEASE; VIRUS.

Injury
See Emergency Medicine, Safety

Kidney

Many patients with kidney disease require *dialysis*—a procedure that filters toxic substances from the blood. The question of just how much dialysis is enough, long troubling to physicians, came under increased scrutiny in 1990 and 1991. Dialysis treatments typically last 3 to 4 hours and take place three times a week. Longer or more frequent treatments can remove more toxins but at greater patient discomfort and expense.

Risk in shortened dialysis. The results of a study comparing death rates to the length of dialysis treatments were published on Feb. 20, 1991, in the *Journal of the American Medical Association*. The three-year study was directed by Philip J. Held, head of renal research at the Urban Institute, a think tank in Washington, D.C.

The team found that patients whose treatments lasted less than $3\frac{1}{2}$ hours had a greater risk of dying than those whose treatments ran longer. If the short treatments had gone on over a period greater than five years, the risk of dying more than doubled.

The study's authors pointed to a possible link between a recent trend toward shortened dialysis treatments and decreasing reimbursement from Medicare, a U.S. government health insurance program. From 1983 to 1988, Medicare reimbursement fell an average of 44 per cent per treatment, after adjustment for inflation.

The study did not include patients treated by a new procedure called *high-flux dialysis*, so the results may not apply to this speedier technique. In addition, the study appears not to have taken patient weight into consideration, though this factor usually helps determine the length of dialysis.

Protein intake and kidney failure.

Limiting the amount of protein in the diet may retard kidney failure in pa-ˈtients with diabetes, researchers reported in January 1991. This finding resulted from a lengthy study of kidney function led by internist Kathleen Zeller at the University of Texas Southwestern Medical Center in Dallas. Permanent kidney failure develops in 30 to 50 per cent of people with diabetes mellitus, a disease in which the body fails to produce or efficiently use the hormone insulin to maintain normal levels of blood sugar.

All the patients studied had Type I diabetes (also known as *insulin-dependent* or *juvenile-onset diabetes*) and early signs of kidney abnormalities that were thought to result from the diabetes. Some of them were put on a low-protein diet, which included 0.6 grams (0.02 ounce) of protein per day for each kilogram (2.2 pounds) of body weight. The rest consumed their usual amount of protein—so long as it equaled at least 1 gram (0.035 ounce) per day per kilogram of body weight.

The patients on the low-protein diet lost kidney function much more slowly than the other patients. The Texas researchers saw the greatest benefit in patients who still had more than 50 per cent of their kidney function when they started the low-protein diet. Despite eating less protein, the patients showed no signs of malnutrition.

How immunosuppressants work.

The success of kidney transplants depends on preventing the immune system from rejecting the transplanted organ. This is done by using *immunosuppressants*—drugs that suppress the body's natural defenses. Recent advances in our understanding of how these drugs work were reviewed in the Jan. 18, 1991, issue of *Science* by Stuart L. Schreiber, a chemist at Harvard University in Cambridge, Mass. Many of these advances came from Schreiber's laboratory.

Immunosuppressants bind to special molecules called *receptors* found within *lymphocytes* (disease-fighting cells). The drug-receptor complex, in turn, interferes with the cell's ability to duplicate the genetic information stored in the cell nucleus. Because of this, the lymphocytes are unable to mount an attack against the transplanted organ. Better understanding of these processes should aid the development of more effective immunosuppressants.

☐ Jeffrey R. Thompson

In WORLD BOOK, see KIDNEY.

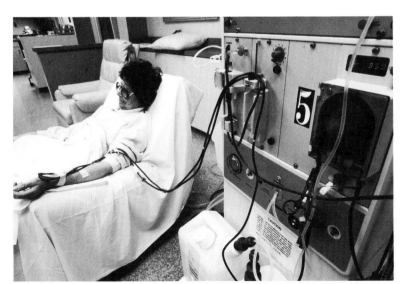

Risks of shortened dialysis treatments
Reducing the length of kidney dialysis treatments can shorten a patient's life, researchers reported in February 1991. Dialysis filters wastes from the bloodstream that the kidneys normally remove. The researchers suggested that cuts in government funding for dialysis may have led to shortened treatment times.

Mental Health

Specific brain abnormalities may play an important role in the hyperactivity and attention problems that affect some adults and children, according to a November 1990 report by researchers at the National Institute of Mental Health in Bethesda, Md. The scientists found that adults who have been *hyperactive* (characterized by an abnormally high level of activity) since childhood had markedly reduced brain activity in areas that regulate movement and attention. The results of the study offered support to researchers who contend that severe hyperactivity stems from an inherited brain disorder, not from a psychological problem.

The characteristics of hyperactivity, also known as *attention-deficit hyperactivity disorder*, include constant fidgeting, an inability to concentrate or complete tasks, and impulsive, often inappropriate behavior. An estimated 4 per cent of school-age children, mainly boys, have the disorder.

Researchers have found that low doses of two types of stimulant drugs help reduce hyperactive symptoms in many children. Critics of drug therapy, however, contend that some children have been misdiagnosed as being hyperactive and that some children have been overmedicated.

The new study focused on 25 adults who had been diagnosed in childhood as being hyperactive and who were

the parents of hyperactive children. Another 50 adults with no symptoms of hyperactivity served as a control group.

The researchers tracked the brain activity of all the adults in the study using *positron emission tomography* (PET) scans, which measure the amount of energy used in different regions of the brain. The PET scans were taken while the participants performed an exercise that required them to press a button upon hearing the softest of three tones.

The researchers found that, in general, the brains of the hyperactive adults were less active than were those of the adults in the control group. Moreover, the level of activity was significantly lower in areas that regulate the ability to pay attention and keep still. If other studies support these findings, doctors may be able to use PET scans to more accurately identify people with the disorder.

Emotional trauma of POW's. Prisoners of war (POW's) exposed to prolonged, brutal treatment continue to suffer from a variety of mental disorders for decades after their release, investigators reported in January 1991. More than 35 years after returning home, as many as 9 out of 10 U.S. servicemen who survived captivity during the Korean War (1950-1953) may live with an anxiety disorder

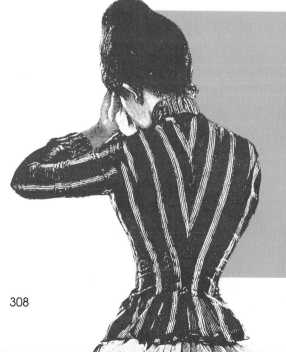

Oppression and depression in women
The experience of being female in modern society largely explains why women are twice as likely as men to develop symptoms of depression, according to a December 1990 report by the American Psychological Association. Among the factors listed were:

- Poverty
- Physical or sexual abuse
- Unhappy marriage
- Stress of having small children
- Job discrimination or other forms of bias
- Infertility
- Social traditions that encourage passive, dependent behavior in women

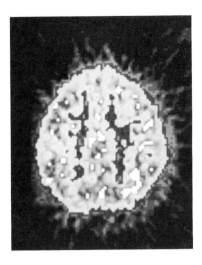

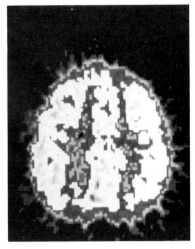

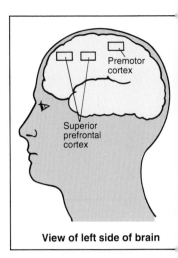

View of left side of brain

called *post-traumatic stress disorder* (PTSD) and other psychiatric problems, said psychologist Patricia B. Sutker of the New Orleans Veterans Administration Medical Center.

Sutker's team analyzed the mental condition of 22 POW's and 22 combat veterans of the Korean War. The POW's had spent an average of 28 months in captivity and endured harsh conditions, including months of solitary confinement, near-starvation, and torture.

Two of the combat veterans and 19 of the POW's exhibited symptoms of PTSD, including recurring memories and dreams of wartime traumas, emotional detachment from family, extreme suspicion of others, and difficulty concentrating. More than half the former POW's with PTSD suffered from *panic attacks*, frightening episodes of anxiety. Six former POW's also experienced severe depression.

For reasons still unclear, better-educated servicemen with middle-class backgrounds—traits more often found among fighter pilots than ground troops—tended to recover more quickly from their ordeal, Sutker said. The ability to psychologically block out trauma may be critical during imprisonment, she added, while confronting POW experiences after release promotes emotional health.

Trauma and young adults. A surprising number of young adults living in urban areas also experience PTSD, according to a March 1991 report by

a research team from Henry Ford Hospital in Detroit. In fact, PTSD ranked fourth among psychiatric disorders affecting these adults, after phobias, severe depression, and addiction to alcohol or illicit drugs.

The researchers reported that about 40 per cent of the 1,007 young adults surveyed said they had experienced at least one extremely traumatic event and 9 per cent had developed PTSD at some time in their lives. Such events included sudden injury or serious accident, physical assault or rape, seeing someone seriously hurt or killed, or receiving news of the sudden death of a close relative or friend. The researchers said their findings challenge the traditional view of mental health workers that only events outside the range of day-to-day human experience, such as captivity or combat, can cause PTSD.

According to the researchers, women were more likely than men to have developed PTSD. Rape was especially traumatic. Of the 16 women who reported having been raped, 13 developed PTSD. Moreover, severe trauma quickly triggered PTSD symptoms in most cases. Only one person in the sample reported that PTSD occurred more than six months after a traumatic event.

Drug treatment for depression. Many people suffering from severe depression can reduce the severity and recurrence of further episodes of the disorder by taking high doses of cer-

Clue to hyperactivity
Hyperactivity may stem from specific brain abnormalities, researchers reported in November 1990. A technique that reveals areas of metabolic activity in the brain showed that brain activity of a hyperactive person, *above far left*, was less than that of a person without the disorder, *above middle*. Activity is decreased most in the *premotor cortex* and *superior prefrontal cortex*, areas used to control movement and attention, *above*.

tain antidepressant drugs for at least three years after their symptoms have eased, according to a December 1990 report. Most physicians currently either reduce the amount of antidepressant medication patients take or stop drug treatment altogether within a few months after an episode of depression lifts.

Psychologist Ellen Frank of the University of Pittsburgh in Pennsylvania and her colleagues studied 230 patients with chronic depression. After four months of treatment with relatively high daily doses of *imipramine,* a common antidepressant, and psychotherapy sessions every week or two, 128 of these patients showed marked improvement.

These patients were then split into five treatment groups for the next three years. The members of the first two groups received either high daily doses of imipramine or daily *placebos* (pills containing inactive substances). The members of the third group received no medication but attended monthly psychotherapy sessions. Those in the fourth and fifth groups received psychotherapy plus either a placebo or high doses of imipramine.

About 80 per cent of the patients on high-dose imipramine—both those receiving the drug alone and those receiving therapy—remained free of depression the entire three years, a much better result than those produced by other treatments that did not include the drug. Treatment consisting of psychotherapy without drugs was also beneficial, however. Half of those attending monthly therapy sessions, while not taking imipramine, stayed free of depression for three years.

Lithium treatment questioned. Psychiatrists have long noted that the drug lithium can diminish the sharp mood swings that affect people with *manic depression* (also called *bipolar depression*). Although lithium is considered a major success story, a study reported in May 1991 by researchers at Michael Reese Hospital in Chicago presented a more pessimistic view of the drug's effectiveness.

Approximately 2 million people in the United States suffer from manic depression. They undergo periods of severe depression alternating with episodes of *mania*—uncontrolled elation, restlessness, and racing thoughts.

The Chicago researchers charted the progress of 35 manic-depressive patients and 35 patients with a form of depression that does not include mania, all of whom had been hospitalized for their condition. The researchers studied the two groups, both of which have periods of severe depression, in order to compare the long-term course of the disorder.

The researchers examined the patients three times after their discharge

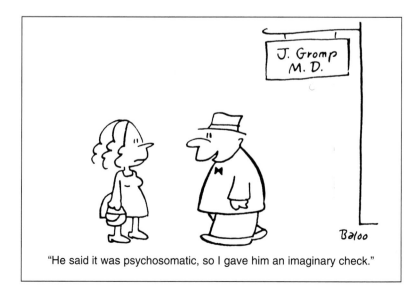

"He said it was psychosomatic, so I gave him an imaginary check."

to outpatient treatment, the last time at $7^1/_2$ years. The outpatient treatment for the patients with manic depression usually consisted of lithium in combination with psychotherapy. The patients with depression received antidepressant drugs other than lithium and, in some cases, psychotherapy.

At the end of $7^1/_2$ years of outpatient treatment, only 12 of 35 people with manic depression functioned well in social situations and displayed no serious psychiatric symptoms. Among those hospitalized for depression alone, 19 of 35 achieved the same level of functioning. Previous research, based on shorter follow-ups of patients, had suggested that twice as many manic-depressive patients on lithium would have displayed good social and emotional functioning.

Another 19 people with manic depression and 13 patients with depression experienced periodic recurrences of their symptoms, social difficulties, and occasional returns to the hospital. Four people with manic depression and three individuals who were depressed did not improve at all after leaving the hospital.

Effects of child abuse. Many children who are exposed to physical abuse at home exhibit unusually aggressive and violent behavior by the time they enter kindergarten, according to a December 1990 report. Even at such a young age, physical abuse apparently encourages a cycle of violence, particularly among boys, said psychologists from Vanderbilt University in Nashville, Tenn.

The researchers conducted physical examinations of 309 kindergartners, all of whom were 4 years old when the project began, and interviewed the children's mothers. In the investigators' opinion, 46 of the children were frequently abused at home.

The researchers found that more than one in three of the abused children continually expressed anger and provoked conflict with teachers and classmates at school. The children often misinterpreted others' intentions as hostile and relied on aggression to resolve problems with peers or adults.

The abused children also tended to be more emotionally withdrawn and socially isolated than were their classmates. These findings held regardless of whether the abused youngsters came from rich or poor families or lived in two- or one-parent homes.

Dodge pointed out, however, that many of the abused children reached kindergarten with no major problems. His team hopes to follow the entire group into adolescence to see if the abused youngsters develop high rates of anxiety, delinquency, depression, and drug abuse.   □ Bruce Bower

In the Special Reports section, see LEARNING TO TREAT SCHIZOPHRENIA. In WORLD BOOK, see DEPRESSION; HYPERACTIVE CHILD; MENTAL ILLNESS.

Nervous System
See Brain and Nervous System

Nursing Homes
See Health-Care Facilities

Eating red meat may increase the risk of developing colon cancer, according to a study published in *The New England Journal of Medicine* in December 1990. Over a six-year period, investigators at the Harvard Medical School and Brigham and Women's Hospital in Boston questioned almost 89,000 women about their eating habits and medical histories.

The researchers found that the women with the highest intake of animal fat were twice as likely to develop colon cancer as the women with the lowest intake. The strongest association was found with beef, pork, and lamb. Women who ate those meats as a main course at least once a day were $2^1/_2$ times more likely to develop colon cancer than women who ate them less than once a month.

Eating chicken or fish, however, lowered the risk. Women who ate chicken without the skin at least twice a week had a risk of developing colon cancer only half that of women who ate it less than once a month.

The researchers noted that it's unclear why red meat may promote colon cancer, as compared with fish and chicken. But they recommended that people generally eat less red meat and more fish and skinless chicken.

Vitamin E and heart disease. Several studies published in January 1991 suggested a possible link between low levels of vitamin E in the blood

Nutrition and Food

and heart disease. Vitamin E is often referred to as an *antioxidant nutrient* because it seems to prevent certain substances in the body from *oxidizing* (combining with oxygen). Scientists theorize that the oxidizing of one type of *cholesterol* (a fatlike substance) sets off events that ultimately build up fatty deposits and form scar tissue in the blood vessels. Such damage contributes to heart disease.

In one study, researchers at the University of Bern in Switzerland surveyed middle-aged men from 16 European countries with different rates of death from *ischemic heart disease*. This disorder is characterized by an insufficient flow of blood to the heart.

The researchers found that men with high blood pressure and high levels of cholesterol in their blood ran a greater risk of dying from ischemic heart disease than other men. But the strongest predictor of such death, researchers found, was a low level of vitamin E in the blood.

In another study, one of the Bern investigators, working with colleagues from the University of Edinburgh in Scotland, examined men who complained of chest pain. The researchers found that men who had low levels of vitamin E had an increased risk of *angina*—chest pain caused by an inadequate flow of blood to the heart. Angina can result when blood vessels to the heart become narrowed by a build-up of fatty deposits.

Finally, researchers at the University of Graz in Austria tested blood samples taken from healthy young volunteers. When they added vitamin E to the samples, they found that the type of cholesterol that damages blood vessels—low-density lipoprotein—was much less likely to be oxidized.

None of these studies, however, proved that low levels of vitamin E cause heart disease nor that higher levels can prevent it. Additional research is needed before any such conclusions can be drawn.

Unhealthy weight fluctuations. A study published in June 1991 in *The New England Journal of Medicine* concluded that large fluctuations in body weight can have negative health consequences. Investigators at Yale University in New Haven, Conn., used data from the Framingham Heart Study, which has monitored 5,000 residents of Framingham, Mass., for several decades.

The Framingham study provided a wide range of information on each individual's history, including information on body weight. In reviewing these data, the researchers found that people with varying weights were more likely to suffer from heart disease and die than were people whose weight remained fairly stable.

Dieting was common among individuals in the study whose weight varied, the investigators observed. But

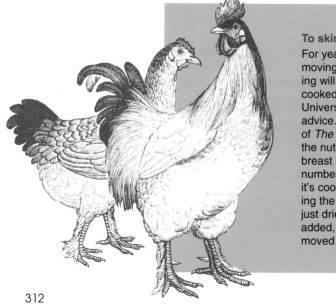

To skin, or not to skin?

For years, experts have advised that removing the skin of a chicken before cooking will reduce the fat content of the cooked meat. But two nutritionists at the University of Minnesota disagree with this advice. Writing in the Sept. 13, 1990, issue of *The New England Journal of Medicine*, the nutritionists reported that a chicken breast has the same fat content and same number of calories after roasting whether it's cooked with the skin or without. Removing the skin before cooking, they noted, just dries out the chicken. The nutritionists added, however, that the skin should be removed before the chicken is eaten.

When in doubt, throw it out
- How long can you store that leftover piece of fried chicken?
- Should you throw out everything in the freezer after a power failure?
- What's the proper cooking temperature for pork?

Knowing the answers to these questions can help you avoid food poisoning, which strikes more than 7 million Americans each year. A brochure prepared by the U.S. Department of Agriculture provides information on storing, preparing, and serving food safely. To order a free copy of *A Quick Consumer Guide to Safe Food Handling*, write to: Consumer Information Center, 574-X, Pueblo, CO 81009.

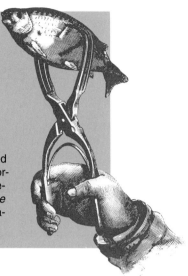

weight can change for a variety of reasons, including illness, smoking, and exercise. In their analyses, the Yale researchers took into account many factors that might affect the risk of heart disease or dying. They further noted that fluctuating body weight seemed to have harmful effects on everyone, whether obese or not.

The researchers were unsure why large or frequent swings in weight would increase the risk of heart disease. But they suggested several possible reasons: Repeated weight gains might allow fat to settle in the abdominal area—which, according to some studies, increases the risk of heart disease. Or, people who jump on and off diets may simply find unhealthful high-fat foods more appealing.

Health experts note that the new findings do not suggest that it's safer to remain overweight than to diet. They generally agree that the best method of dieting is to lose weight slowly so that it stays off. See also WEIGHT CONTROL.

Children's food choices. Two studies published in 1991 provided insights into what children eat when left to themselves. Researchers at the University of Illinois at Urbana-Champaign found that the number of calories children consume remains fairly constant from day to day, though it

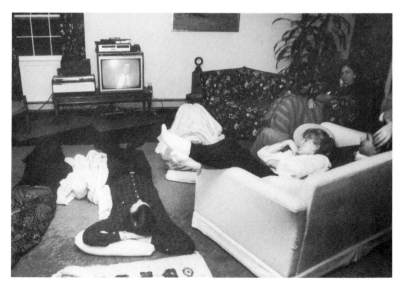

Cholesterol and the couch
Young people who watch a lot of television are more likely to have high blood-cholesterol levels than those who watch less TV, pediatric researchers at the University of California at Irvine reported in November 1990. Couch potatoes generally exercise less than others do, and they tend to eat more unhealthful high-fat snacks.

may vary widely from meal to meal. They reported their findings in *The New England Journal of Medicine*.

The researchers measured the total food intake of 15 children aged 2 to 5, twice a week for three weeks. The children appeared to adjust their calorie intake so that a low-calorie meal would follow a meal very high in calories. The researchers suggested that this finding might persuade parents to stop forcing food into finicky eaters at every meal.

Left on their own, however, children tend to make poor nutritional choices, according to research published in *The American Journal of Clinical Nutrition*. Investigators at Memphis State University in Tennessee directed 53 five-year-olds to choose whatever they wanted for lunch from a variety of foods at a cafeteria. Next, the children were told to select a lunch that their mothers would later inspect. Each mother could then make changes in her child's food choices.

Children chose more foods that were low in nutrition—low in minerals and vitamins and/or high in salt, sugar, or fats—when on their own than when they knew their mothers would inspect their choices. The lunches the mothers selected contained fewer foods that were low in nutrition.

□ Jeanine Barone

In WORLD BOOK, see NUTRITION.

Occupational Health

See Safety

Pregnancy and Childbirth

Pregnant women who work at a video display terminal (VDT) are no more likely to miscarry than are women who do not work with the machines, according to a large-scale United States government study reported in March 1991. The study addresses a concern expressed for more than a decade by health experts and office-worker advocacy groups about the potentially harmful effects of VDT's on pregnant women and their fetuses.

Debate over the safety of VDT's has centered on the *electromagnetic fields* (EMF's) emitted by these machines. Since 1980, there have been several reports of clusters of miscarriages and fetal birth defects among women who worked with VDT's in offices. Most studies analyzing the connection between VDT use and miscarriage rates have produced either unclear results or no evidence of harm, though two small studies suggested an increased risk of miscarriage.

The government study was conducted by researchers at the National Institute for Occupational Safety and Health (NIOSH) in Cincinnati, Ohio. The researchers studied 882 pregnancies in telephone operators. They found that 14.8 per cent of operators who spent their entire workday in front of a VDT screen miscarried during the

VDT's and miscarriages

Working at a video display terminal (VDT) apparently does not increase the risk of miscarriage for pregnant workers, according to a United States government study reported in March 1991. Over the past decade, many health experts have expressed concerns about the potentially harmful effects of the electromagnetic fields (EMF's) emitted by VDT's near pregnant women and their fetuses.

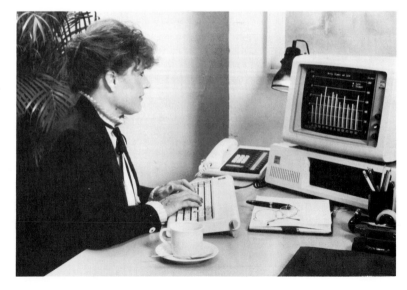

first three months of pregnancy, compared with 15.9 per cent of a comparable group of women operators who used other types of equipment.

The NIOSH results were more accurate than those of previous studies because the researchers used telephone company records of hours worked and actual measurements of the EMF level at sample workstations to calculate the level of exposure. Earlier research was based largely on estimated VDT use and EMF exposure.

But some health experts and office-worker advocacy groups criticized the study as flawed. They argued that the NIOSH researchers did not conduct blood tests of the women to determine if any of them were in the very earliest stage of pregnancy—before the women themselves knew they were pregnant—and so did not determine whether working on a VDT can harm fetuses in the first few weeks after conception.

The NIOSH researchers cautioned that the study provided no new information on the overall potential health risks of EMF's from other sources. This is because both groups of women in the study had similar levels of exposure to the radiation outside the workplace in the form of EMF's emitted by electric appliances, electrical wiring in homes, and power transmission lines.

Folic acid and birth defects. Women who take folic acid, a B vitamin, before they conceive and throughout their pregnancy greatly reduce their risk of giving birth to a baby with a serious defect of the central nervous system. That conclusion was reported in July 1991 by a team of medical researchers from the Medical College of St. Bartholomew's Hospital in London.

From 10 to 20 babies in every 1,000 are born with serious defects of the central nervous system that cause varying degrees of mental and physical disability. These so-called *neural tube defects* include *anencephaly*, a lethal condition in which nearly all the brain is missing, and the most serious form of *spina bifida*, in which the spinal cord is exposed through a gap in the backbone.

Several previous studies had suggested that taking multivitamins, in-

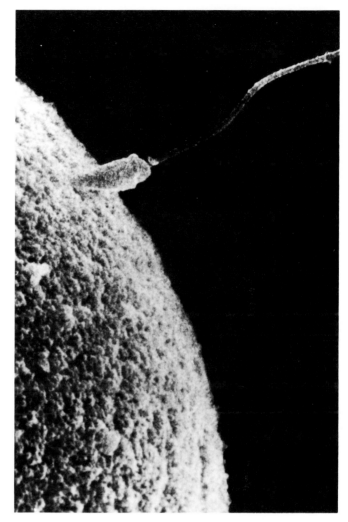

cluding folic acid, reduced the risk of giving birth to a child with a neural tube defect. The British study, however, is the first to determine that folic acid, in particular, is the protective substance.

The researchers studied the pregnancies of more than 1,800 women. The women, who were divided into four groups, took either folic acid alone, folic acid with other vitamins, other vitamins without folic acid, or a *placebo* (pill containing an inactive ingredient).

Twenty-seven of the women gave birth to a child with a neural tube defect. Of this number, 21 had not taken folic acid. The researchers were unable to explain why some women who took folic acid still gave birth to babies

A "come hither" signal
A human sperm combines with a human egg. The first evidence that human eggs communicate with sperm before the two combine during fertilization was reported in April 1991 by American and Israeli scientists. A still-mysterious chemical in the fluid that surrounds a maturing egg may alert sperm to the presence of the egg and beckon the sperm to swim up a Fallopian tube, where fertilization occurs.

with nervous system defects. Nevertheless, United States health officials said the findings indicated women should begin taking folic acid supplements before they try to become pregnant.

Hard work doesn't hurt. Women who work long hours at physically demanding, highly stressful jobs are just as likely to carry their pregnancy to term as are women with less demanding occupations, according to a large study of women physicians by the National Institute of Child Health and Human Development in Bethesda, Md. The researchers said the results of the study, released in October 1991, suggested that a woman whose pregnancy is progressing normally could continue to work as long as she wants.

The government researchers compared the pregnancies of 1,293 physicians during the residency part of their medical training with the pregnancies of 1,494 women who were not doctors. The researchers found no statistically significant problems in the doctors' pregnancies, even though the residents worked an average of 70 hours per week—almost twice as many hours as did the other women. Both groups experienced similar rates of miscarriages, *tubal pregnancies* (in which the embryo is implanted in a Fallopian tube rather than the uterus), stillbirths, premature deliveries, and low-birth-weight babies.

Prenatal technique questioned. A European study published in June 1991 suggested that a technique used to diagnose fetal defects at an early stage may be more risky to the fetus than was previously believed.

The diagnostic technique is *chorionic villus sampling* (CVS), which is usually performed in the 8th to 12th week of pregnancy. In this technique, cells from hairlike projections of a membrane that surrounds the fetus are removed and examined for abnormalities. The cells are identical to the fetus's genetic material.

Some women chose CVS over *amniocentesis*, in which fluid is removed from the womb, because amniocentesis is usually not performed until the 16th week of pregnancy. Doctors have generally not performed amniocentesis earlier because they believed that there would be too few fetal cells to examine at that stage. They also feared that removing fluid from the womb before the 16th week of pregnancy could damage the fetus.

The studies found that the miscarriage rate among women who underwent CVS was 5 per cent higher than that in women who underwent amniocentesis. The miscarriage rate associated with amniocentesis is from 0.5 to 1.0 per cent.

☐ Cristine Russell

In the Special Reports section, see HEALTHY MOTHERS, HEALTHY BABIES. In WORLD BOOK, see CHILDBIRTH.

Respiratory System

A January 1991 report by medical researchers from Argentina and Canada suggests that the primary cause of death in patients with severe asthma is *asphyxiation* (suffocation) due to the disease process itself. This study disputes the belief held by many medical experts that overuse of *bronchodilators*—commonly prescribed asthma drugs that relax and expand airways in the lungs—contributes to asthma deaths by causing irregular heartbeats in patients.

Asthma causes inflammation of the *bronchi*, airways to the lungs. This inflammation narrows the bronchi. During acute attacks, muscles around the bronchi tighten, which narrows the breathing passage, and the airways fill with mucus and fluid. This creates potentially fatal breathing difficulties. According to the National Center for Health Statistics in Hyattsville, Md., approximately 10 million Americans suffer from asthma. Annual asthma deaths have risen in the United States from 2,600 in 1980 to about 4,600 in 1987, the latest year for which statistics are available.

In the study of 10 asthma patients who had stopped or nearly stopped breathing when admitted to the hospital, the researchers discovered that these near-fatal episodes were due to breathing difficulties, not heart irregularities. They suggested that asthma is usually undertreated, partly out of fear that bronchodilators will worsen patients, and that such undertreatment may contribute to asthma deaths.

Overuse of asthma drugs. A German pharmaceutical company told the U.S. Food and Drug Administration (FDA) in August 1991 that people who exceed the recommended dosage of *beta-2 agonists*, types of bronchodilators found in inhalers used by many asthma patients, may increase their risk of fatal asthma attacks. The U.S. subsidiary of the company told the FDA that preliminary results from a study of 12,300 Canadian asthma patients from 1978 to 1987 showed that people who used two inhalers (a two-month supply of the drug's recommended daily dose) in just one month faced twice the risk of fatal or near-fatal asthma attacks as people who used only one inhaler per month. The report noted that further research was needed to tell whether the increased asthma deaths were caused by the drugs themselves.

Asthma guidelines. In February 1991, a federal panel of scientists and health experts convened by the National Heart, Lung, and Blood Institute in Bethesda, Md., issued the first-ever national guidelines for the diagnosis and treatment of asthma. The new guidelines emphasized treatment with inhaled steroids in order to prevent inflammation of the lungs. These anti-inflammatory drugs offer long-term prevention rather than just treating short-term, immediate symptoms of asthma, as bronchodilators do, according to the panel.

The report also urged doctors to test suspected asthma patients with a machine called a *spirometer*, which measures how much air a patient exhales. In addition, the panel urged doctors to teach asthmatics how to use a spirometer and interpret its results in order to determine whether an asthma attack is impending.

Smoking trends and lung cancer. Although lung cancer continued as the leading cause of cancer death in the United States, deaths from the disease have decreased since 1983, according to a May 1991 report. Lawrence Garfinkel, a special consultant in epidemiology and statistics for the

Can toothpaste take your breath away?
A 21-year-old woman with a history of asthma had been wheezing and having trouble breathing for approximately six weeks. But her doctors in Santa Clara, Calif., were at a loss to explain why. Various medications had failed to eliminate her symptoms, and a chest X ray turned up no clues. Then their patient's breathing difficulties improved dramatically after she switched from a paste-based toothpaste to a gel-type brand. This, the physicians wrote in a letter to *The New England Journal of Medicine,* ended the mystery. The woman's toothpaste had been the source of her trouble, they theorized. To test their theory, the doctors exposed the woman to various brands of toothpaste and found that the paste-based types invariably triggered her wheezing. According to the toothpaste manufacturer, the only difference in ingredients between the paste and gel types of toothpastes was the type of artificial flavoring. The culprit turned out to be the artificial spice-mint or wintergreen flavoring in paste-based toothpaste. The gel-based type, which had no effect on her breathing, contained a mild spice-blend flavoring. The patient then revealed to her doctors that chewing gum flavored with wintergreen or peppermint also made her wheeze. The physicians concluded that doctors should look for unusual causes of asthma attacks when patients have breathing difficulties that fail to clear up.

American Cancer Society in New York City, and Edwin Silverberg, a former epidemiologic research associate with the American Cancer Society, analyzed smoking habits and the incidence of lung cancer in the United States over the past 25 years.

According to their report, the total number of lung cancer deaths in men increased steadily from 1940 to 1982 and then leveled off. In women, the number of lung cancer deaths continued to increase, except for women in the 35 to 44 age group. There has been a decrease in the *incidence* (percentage of people who develop the disease) of lung cancer in both men and women since 1983, according to the report.

Respiratory distress syndrome. Researchers from three medical institutions in New York state reported in March 1991 on the relative effectiveness of two treatments for *respiratory*

distress syndrome, a condition in premature infants in which the lungs are imperfectly expanded. This is caused by the inability of the premature lung to secrete enough surfactant, a substance that prevents the walls of the lungs' air sacs from sticking together and collapsing.

There are two types of surfactant treatment. One type involves giving early, preventive doses to premature infants at risk for developing the syndrome. The other type involves treating with surfactant only after the development of the syndrome.

In the study, the researchers gave a calf-lung surfactant extract to 479 premature infants, each with a gestational age (growth time in the womb before birth) of less than 30 weeks. Some of the infants were treated before they developed the syndrome, and some after. Researchers reported an 88 per cent survival rate with the preventive surfactant therapy, compared with an 80 per cent survival rate with therapy given after the syndrome developed. The greatest benefits of preventive therapy occurred in very premature infants, delivered at 26 or fewer weeks of gestation, according to the study.

Chronic lung disease. In addition to surfactant treatment, respiratory distress syndrome can be treated with mechanical ventilators that supply oxygen to the infant. However, this method of treatment has been linked to another disease—bronchopulmonary dysplasia, the most common chronic lung disease in infants in the United States. This illness is marked by abnormal cell growth and cell loss in the lungs. Medical researchers at Stanford University Medical Center in Stanford, Calif., reported in December 1990 that most children who develop bronchopulmonary dysplasia as infants continue to suffer lung problems into adulthood. The researchers studied 26 young adults born between 1964 and 1973 who had bronchopulmonary dysplasia in infancy and found that 76 per cent still experienced reduced lung function. The reduced function was marked by an inability to expel air fully and an added susceptibility to wheezing.

Medical experts suspect that the damage that leads to bronchopulmonary dysplasia is caused by the concentrated doses of oxygen or the pressure of air from the ventilator treatment they received as infants. Because surfactants offer an alternative to mechanical ventilators for the treatment of respiratory distress syndrome, their use may reduce the incidence of bronchopulmonary dysplasia. But it is too early to determine the long-term outcome of the surfactant-treated infants, experts noted.

☐ Robert Balk

In WORLD BOOK, see RESPIRATION; ASTHMA.

Safety

Most warning labels on toys do not clearly inform buyers about potential choking hazards to young children, researchers from Johns Hopkins University in Baltimore concluded in June 1991. Although these toy labels are intended to warn consumers about small parts that may choke children under 3 years of age, they often do not specify that the toy presents a potential choking hazard. Instead, the labels commonly indicate whether a toy is recommended for children under or over 3 years of age.

The researchers surveyed 200 toy buyers in a shopping mall. Many of those questioned did not recognize that such labels are intended as warnings. On the contrary, parents and other toy buyers incorrectly interpreted the labels as a guide to the age at which children might find a toy interesting or intellectually stimulating.

The researchers recommended that the United States government require toy manufacturers to use a more explicit warning. They suggested using a label that would state, for example: "Not recommended for children under 3 due to danger of choking from small parts."

Reducing accidents. Increased public awareness about safety helped reduce the death rate from accidents in the United States by 19 per cent during the 1980's, according to figures reported in August 1990 by the

Decline of fatal accidents
During the 1980's, the United States made greater progress in reducing accidental deaths than in any other decade in its history, according to figures released in August 1990 by the National Safety Council. The nation recorded a 19 per cent drop in the overall fatal accident rate (number of deaths per 100,000 people), which included deaths from motor vehicle accidents, falls, drownings, and fires. Accidents still ranked as the fourth leading cause of death, however, following heart disease, cancer, and stroke.

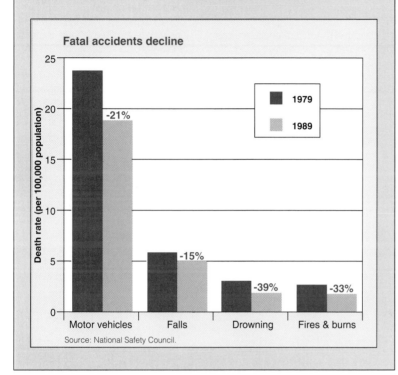

Fatal accidents decline

Source: National Safety Council.

National Safety Council, a nonprofit agency based in Chicago. Accidents are the fourth leading cause of death, exceeded only by heart disease, cancer, and stroke.

The rate of motor vehicle deaths, which account for about half of all accidental deaths, declined by just over 20 per cent. The biggest decrease occurred among young drivers, aged 15 to 24. The death rate for falls, fires, poisonings, and other accidents in the home decreased by 16 per cent. This decline would have been even greater, however, had it not been for a big increase in deaths from drug overdoses. The rate of accidental deaths occurring in the workplace was down 29 per cent, while the rate for drownings, plane crashes, and other accidents in

public places dropped by 22 per cent.

Experts said that a number of factors probably were involved in the trend toward a safer society. These included campaigns against drunken driving; greater use of automobile seat belts, airbags, and infant safety seats; the wide use of home smoke detectors; and greater overall public awareness about accident prevention.

Preventing accidental shootings.
About 1 out of every 3 deaths from the accidental discharge of firearms could be prevented by installing two safety devices on guns, a study conducted for the U.S. Congress concluded in March 1991. About 1,500 Americans are killed each year in accidents involving firearms. The weapons

are the fourth leading cause of accidental deaths among children aged 5 to 14 years and the third leading cause among people aged 15 to 24.

The study was conducted by Congress's investigative and auditing agency, the U.S. General Accounting Office (GAO). It analyzed the circumstances surrounding 107 accidental shootings to determine what kinds of safety devices might have prevented the firearm from discharging.

One of the proposed safety devices makes it difficult for children under age 6 to pull the trigger on a firearm. The GAO estimated that the childproof safety device could prevent 113 accidents each year in which children under age 6 kill themselves or others.

The other device provides a clear indication that a gun is loaded. The loading indicator could prevent about 345 additional deaths. Experts noted that many firearm accidents occur when gun owners unload a weapon but forget that a round of ammunition remains in the firing chamber.

The GAO study also noted that many more lives could be saved if gun owners followed sensible practices, such as unloading firearms and locking them up for storage and refraining from horseplay and the use of alcohol when handling firearms.

All out for buckling up. Citing the importance of seat belts in preventing injury and death, the National Highway Traffic Safety Administration (NHTSA) in May 1991 started a nationwide campaign to encourage Americans to buckle up. The campaign's goal was to get 70 per cent of motorists to use seat belts by 1992, up from about 50 per cent in 1991.

NHTSA said that overall use of seat belts had tripled between 1984 and 1987, from about 14 per cent of all motorists to 42 per cent. Since then, the rate of increase has slowed, even though 38 states that contain 90 per cent of the nation's population have passed laws requiring motorists to buckle up. Usage was especially low among younger drivers, with only about 30 per cent of teen-agers wearing seat belts.

NHTSA said the campaign will involve public education and efforts to encourage police to enforce seat belt and child restraint laws by issuing motorists warnings or citations. Officials said that a similar emphasis on enforcement in Canada had increased seat belt usage from 36 per cent of motorists in 1980 to 82 per cent in 1990.

Regulation for trucks and vans. The U.S. Department of Transportation (DOT) in March 1991 ordered automobile manufacturers to begin installing front-seat airbags or automatic seat belts in vans, light trucks, and utility vehicles in 1994. The vehicles previously were required to have only manually operated seat belts.

DOT said that the new regulation could prevent about 2,000 deaths each year when fully in effect. It would be phased in over a period of three years. After 1997, airbags or automatic seat belts would be required in all trucks and vans manufactured in the United States.

Don't drink the lead
A lead compound gives lead crystal its characteristic heavy weight. But lead is also a poison. If wine or another beverage sits in a crystal glass or decanter long enough, the liquid can absorb some of the lead from the crystal, researchers recently found. The scientists believe that the amount of lead that dissolves in a short time—during a meal, for example—is unlikely to cause problems. The finding, however, suggests that people should avoid long-term storage of beverages in lead-crystal containers. Further investigations are underway.

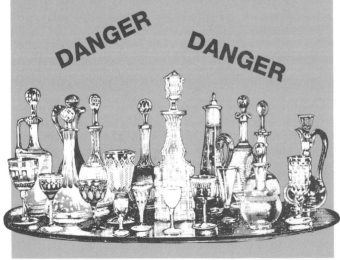

Lead crystal hazard. Scientists at Columbia University in New York City warned in January 1991 that wine or liquor kept in lead crystal decanters or glasses for long periods of time may become contaminated with high levels of lead. But they said additional studies were needed to determine if use of lead crystal actually causes health problems in adults or unborn children. Lead poisoning can cause damage to the nervous system and other health disorders.

Lead crystal contains up to 32 per cent of a lead compound, lead oxide, which gives crystal glassware its characteristic heavy weight. The scientists found that tiny amounts of this lead *leaches* (dissolves) out of the glass into wine or liquor. In many lead crystal glasses tested, leaching began within the first hour after pouring wine or liquor into them. The levels of lead remained low, however, and did not pose a risk of lead poisoning.

But leaching continues over time. Researchers found more worrisome lead levels in brandy and other spirits that had been stored in lead crystal decanters for long periods of time. Some brandies stored in crystal decanters for several years contained 50 times more lead than normal. As a result, the Food and Drug Administration recommended against long-term storage of food and beverages in crystal containers.

Seafood safety. A panel of experts on the safety of seafood in January 1991 called for greater public awareness of the hazards of eating raw or undercooked clams, oysters, and mussels. The panel warned that raw shellfish may carry disease-causing microorganisms that thrive in polluted offshore waters. Consumers of raw shellfish thus risk a variety of ailments, ranging from mild gastrointestinal upsets to hepatitis, a potentially serious liver disorder.

Most cooked seafoods are unlikely to cause food poisoning or other illness, the panel concluded following the two-year study organized by the National Academy of Sciences in Washington, D.C. Even though consumption of seafood had increased by almost 60 per cent during the 1980's, the panel found no evidence of a par-

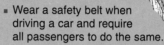

Preventing head injury
Head injuries are potentially serious because they can result in damage to the brain. Each year, more than half a million Americans suffer brain injuries as the result of a blow or fall. Following the rules below can help prevent head injuries.

- Wear a safety belt when driving a car and require all passengers to do the same.
- Use infant and child safety seats in cars and make sure they fit the child properly.
- Don't drink and drive. Car accidents are a primary cause of head injury. And many car accidents are caused by drunk driving.
- Ride a bicycle that is the right size for you and obey all traffic laws. They apply to cyclists, too.
- Wear a helmet when riding a bicycle or motorcycle and when skateboarding.
- Before diving into a pool or lake, jump into the water feet first to check the water depth.

Source: National Head Injury Foundation.

allel increase in seafood-related illness, as some experts had feared.

Cost of nonfatal accidents. About 41 million Americans suffer some economic loss from a nonfatal injury each year, a study requested by the U.S. Congress concluded in April 1991. The study found that accidents affect on average 1 of every 6 people each year and cost the economy more than $175 billion. The economic losses result from medical expenses, the cost of additional household help or equipment, and time from missed work.

Most of the accidents reported in the study were not very serious. They involved strains, sprains, cuts, bruises, and fractures. Almost 40 per cent of the accidents resulted from slips and falls. About 30 per cent involved toys, sports equipment, tools, and various other products. Motor vehicles were involved in about 20 per cent of non-fatal accidents.

One-third of the accidents occurred while people were engaged in sports or other leisure-time activities. About one-fourth took place while people were working around the house, and another fourth occurred while people were either on the job or commuting to work.

The study was conducted for Congress by the Rand Corporation, a nonprofit research organization based in Santa Monica, Calif. Researchers said the study, which included 26,000 households, was one of the most comprehensive ever conducted on the costs of nonfatal injuries.

Slap with care. Parents should caution their children about a popular toy called a *slap wrist bracelet*, the U.S. Consumer Product Safety Commission (CPSC) announced in October 1990. The bracelet consists of a thin strip of metal, about 9 inches (23 centimeters) long, covered by fabric or paper. When slapped against the wrist, the flat strip snaps into a cylindrical bracelet and encircles the wrist.

CPSC expressed concern that the bracelet's fabric or paper covering may tear or come apart after repeated use, exposing a sharp metal edge that could cut the skin. CPSC advised parents to alert their children to the potential hazard. Parents also should inspect slap bracelets being used by young children to ensure that the metal strip is covered. CPSC also said that it would urge manufacturers to modify the bracelets to prevent possible injuries.

Electromagnetic fields and cancer. Concern about the possible health effects of electromagnetic fields generated by high-voltage electric power lines and other electric equipment intensified in December 1990. After reviewing scientific studies, the U.S. Environmental Protection Agency (EPA) concluded that low-level electromagnetic fields are "a possible, but not proven, cause of cancer in humans." The EPA found evidence of a possible link between the fields and some forms of cancer, including leukemia (a blood cancer) and brain cancer.

Electromagnetic fields are generated by electric current passing through wires or other conductors. A wide variety of electrical devices—including power transmission lines, broadcast antennas, personal computers, and household appliances—generate such fields.

Many experts expressed skepticism about the findings. The EPA said that additional research would be needed to determine the seriousness of the health risk. ☐ Michael Woods

In WORLD BOOK, see SAFETY.

Sexually Transmitted Diseases

The number of reported cases of infectious syphilis in the United States in 1990 reached its highest level in 40 years, according to a report issued in November by researchers from the Centers for Disease Control (CDC) in Atlanta, Ga. More than 50,000 cases of the disease were reported in 1990. The cities with the highest rates of syphilis were Atlanta; Washington, D.C.; and Miami, Fla.

The increase in syphilis, a sexually transmitted disease (STD), began in the mid-1980's and occurred chiefly among minority heterosexual men and women in metropolitan areas. According to the CDC, the infection rate for black and Hispanic Americans in 1990 was 39 times and 9 times higher, respectively, than the infection rate for white Americans.

The CDC researchers suggested a number of factors contributing to the syphilis increase among minority heterosexuals. These included poverty, the practice of exchanging sexual services for drugs (especially crack cocaine), limited access to health care, homelessness, and residence in areas where syphilis rates are high.

The increasing syphilis rate has important implications, health officials said. As the number of heterosexual adults with syphilis increases, so too does the number of babies born with the disease. The rising syphilis rate also indicates that community education programs intended to reduce sexual behavior that increases a person's risk of contracting an STD—including AIDS—have apparently not reached many inner-city heterosexuals. Finally, health experts fear that because syphilis produces genital ulcers that may help increase the risk of contracting the virus that causes AIDS, the rise in syphilis may hasten the spread of AIDS among groups who are at high-risk of contracting the virus.

Detecting human papillomavirus.
A study of female college students comparing a new technique for identifying human papillomavirus (HPV) with the most commonly used test for that purpose has revealed a much higher rate of infection than researchers had suspected. The study, reported in January 1991, was conducted by researchers at the University of California at Berkeley.

HPV, which causes genital warts, is a common sexually transmitted virus. Studies have also linked some forms of the virus with cancers of the reproductive tract, including cancer of the *cervix,* the lower opening of the *uterus* (womb).

The researchers tested the students with a commonly used test, which detects the presence of *antibodies* (disease-fighting proteins) formed against HPV, and a more sensitive, experimental test, which detects material from the virus itself. Using the new technique, the researchers found that 46 per cent of the women were infected with HPV. In contrast, the commonly used test revealed the presence of HPV in only 11 per cent of the women. The researchers also found that the more sexual partners a woman had, the more likely she was to be infected with HPV.

Pelvic inflammatory disease (PID), apart from AIDS, is the most serious and most costly common sexually transmitted disease affecting women, researchers at the National Institutes of Health and the CDC reported in April 1991. PID refers to infections of the female upper reproductive tract. It can result in severe complications, such as chronic pelvic pain and *ectopic pregnancy.* (In an ectopic pregnancy, the fetus usually implants in one of the two *Fallopian tubes,* which

STD hot lines
Confidential information about sexually transmitted diseases is available from several national hot lines.

☎ **The National AIDS Hot line (800-342-AIDS)** is open 24 hours a day, 7 days a week. Callers can obtain information on HIV infection (infection with the AIDS virus) and AIDS, as well as referrals for treatment, counseling, and legal services. Spanish-language information on HIV infection and AIDS is available at 800-344-7432, 7 days a week, from 8 a.m. to 2 a.m. Eastern time. People who are hearing-impaired can obtain this information by calling 800-243-7889, Monday through Friday, from 10 a.m. to 10 p.m. Eastern time.

☎ **The National Sexually Transmitted Diseases Hot line (800-227-8922)** is open Monday through Friday from 8 a.m. to 11 p.m. Eastern time. Trained counselors provide information, printed literature, and referrals, mainly to public health clinics.

☎ **The Herpes Resources Hot line (919-361-8488)** is open Monday through Friday from 9 a.m. to 7 p.m., Eastern time. Callers can obtain information, printed literature and audio tapes, and referrals to health clinics and support groups.

connect the ovaries and uterus, rather than in the uterus.)

Up to 1 million new cases of PID are reported each year. The condition is most common among sexually active women aged 15 to 19 years. Almost 300,000 American women are hospitalized for PID annually. The cost of medical care for women with PID reached $4.2 billion in 1990.

The researchers said that if current trends continue, 50 per cent of the women who were 15 years old in 1970 will have experienced at least one episode of PID by the year 2000. They also estimated that the annual cost of treating women with PID will total almost $10 billion by the year 2000.

Contraception and STD's. Barrier methods of contraception not only help prevent unplanned pregnancy but also significantly reduce the risk of contracting an STD. That conclusion was reported in April 1991 by researchers at the University of Southern California in Los Angeles who reviewed published studies of the effectiveness of various contraceptive devices in preventing the spread of STD's.

The researchers found that, in general, condoms, when used appropriately, effectively reduce the risk of transmitting STD's. Vaginal spermicides also appear to decrease women's risk of contracting a cervical infection by chlamydial or gonococcal bacteria.

In contrast, intrauterine devices (IUD's) may increase the risk of contracting an upper genital tract infection. Hormonal contraception, particularly oral contraceptives, are ineffective in preventing infections of the lower genital tract.

One of the problems facing couples making choices about contraception is that the methods providing the best protection against pregnancy are the least effective in preventing the transmission of STD's. In contrast, those contraceptive methods with the best record against STD's provide only moderate protection against pregnancy. Some experts recommend that couples use two contraceptive methods—one method to reduce the risk of transmitting or contracting an STD and the other to prevent an unplanned pregnancy. □ Willard Cates, Jr.

In the Special Reports section, see THE SPECTER OF AIDS; SEXUALLY TRANSMITTED DANGER. In WORLD BOOK, see VENEREAL DISEASE.

Skin

A new technique for removing tattoos was announced in April 1991 by researchers at Harvard University Medical School in Boston. The technique uses a *laser* (light-amplifying device) to remove the tattoo pigments permanently while causing little or no scarring or change in skin texture.

The type of laser used by the Harvard researchers, called a *ruby laser*, amplifies light at a wavelength that is absorbed only by the tattoo pigments deposited in deeper layers of the skin. Blood cells and other important tissues in the skin remain unaffected.

The investigators theorized that the laser energy fragments the pigments and metal granules that make up the tattoo. Once the particles become small enough and scatter, they are no longer visible. The body then gradually disposes of these tiny particles.

The number of treatments needed to remove a tattoo depends on its size, color, and location, though the average is four to six. People who have undergone the tattoo-removal treatments describe the sensation of the laser as resembling the snapping of a rubber band against the skin.

Before the development of the laser technique, tattoos were removed by such methods as surgical excision, *dermabrasion* (taking off layers of skin

Halting hair loss
By bathing the scalp in an electric field, a device that looks like a hairdrier may help stop hair loss and restore thinning hair on balding heads, according to a 1990 report by researchers at the University of British Columbia in Vancouver, Canada. To be successful, however, the treatments must continue for life. Moreover, they work only on people who have been bald a short time and still retain hair roots.

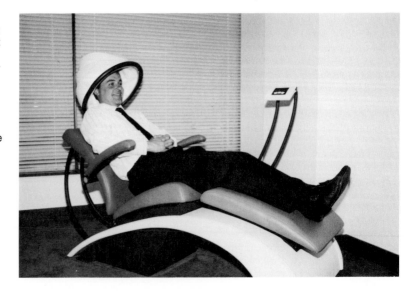

with a high-speed rotary tool), skin grafts, or the application of chemicals to the skin. A tattoo can also be partially hidden by tattooing flesh-colored pigments over the original design.

Regulating tanning salons. By 1991, more than half of the states in the United States had passed laws—or were in the process of passing laws—that regulated tanning parlors. The safety of such facilities has come into question because of the long-term harmful effects of ultraviolet (UV) light—a form of electromagnetic radiation released by the sun and by the salon's tanning lamps. More than 1 million people patronize tanning salons each year, according to estimates by dermatologists.

Tanning is the skin's response to injury caused by UV radiation. In excessive doses, this radiation can cause acute sunburn, aging of the skin, and skin cancers. Although many tanning salons advertise that their equipment is safer than sunlight, critics say that the salon lamps can generate five times the amount of UV-A radiation—the longest wavelengths of UV light—that a person would receive at the equator. In addition, some people may sustain severe burns if they are taking certain medications (including some types of antibiotics and diuretics) in combination with exposure to large doses of UV radiation.

The American Academy of Dermatology favors requiring all tanning salons to do the following: inform patrons about the risks of UV radiation; check all medications taken by patrons; require goggles to prevent eye damage; keep treatment records; and require parental consent before allowing minors to use tanning equipment.

Dangers of tanning pills. A previously healthy woman died after taking "tanning" pills provided by a tanning salon, according to a report in the *Journal of the American Medical Association* in September 1990. Researchers from Vanderbilt University in Nashville reported that the cause of death was *aplastic anemia*, a condition that can result when a *toxic* (poisonous) substance destroys the bone marrow's ability to produce blood cells. If untreated, a patient who has

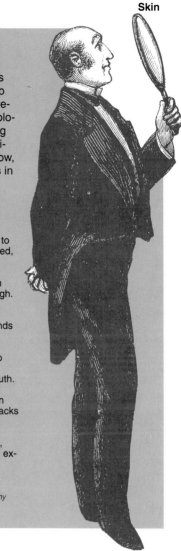

The skin as a mirror
What happens on the body's surface may provide clues to medical conditions hidden beneath. According to dermatologists, a number of underlying problems, including the nutritional deficiencies listed below, can be signaled by changes in the skin and hair.

Protein: Deficiency causes dry skin, loss of skin color.

Essential fat: Deficiency leads to patches of baldness, eczema (red, itchy skin).

Vitamin A: Deficiency results in thickened skin that is dry or rough.

Vitamin C: Deficiency causes bleeding gums, inability of wounds to heal quickly.

Vitamin B_6: Deficiency leads to flaky skin, sores in the mouth, cracks at the corners of the mouth.

Riboflavin: Deficiency results in oily skin, sores in the mouth, cracks at the corners of the mouth.

Niacin: Deficiency causes dark, round spots in areas of the skin exposed to the sun, sores in the mouth and rectum.

Source: *Journal of the American Academy of Dermatology.*

aplastic anemia may die from bleeding or infection.

The pills that the woman took contained *canthaxanthin*, a substance that colors the skin a shade of orange-brown through its accumulation in various layers of the skin and fat. The researchers speculated that the woman took a large dose of the substance because her skin had turned deep orange rather than "tanned."

Canthaxanthin has been known to cause severe itching of the skin, problems with vision, and *hepatitis* (inflammation of the liver). Although there was no direct proof that the pills caused the woman's death, the Vanderbilt physicians noted that no other cause was apparent. The fact that the patient's symptoms began several

325

weeks after she took the pills suggested they were responsible for her illness, the physicians concluded.

Canthaxanthin is sold under several names, including Orobronze, Darker Tan, and BronzGlo. These preparations, which are advertised as harmless, are available through tanning salons, health stores, and mail order houses. None of these products, however, has been approved as either a prescription or over-the-counter medication by the U.S. Food and Drug Administration, the agency that monitors drug safety.

Smoking and the skin. Smoking increases the likelihood of developing premature facial wrinkles, researchers at the University of Utah reported in May 1991. The scientists studied 109 smokers and 23 nonsmokers aged 35 to 59.

The risk of premature wrinkling doubled, the researchers found, for people who had smoked from 1 to 49 *pack-years*. (A pack-year was defined as equal to smoking one pack a day per year.) Those who smoked 50 or more pack-years had 4.7 times the risk. For the average smoker, the researchers reported, the risk of premature wrinkling at least tripled. See also SMOKING.

☐ Kathryn E. Bowers and Kenneth A. Arndt
In WORLD BOOK, see SKIN.

Smoking

More Americans are quitting smoking, but the death toll from the addictive habit has continued to rise dramatically, United States health officials reported in January 1991. In 1988, the latest year for which figures were available, 434,175 Americans died of smoking-related illnesses, according to William L. Roper, director of the federal Centers for Disease Control (CDC) in Atlanta, Ga.

That death toll is the highest ever attributed to smoking, marking an 11 per cent rise since 1985 and a 131 per cent rise since 1965. The steady upward trend, Roper said, reflected a delayed effect on the health of large numbers of people who had smoked heavily in the 1950's and 1960's.

Health officials hope the trend will reverse as more people quit the habit. An estimated 50 million Americans smoked in 1991. This constituted 29 per cent of the adult population, down from 30 per cent in 1985 and 40 per cent in 1964—the year of the U.S. surgeon general's first report on the dangers of smoking. Even so, health officials need to continue warning about the dangers of smoking, Roper said, reaching out especially to young people and women, who together make up the largest percentage of smokers.

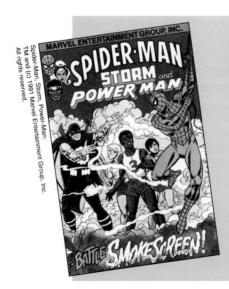

Don't go up in smoke
Smoking is too big a burden for even a superhero to handle. This is the message of a comic book that explains the risks of smoking to youngsters. The American Cancer Society estimates that 12 per cent of Americans aged 12 to 17 already have this potentially fatal habit. For a free copy of *Spider-Man, Storm, and Power Battle Smoke Screen*, contact your local chapter of the American Cancer Society, listed in the white pages of the telephone book.

Passive smoking risks. Evidence of the health threat posed by second-hand smoke continued to mount in 1991. *Passive smoking*, as it is called, occurs when a nonsmoker breathes smoke from someone else's cigarette.

In January, researchers at the University of California at San Francisco reported that passive smoking causes an estimated 53,000 deaths each year in the United States. This makes it the third leading preventable cause of death, behind active smoking and alcohol abuse. Passive smoking causes 37,000 deaths from heart disease each year, almost 4,000 lung-cancer deaths, and 12,000 deaths from other cancers, the researchers said.

Exposure to second-hand smoke had previously been linked to lung cancer and other forms of cancer. The California researchers surveyed a wide range of medical studies and found an even stronger link between passive smoking and heart disease. They discovered that nonsmokers married to smokers had a 30 per cent greater chance of dying of heart disease than other nonsmokers.

Children and passive smoking. Two reports published in January 1991 highlighted the dangers to children of passive smoking. One study, by researchers at the University of North Carolina in Chapel Hill, suggested that if a father smokes even before a child's birth, that child's risk of brain cancer and leukemia is increased. The researchers speculated that smoking may have harmful effects on the father's sperm.

Another study, by researchers at Yale University in New Haven, Conn., indicated that children exposed to second-hand smoke are four times as likely as other children to develop serious infectious diseases. The researchers suggested the smoke may lower a child's defenses against infection.

Smoking and depression. In the first extensive study of smoking and depression, researchers at the New York State Psychiatric Institute in New York City found that smokers are more than twice as likely as nonsmokers to suffer from serious depression. Their study of more than 3,000 people in St. Louis, Mo., was reported in the

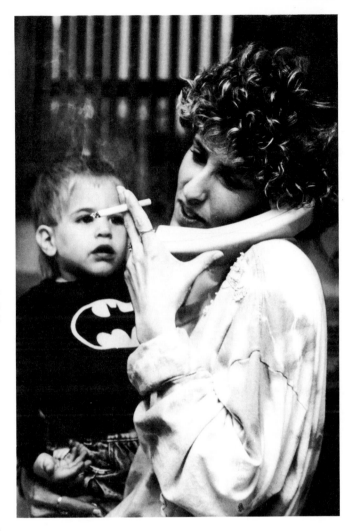

Sept. 26, 1990, issue of the *Journal of the American Medical Association*.

The survey showed that 6.6 per cent of smokers had experienced major depression, defined by the researchers as a depressed mood that lasted at least two weeks and had at least four other symptoms, such as sleep disturbance and loss of appetite. Among people who had never smoked, 2.9 per cent had suffered from major depression.

A study by CDC researchers in the same issue of the journal concluded that depressed smokers were 40 per cent less likely to kick their habit successfully than nondepressed smokers. Using data from two national health surveys, the scientists found that smoking rates rose—and the ability to

Smoke hurts kids
Parents who smoke may be endangering the health of their children. Children of smokers have a greater chance of developing lung cancer than children of nonsmokers, according to a 1990 report. Furthermore, a study published in 1991 found that children who live in households with smokers are more susceptible to infectious diseases.

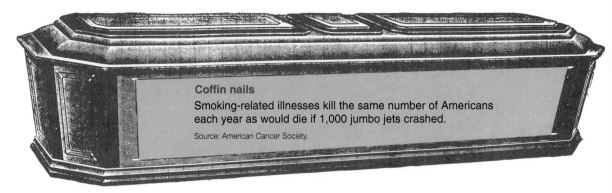

Coffin nails

Smoking-related illnesses kill the same number of Americans each year as would die if 1,000 jumbo jets crashed.

Source: American Cancer Society.

quit smoking fell—as a person's score increased on a standardized survey of symptoms of depression.

One-fifth of those who smoked at least a pack of cigarettes daily scored high on symptoms of depression. When questioned nearly a decade later, 17.7 per cent of the nondepressed smokers said they had successfully stopped smoking, while only 9.9 per cent of the depressed smokers said they had quit.

In both studies, the researchers noted, the results supported the idea that some people may seek relief from painful feelings by becoming addicted to drugs, including *nicotine*, a habit-forming substance in tobacco smoke. They said more research was needed to understand the relationship between depression and smoking and to determine whether treating depression might help smokers kick their habit.

Hiding chest pain. A study reported in November 1990 suggested that cigarette smoking may mask chest pain, an important warning signal of heart disease. Researchers at the University of North Carolina in Chapel Hill, who conducted the study, said that the higher tolerance for pain they found in male smokers may explain the higher rate of "silent," or painless, *ischemia* (insufficient blood flow to the heart) among smokers.

Previous studies had shown that the nicotine in cigarette smoke lessened the perception of pain in animals. To test the effect of nicotine on humans, the North Carolina researchers put heat probes on the forearms of 20 men aged 19 to 44 who smoked an average of 23 cigarettes a day, and on 5 men who did not smoke. The heat probe was gradually heated until each man first felt pain and then until

Smoking increases the likelihood that a person's face will wrinkle prematurely, according to a 1991 report by researchers at the University of Utah. The researchers found that people who smoked the most and the longest were at greatest risk.

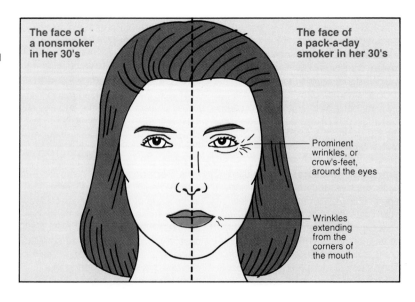

The face of a nonsmoker in her 30's

The face of a pack-a-day smoker in her 30's

Prominent wrinkles, or crow's-feet, around the eyes

Wrinkles extending from the corners of the mouth

he could no longer tolerate the pain.

Before the men were tested a second time, the smokers smoked three cigarettes. Although the nonsmokers showed no change in their sensitivity to pain, the smokers' tolerance rose significantly. The researchers speculated that nicotine may bind to nerve cells, interfering with pain messages to the brain.

Health benefits of quitting. People can achieve "major and immediate" improvements in health by quitting smoking, U.S. Surgeon General Antonia Novello said in September 1990, when she released her office's 21st annual report on the health effects of smoking. Although the benefits of stopping smoking were well known for individual diseases, the report was the first to provide an analysis of overall health benefits.

The likelihood of developing heart disease dropped by 50 per cent after one smoke-free year, and after 15 years, it approached the level of nonsmokers, Novello said. The risk of lung cancer dropped by 50 per cent over 10 smoke-free years. The risk also dropped for cancers of the larynx, mouth, throat, pancreas, bladder, and cervix, as well as for pneumonia, bronchitis, and ulcers.

☐ William H. Allen

In WORLD BOOK, see SMOKING.

Stroke

The results of two important studies reported in 1991 demonstrated that a once-controversial operation can help prevent stroke in high-risk patients. The operation, *carotid endarterectomy*, involves opening the *carotid arteries* (the major vessels carrying blood to the brain) and removing deposits of fat and calcium that are obstructing the vessels.

Although vascular surgeons perform tens of thousands of endarterectomies in the United States every year, there has been no scientific evidence that the operations actually prevent stroke. In addition, an estimated 3 to 6 per cent of patients undergoing this type of surgery suffer strokes during or shortly after the operation. Thus, the two studies were designed to determine whether the benefits of the procedure outweighed the risks.

Researchers at 50 medical centers in the United States and Canada participated in one study. They reported that of 300 patients with severe arterial blockages who received endarterectomies, 7 per cent suffered strokes within 18 months. This compares with 24 per cent of the study's 295 patients who received more standard drug treatment—aspirin and other drugs to prevent blood clots and, if needed, drugs to lower cholesterol,

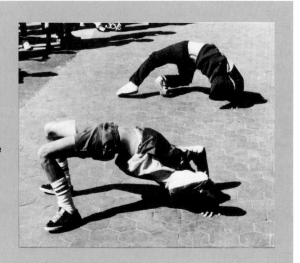

Break dancing: stroke risk?

Break dancers run the risk of straining their back or pulling a muscle, but they may also be courting a much more serious risk: stroke. In August 1990, physicians in London reported treating a 27-year-old man who suffered bleeding in the brain after break dancing and consuming a large quantity of alcohol. The doctors said the man's drinking may have contributed to the stroke by increasing blood flow in the brain. They added, however, that the vigorous head shaking involved in break dancing was the probable cause of the stroke. The doctors advised caution for those who want to break dance, especially when drinking.

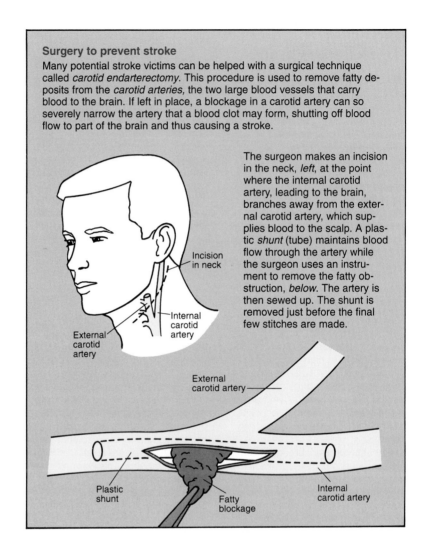

Surgery to prevent stroke

Many potential stroke victims can be helped with a surgical technique called *carotid endarterectomy*. This procedure is used to remove fatty deposits from the *carotid arteries,* the two large blood vessels that carry blood to the brain. If left in place, a blockage in a carotid artery can so severely narrow the artery that a blood clot may form, shutting off blood flow to part of the brain and thus causing a stroke.

The surgeon makes an incision in the neck, *left*, at the point where the internal carotid artery, leading to the brain, branches away from the external carotid artery, which supplies blood to the scalp. A plastic *shunt* (tube) maintains blood flow through the artery while the surgeon uses an instrument to remove the fatty obstruction, *below*. The artery is then sewed up. The shunt is removed just before the final few stitches are made.

Incision in neck

Internal carotid artery

External carotid artery

External carotid artery

Plastic shunt

Fatty blockage

Internal carotid artery

blood pressure, or blood *glucose* (sugar) levels.

In May 1991, the results of another, larger study also indicated a benefit from carotid endarterectomy. Physicians at 80 medical centers in 14 nations performed the procedure on 455 patients, while 323 received the more standard drug treatment. Three years later, 12 per cent of the endarterectomy patients had suffered strokes compared with 24 per cent of patients who had received drugs—a 12 per cent reduction in stroke risk.

Blood test helps predict stroke. In February 1991, medical researchers at the Oregon Health Sciences University in Portland said that they had combined results from three blood

tests to identify patients who may be in danger of stroke. One test measures *albumin* (a protein found in most tissues), which appears to "leak" into the blood from arterial walls damaged by *atherosclerosis*, a narrowing of the artery caused by fat deposits. The other two tests measure levels of glucose and *fibrinogen* (a protein that assists blood clot formation). High levels of glucose or fibrinogen increase blood *viscosity* (thickness and stickiness), a factor linked with increased stroke risk.

In February 1991, the Oregon researchers reported that they tested blood samples from 129 patients who had suffered strokes, measuring albumin, glucose, and viscosity. By using the combined results of the tests, they correctly identified 24 of the 32 patients who had suffered a second stroke within a year. The blood test may eventually be used to help prevent strokes by identifying high-risk patients so that they can be treated.

Stroke-preventing drug. Low doses of *warfarin*, a drug that prevents blood from clotting, can prevent stroke in patients who have *atrial fibrillation*. Researchers for the National Heart, Lung, and Blood Institute reported this finding in November 1990.

Atrial fibrillation is a condition in which the contractions of the atrium, or upper chamber, of the heart are too rapid and weak to pump all the blood

into the heart's lower chamber. As a result, some blood collects in the atrium, where it has a tendency to clot. These clots can lodge in vessels leading to the brain, causing strokes.

The researchers studied 420 patients with atrial fibrillation, 212 of whom received low doses of warfarin, and 208 of whom were in a control group that received no warfarin. After two years, 2 people in the warfarin group had suffered strokes compared with 13 people in the control group. Researchers calculated that the warfarin patients reduced their risk of stroke by 86 per cent.

☐ Beverly Merz
In WORLD BOOK, see STROKE.

Teeth
See Dentistry

Studies during 1991 showed that microwave therapy may be an effective treatment for an enlarged prostate gland. The treatment involves bombarding the gland with microwave energy, which then generates heat. The heat destroys excess prostrate tissue, which may help improve urine flow.

About 75 per cent of men over the age of 50 develop an enlarged prostate. The gland, which is normally about the size of a walnut, lies beneath the bladder and surrounds the *urethra*, the tube that carries urine from the bladder. The prostate produces a substance used to transport sperm cells.

As the prostate grows, it can press against the urethra and obstruct it. Symptoms of such obstruction of the urethra may include slowing of the urinary stream, a burning sensation while urinating, blood in the urine, a feeling of incomplete emptying, and an increased frequency of urination.

The microwave heat treatment takes about an hour and can be given as an outpatient procedure using no general anesthesia. It causes little discomfort or blood loss and may allow the patient to return to normal activities within 48 hours.

In microwave treatment, doctors insert a probe into the urethra. The

Urology

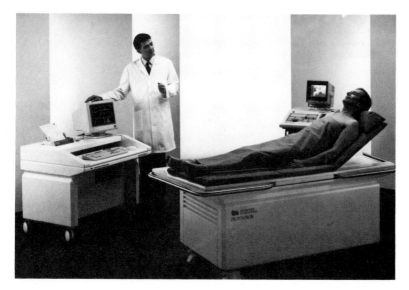

New prostate treatment
An experimental machine called the "Prostatron" uses microwave energy as an alternative to surgery for the treatment of enlarged prostate glands. The technique, which doctors in the United States were studying in 1991, transmits microwave energy through a probe inserted into the patient's urethra. The microwaves generate heat, which destroys extra tissue in the gland and reduces its size.

probe contains wires that generate microwaves, which heat the prostate tissue. A cooling mechanism surrounding the probe protects the urethra and nearby tissues. The doctors also monitor the patient's rectal temperature so that damage to the rectum does not occur as a result of the procedure. After treatment, some of the patients will go into *urinary retention* (inability to urinate), which requires a *catheter* (tube) to drain the bladder for a few days.

Five medical centers in the United States have begun studies on the experimental technique using a machine called the "Prostatron," made by a French company. The goal of these studies is to determine if the therapy is safe and effective.

New prostate drug. An experimental drug called Proscar reduces the size of enlarged prostate glands, according to a June 1991 study by the drug's developer. The firm Merck Sharp & Dohme Incorporated of Rahway, N.J., found that Proscar reduced prostate size by approximately 20 per cent in 57 per cent of the 1,600 men who took the drug for a year.

Proscar works by blocking the effect of a certain form of *testosterone* (the male sex hormone) on the prostate. This form of testosterone—dihydrotestosterone—contributes to the swelling of the gland, according to medical experts.

New use for an old drug? Clinical studies completed in June 1991 show that a drug commonly used to treat high blood pressure may also relieve some symptoms of an enlarged prostate. In a study involving 314 men with enlarged prostates, the drug terazosin hydrochloride (marketed as Hytrin) improved urinary flow in 70 per cent of patients compared with 38 per cent of the men who took a *placebo* (inactive substance). The study was conducted by Abbott Laboratories, North Chicago, Ill., the manufacturer of Hytrin. The drug company hopes to have approval from the United States Food and Drug Administration to sell Hytrin as a medication for enlarged prostates by the end of 1991.

Hytrin belongs to a class of drugs called *alpha blockers*. These drugs block the activity of certain nerve cells, some of which control muscle tension. Medical experts say that Hytrin causes the muscles in the prostate and urethra to relax, which allows better urine flow.

Hytrin is used for patients who cannot tolerate or who do not wish to have surgery. Because Hytrin does not reduce the size of the prostate, but only relieves symptoms, the drug must be taken indefinitely to prevent symptoms from reappearing.

□ Dennis Pessis

In the Special Reports section, see Combating Prostate Cancer. In World Book, see Prostate gland.

Venereal Diseases

See Sexually Transmitted Diseases

Veterinary Medicine

A vaccine to prevent Lyme disease in dogs was made available to veterinarians in late 1990. Lyme disease, a serious bacterial infection transmitted to people and animals by certain types of ticks, has been reported in human beings in 44 states. Experts estimate that the disease may be equally serious and widespread in animals. The infection, which is caused by a bacterium called *Borrelia burgdorferi*, can lead to chronic arthritis.

Fort Dodge Laboratories in Fort Dodge, Iowa, distributed the vaccine after the United States Department of Agriculture granted the company a conditional license in mid-1990. The vaccine limits the bacteria's ability to multiply in the dog's bloodstream by stimulating the dog's infection-fighting immune system to produce antibodies that attack the bacteria. Two injections are given three weeks apart, followed by a booster shot every year.

The Lyme disease vaccine should be especially beneficial for dogs that live in tick-infested areas. Researchers at several institutions are working to develop Lyme disease vaccines for cats, horses, cattle, and other animals—including human beings.

Unfortunately, because the dog vaccine stimulates the production of antibodies, it also interferes with the only available tests to diagnose Lyme disease. These tests detect antibodies to *B. burgdorferi* rather than the bacteri-

Hot line help for poisoned pets
Pets can be a lot like little children—always putting things into their mouths. People who are unable to reach a local veterinarian when their pets have swallowed something that might be poisonous can get help by calling:

**National Animal Poison Control Center:
1-800-548-2423.**

The center's professional staff answers calls at this number 24 hours a day, 7 days a week; the $25.00 fee must be charged to a major credit card. Any follow-up calls for the same incident are free.

Source: *Journal of the American Veterinary Medical Association.*

um itself. If the antibody levels are high, veterinarians assume that the dog has been infected. Once a dog has been vaccinated, however, a diagnostic test will also show high levels of antibodies in the dog's blood. A veterinarian testing such an animal will not know whether the high antibody levels indicate that the vaccine was successful—or that the animal became infected despite the vaccine and now requires treatment.

Experts say that the reliability of the diagnostic tests is questionable even without the complication presented by vaccination. It takes weeks for an animal's body to develop antibodies after infection, so the tests are not dependable in early stages of the disease. Moreover, if a pet does test positive, it is difficult to determine the stage of infection or whether the animal has already recovered. To make diagnosis more reliable, scientists in mid-1991 were attempting to develop a test to detect the bacterium itself in blood or urine.

Outbreaks of rabies in raccoons and other wild animals concerned residents of the Northeastern United States in spring 1991. More than 15 rabid foxes, raccoons, and skunks were reported in a single New York county. Rabid animals were found in Connecticut and New Jersey as well.

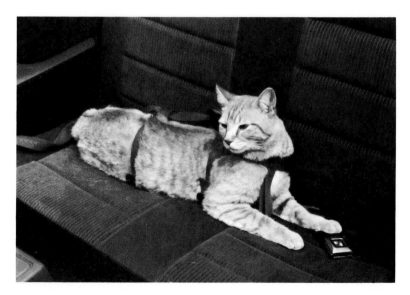

Pet seat belt
A cat rides securely in the back seat of a car thanks to a harness fastened around its shoulders and abdomen. The National Highway Traffic Safety Administration and the American Veterinary Association suggest that pet owners use harnesses because an unrestrained pet can act as a missile during an accident or sudden stop, endangering its own safety and that of others.

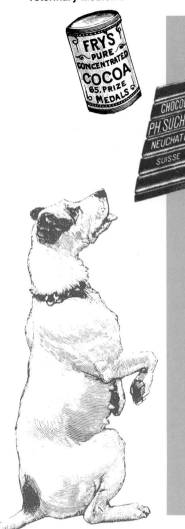

A sweet tooth could be deadly

Many dogs, and some cats, enjoy sharing their owners' candy bars or pieces of chocolate. But chocolate contains *theobromine,* a chemical that can cause reactions ranging from diarrhea to seizures and death. A large amount of chocolate can be fatal, especially when eaten by small dogs, puppies, or cats. Side effects include restlessness, frequent urination, irregular heartbeat, overactivity, and tremors. These symptoms may not occur until several hours after an animal has eaten a large amount of chocolate. If you suspect your pet overdosed on chocolate, call your veterinarian immediately.

How much chocolate is dangerous to your pet?

If your dog is...	...how many pieces from a 30-piece, 16 oz. box of chocolates are risky?
under 10 pounds (e.g., Chihuahua or Pekingese)	more than 4 pieces
10 to 20 pounds (e.g., pug or Shih Tzu)	more than 8 pieces
20 to 30 pounds (e.g., beagle or cocker spaniel)	more than 12 pieces
30 to 40 pounds (e.g., Kerry blue terrier or standard schnauzer)	more than half a box
40 to 50 pounds (e.g., bulldog or Dalmatian)	more than half a box
50 pounds and up (e.g., Doberman pinscher or golden retriever)	more than half a box

Source: Thomas J. Lane, Extension Veterinarian, University of Florida.

Rabies is a fatal viral infection of the central nervous system. The rabies virus can be transmitted to people through the saliva of infected animals. According to the U.S. Centers for Disease Control (CDC) in Atlanta, Ga., 13 cases of rabies in human beings were reported from 1980 through 1990. Some cases of the disease occur when a household pet comes into contact with a rabid wild animal, becomes infected, and transfers the virus to people.

The CDC recommends that people avoid contact with wild animals and have their pet cats as well as dogs vaccinated against the rabies virus. In 1991, several municipalities in the Northeast enacted laws requiring such vaccination.

Early neutering of pets. Long-term studies of pets neutered at unusually young ages were underway in 1991 at several U.S. facilities that have animal adoption programs. A survey of the results was expected by the end of the year.

Many veterinarians hope that early neutering will help solve the pet overpopulation problem by enabling animal shelters to neuter animals before they are adopted. A preliminary study had concluded in 1990 that there is little difference between the biological and behavioral development of dogs neutered at 7 weeks of age and those neutered at 7 months.

☐ Thomas J. Lane

In WORLD BOOK, see VETERINARY MEDICINE.

Health experts have long recognized that the most important risk factor for obesity in a child is parental obesity. (Obesity is defined as a weight more than 20 per cent above the ideal weight for age, height, and sex.) A parent may pass along a genetic predisposition to obesity to a child. A parent also may provide a negative role model for the child by overeating. But, according to the results of a 10-year study published in November 1990, obese parents can help obese children control their weight.

Psychologist Leonard Epstein of the University of Pittsburgh in Pennsylvania and his colleagues studied 76 obese children, ages 6 through 12, who had at least one obese parent. The families were divided randomly into three groups and given training on diet, exercise, and behavior change in eight weekly meetings followed by six meetings spread over the following six months. All the groups were instructed to maintain a 1,200 to 1,500 daily calorie limit, and they also were given sample menus.

The first group received rewards (money for the adult, a special outing for the child) at each session if both parent and youngster lost weight. In the second group, the parent received the money reward and the child received a special outing if only the child lost weight. In the third group, the parent received money just for attending the meeting with the child. Participants in the first two groups also received training on how to reinforce good eating and exercise habits in other family members.

Initially, parents and children both lost weight. But after 10 years, all the parents were heavier than when the study began. However, after 10 years, the weight of children in the first group dropped from 42 per cent overweight to 35 per cent overweight, on the average. The weight of children in the second group rose from 44 per cent overweight to almost 50 per cent overweight. Children in the third group went from being 46 per cent overweight to 65 per cent overweight.

Epstein's conclusion was that, even though parents in the first group regained weight themselves, their involvement at the beginning of the pro-

gram and their reinforcement of new behaviors helped alter their children's eating habits in the long term.

Fatal cycles. Cycles of losing weight followed by regaining weight can have serious and even fatal consequences, according to a report by psychologist Kelly D. Brownell and his colleagues at Yale University in New Haven, Conn., published in June 1991. The researchers analyzed the weight fluctuations and health of 3,130 men and women who participated in the Framingham Heart Study (a decades-long study of risk factors, including obesity, for heart disease) in Massachusetts. Brownell discovered that the risk of heart disease, death from heart disease, and death from all causes was 25 to 100 per cent higher in the group whose weight fluctuated the most.

The risk was the same no matter how much each person in this group weighed at first, whether or not they smoked, what blood pressure and cholesterol levels they had, or how much they exercised. Brownell said that the dangers may be equal for repeatedly losing and regaining 5 pounds (2 kilograms) as for losing and regaining 50 pounds (20 kilograms) one time.

Diet pill danger. Experts are concerned about an ingredient in diet pills, *phenylpropanolamine* (PPA), a drug that can cause high blood pressure, dizziness, seizures, and strokes. In a report to a congressional subcommittee in September 1990, the U.S. Public Health Service said that dieters between 10 and 19 years of age account for the greatest number of adverse reactions to PPA. Adolescents, particularly girls in their teens and preteens, often are greatly concerned with weight control. Health experts worry about the preoccupation with dieting and use of diet pills in this young group. A 1990 poll conducted by a popular magazine for teen-agers found that 49 per cent of the teen-age girls surveyed used over-the-counter diet pills, and 13 per cent used laxatives or diuretics to lose weight.

Although no clinical studies have been conducted on PPA's effects on people under 18, several brands of

The New Way to Weigh In

Many health experts say that if a person is too fat, his or her odds of developing health problems go up. Experts say that an unhealthy weight can lead to such problems as heart disease, high blood pressure, and diabetes. So what constitutes a healthy weight?

According to new federal recommendations, a healthy weight "depends on how much of your weight is fat, where in your body the fat is located, and whether you have weight-related medical problems." The recommendations, "Nutrition and Your Health: Dietary Guidelines for Americans," were published jointly by the United States Department of Agriculture and the Department of Health and Human Services in November 1990.

The new guidelines suggest ideal weights that are higher than those the government published in 1980 and 1985. Also, the new weights suggested for older people are higher than those for young adults. This upward adjustment reflects recent research that, according to the federal experts who drew up the new recommendations, "suggests that people can be a little heavier as they grow older without added risk to health."

However, some authorities dispute that idea. "The impact of weight on health is more severe when one is older than when one is younger," said William P. Castelli, medical director of the Framingham Heart Study. This study, which began in 1948, is an ongoing investigation of risk factors—including overweight—for coronary heart disease of people living in Framingham, Mass.

Another change from previous federal weight tables is that the new table does not distinguish between men and women. It just lists suggested weight ranges for two age groups according to height. People of equal height may have equal amounts of fat, but have different amounts of bone and muscle (which weigh more than the same volume of fat). For this reason, the higher end of each weight range generally applies to men, who usually have more muscle and bone than do women of the same height. The lower weights generally apply to women.

The weight guidelines also provide a simple method for checking how fat is distributed in the body. Recent research has suggested that excess fat in the abdomen is a greater

Suggested Adult Weights		
Height	**Weight in pounds**	
	19 to 34 years	35 years and over
5' 0"	97-128*	108-138*
5' 1"	101-132	111-143
5' 2"	104-137	115-148
5' 3"	107-141	119-152
5' 4"	111-146	122-157
5' 5"	114-150	126-162
5' 6"	118-155	130-167
5' 7"	121-160	134-172
5' 8"	125-164	138-178
5' 9"	129-169	142-183
5' 10"	132-174	146-188
5' 11"	136-179	151-194
6' 0"	140-184	155-199
6' 1"	144-189	159-205
6' 2"	148-195	164-210
6' 3"	152-200	168-216
6' 4"	156-205	173-222
6' 5"	160-211	177-228
6' 6"	164-216	182-234

*Higher weights in ranges generally apply to men.

Source: Derived from the National Research Council, 1989.

health risk than fat in the hips and thighs. According to the method, measure the waist near the navel while standing relaxed. Then measure the hips over the buttocks. Finally, divide the waist measurement by the hip measurement to arrive at the ratio. People with a waist-to-hip ratio near or above one may be at greater risk of several diseases, particularly cardiovascular disease.

The 1990 guidelines—unlike those issued in the past—recommend limits for consumption of fat and saturated fat. The report noted that dietary fat should not exceed 30 per cent of calories, and saturated fat should amount to less than 10 per cent of total calories eaten each day. The average American diet now is 37 per cent fat.

The report reaffirmed five dietary recommendations published in 1985:

- Eat a variety of foods, choosing different foods each day from each of five groups. These groups include vegetables; fruits; grains (breads, cereals, rice, and pasta); dairy products (milk, yogurt, and cheese); and proteins (meats, poultry, fish, dry beans, eggs, and nuts).
- Eat plenty of vegetables, fruit, and grain products.
- Use sugars in moderation.
- Use salt and sodium only in moderation.
- Drink alcoholic beverages only in moderation, if at all.

The guidelines are available free from the Consumer Information Center, Department 514-X, Pueblo, CO 81009.

□ William H. Allen

diet pills containing PPA carry warning labels stating that they should not be used by those under 18 without consulting a doctor. Other diet products with PPA say children under 12 years of age should not take the pills. The U.S. Food and Drug Administration has said, however, that it will continue to approve PPA in over-the-counter products.

Where's the fat? Several studies reported in October 1990 focused on fat, both in human beings and animals. A mammal's body, whether that of a human being or a sleek, wild animal, has pockets of fat in similar locations rather than layers of uniform thickness, according to biologist Caroline M. Pond of the Open University in Milton Keynes, England. She discovered that a large amount of fat surrounds the hearts of many mammals, not only of human beings, as was previously thought. She found that this fat has the ability to take up fatty acids in the blood and to generate *lipids,* the fatty substances that fuel the heart.

The other studies also suggested that fat deposits in specific areas serve different functions. Fat on the thighs and hips in women is an energy source needed for pregnancy and breast-feeding, according to nutritionist M. R. C. Greenwood of the University of California at Davis. Abdominal fat is mobilized by stress hormones, reported Marielle Rebuffe-Scrive, a psychologist at Yale University. She speculates that this fat probably evolved early in prehistoric people to allow them to react quickly—to fight or flee—when hunting dangerous prey. But research suggests that in modern human beings, who live in conditions vastly different from those of prehistoric people, this abdominal fat may be the type that raises the risk of heart disease.

Help for the severely overweight. For the estimated 1 million severely obese people in the United States— men more than 100 pounds (45 kilograms) overweight and women more than 80 pounds (36 kilograms) overweight—the National Institutes of Health in Bethesda, Md., endorsed two operations in March 1991. In one

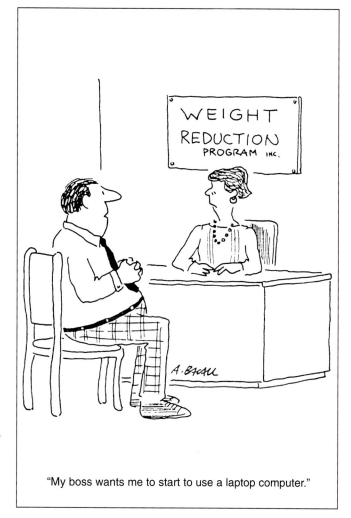

"My boss wants me to start to use a laptop computer."

procedure, a large part of the stomach is stapled shut, leaving a small pouch that is quickly filled, making the patient feel full. In the other operation, the surgeon also makes a stomach pouch but attaches a Y-shaped section of small intestine so that some food bypasses the small intestine and goes directly to the large intestine.

People undergoing these procedures lose more than 100 pounds (45 kilograms) in 18 to 24 months. However, studies show that up to 10 per cent of the patients who have this surgery suffer side effects, which include diarrhea, persistent vomiting, and even aversion to food.

☐ Ricki Lewis

In WORLD BOOK, see WEIGHT CONTROL.

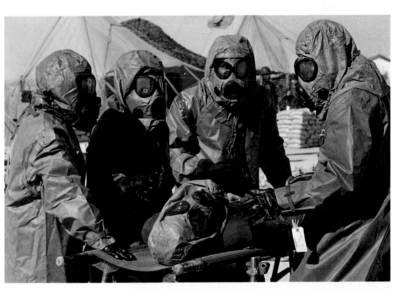

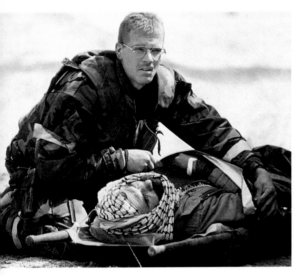

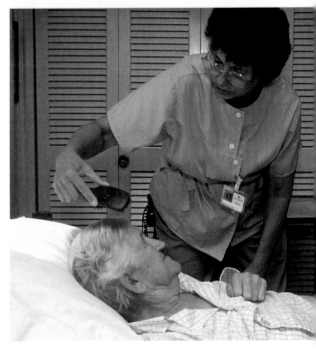

People in Health Care

Two articles spotlight health-care professionals in action.

Medicine at the Front   340
by Marc S. Micozzi
Military planners mobilized thousands of medical workers during
the Persian Gulf War. And these medics brought to the desert
battlefield the lifesaving technology of modern medicine.

Caring for the Terminally Ill   354
by Paul Galloway
Hospices help make the final days of people with incurable diseases
as comfortable as possible..

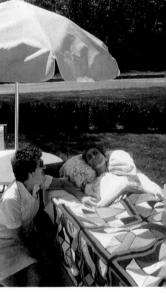

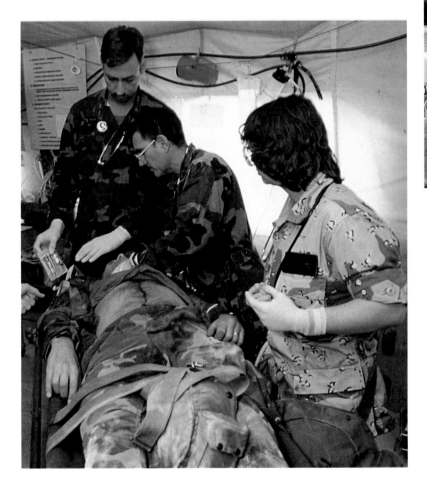

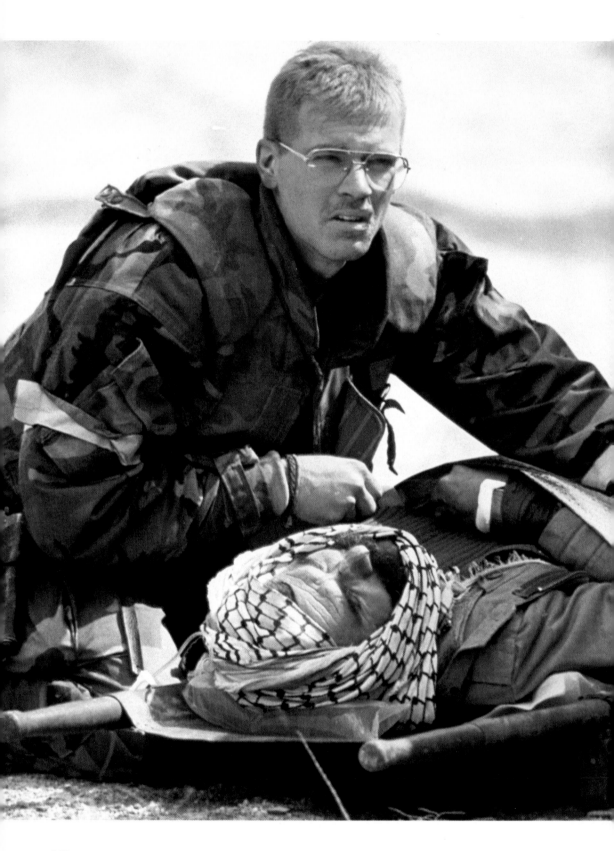

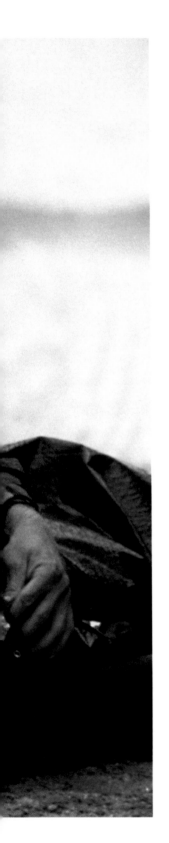

Thousands of medical workers
served in the Persian Gulf War.
Their mission: to provide lifesaving
care in a hostile environment.

Medicine at
the Front

By Marc S. Micozzi

When the United States and its allies launched Operation
Desert Storm in January 1991 to liberate Kuwait from Iraq, the
most elaborate medical establishment ever put onto a battlefield
was ready to treat the wounded. From combat soldiers able to
provide basic lifesaving techniques at the battlefront, to highly
trained surgeons and other specialists offering their skills in
state-of-the-art hospitals, the medical services available to the
more than 500,000 allied troops were varied and complex
enough to support a city the size of Seattle.

In all, 3,100 U.S. medical doctors served in the Gulf, offering
specialties ranging from orthopedists to *otolaryngologists* (ear,
nose, and throat specialists), from psychiatrists to plastic surgeons. They were joined by approximately 30,000 nurses,
medics, laboratory technicians, respiratory technicians, order-
lies, dental assistants, and other health-care workers. Although
the war ended quickly with few allied casualties, the medical
presence in the Gulf region was a dramatic demonstration of the
ability of today's military planners to organize and implement a
complex system of health care designed to cope with thousands
of U.S. and allied casualties. As it was, most of the soldiers

treated at U.S. military medical facilities were Iraqis who had surrendered or had been captured.

The logistics of setting up such a massive health-care system were nearly as complicated as planning for the military operation itself. The allied forces made history in the Gulf by deploying, or distributing, more sophisticated medical resources at greater distances more rapidly than ever before.

The armed forces called up about 3,500 reserve physicians and approximately 20,000 other reserve medical workers to prepare for the conflict, though not all of them served in the Persian Gulf. The surgeon general's office of the U.S. Central Command—the basic group responsible for providing medical care for troops in the Middle East—decided on the quantities of medical equipment and workers that were needed, based on the number of U.S. troops sent. The office also ordered the equipment and coordinated its delivery to the area of combat. In all, the military bought approximately $500 million worth of medical equipment and supplies in preparation for the Persian Gulf War, according to Colonel Ben Knisely, deputy command surgeon for Desert Storm Central Command.

Medical preparations for war

To prepare for any war, medical planners have to consider a number of factors, including conditions peculiar to the locale in which the fighting takes place. Besides the enemy, the harsh conditions of the Arabian Desert presented many possible medical problems. Dehydration was a concern in the hot, dry environment of the Gulf. Sunstroke, sunburn, burns from contact with metal objects heated by the desert sun; toxic fumes from burning tanks and oil wells; and bites from venomous snakes, scorpions, and spiders were problems for which medical organizers had to plan. Medical officers predicted that at least 10 per cent of casualties would come from burns.

Medical officials also considered the kinds of weapons the allied troops were likely to encounter, the nature of the injuries those weapons could inflict, and the type of treatment these injuries would require. High-impact bullets from modern assault weapons create gaping wounds and send shock waves through the body, damaging internal organs. Some projectiles may burst organs and blood vessels and shatter bones while leaving nearly invisible entrance wounds, thus creating hidden injuries that physicians at the front would need to look for. The frightening prospect of chemical weapons—fortunately not realized—also required special training and equipment to deal with chemical burns and poisonous gases.

Many soldiers received varying degrees of extra medical training, in many cases before arriving in the Gulf region. All troops were given some first-aid instruction during basic training, such

The author:

Marc S. Micozzi is director of the National Museum of Health and Medicine and associate director of the Armed Forces Institute of Pathology, both in Washington, D.C. He is also a physician.

as how to perform *cardiopulmonary resuscitation* (CPR) and how to stop bleeding. Soldiers called *combat lifesavers* received an extra 24 hours of instruction in more advanced first-aid techniques. Combat lifesavers are taught how to start an IV (an *intravenous solution* with essential body fluids containing sugar and salt inserted directly into the veins), splint broken bones, bandage wounds, and apply a tourniquet.

Training medical personnel

Traditional Army "medics," called corpsmen in the Navy, Air Force, and Marines, take a 10-week course in advanced first aid. All four branches of the service send their medics and corpsmen to the Army's Academy of Health Sciences in San Antonio, Tex., for training. Medics learn advanced ways to stop bleeding, how to administer medications such as morphine, and how to suture wounds. They also learn how to determine the proper amount of IV solution a wounded soldier should receive and how to open an airway by installing a temporary emergency breathing passage in the throat.

Corpsmen carry 30-pound backpacks containing about 70 pieces of equipment, including a stretcher, bandages, sutures, needles and scalpels, bags of IV solutions, and containers of Valium, morphine, and codeine painkillers. These are enough supplies to treat as many as three severely wounded and two lightly wounded soldiers.

In preparing for the Gulf War, special training and equipment were needed to cope with the risk of chemical weapons. Of greatest concern to planners were *mustard gas* (which causes burns, blindness, and death) and *nerve gas* (which attacks the central nervous system to cause extreme weakness and death).

Soldiers and medics alike were equipped with and taught how to use gas masks and special suits designed to seal off contact with the air and prevent breathing the gas. Soldiers also carried three doses each of two drugs—*atropine* and *pralidoxime*, which neutralize and counter the effects of nerve gas. These drugs were packaged in spring-loaded, self-injection kits designed to be administered by tapping a container carrying the drug and a needle against the body.

Each soldier also carried a self-injection kit containing a single dose of Valium to control convulsions that result from exposure to nerve gas. Medics carried additional doses of each of these three drugs and were trained to administer them. Troops also had a new antidote to nerve gas—*pyridostigmine*. This drug had not been used before in war and was meant to be taken in tablet form several hours before an expected gas attack to enhance the effectiveness of the other nerve gas antidotes.

Troops were also trained to use decontamination kits containing a resin bag for absorbing mustard gas residue from their

Levels of care in combat

The U.S. military provides four basic levels of medical care for wounded soldiers, starting with the medic in the field and progressing through field hospitals and hospital ships to full-scale medical centers hundreds or thousands of miles from the front. Helicopters, planes, or land ambulances transport the wounded to where they can receive the appropriate level of care, depending on how seriously a soldier is injured.

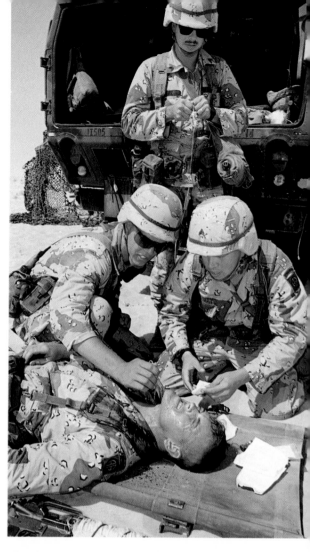

Battlefield first aid
An injured soldier receives care in the field during the 1991 military operations in the Persian Gulf, *right*. "Buddy" teams trained in first aid, as well as combat lifesavers and medical corpsmen (medics) with more advanced training, provide such care.

Emergency care in field hospitals
Highly mobile field hospitals, *below*, are located farther away from the fighting. The field hospital staff can perform simple but lifesaving emergency surgery. These doctors and medics provide a level of care between that available immediately on the battlefield and the more sophisticated care available at full-scale hospitals.

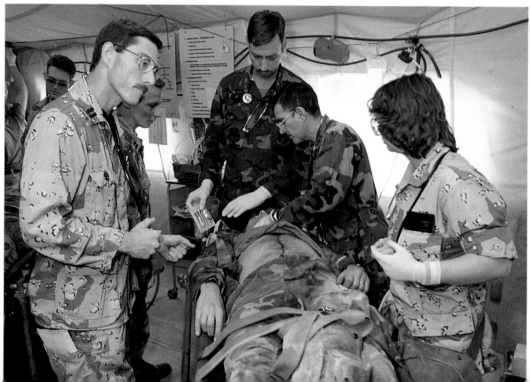

Caring for the wounded at sea

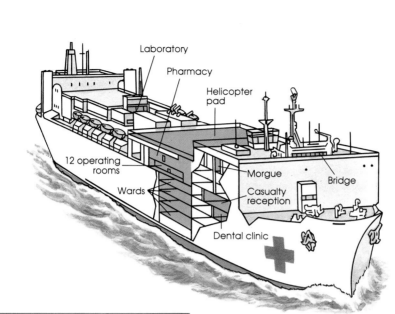

Laboratory

Pharmacy

Helicopter pad

12 operating rooms

Wards

Morgue

Bridge

Casualty reception

Dental clinic

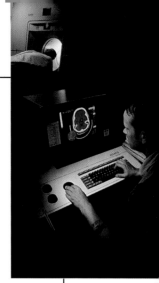

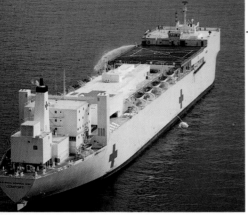

Hospital ships, such as the *Comfort, left*, are operated by the U.S. Navy. The *Comfort* is a 1,000-bed floating hospital, *above*, 10 stories high from the water line and equipped with operating rooms, laboratories, and sophisticated devices such as a computerized tomography (CT) scanner, *above right*. CT scans, which combine a large number of X rays to provide detailed cross-sectional images of the body, can be used, for example, to locate bullets or pieces of shrapnel lodged in a soldier's body.

Medical evacuation
During the Gulf War, Air Force planes equipped with hospital beds and staffed by flight nurses and medics, *left*, evacuated soldiers to medical centers in Europe and the United States.

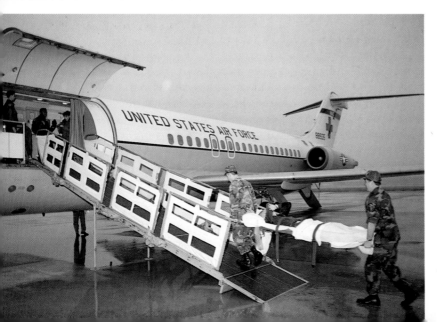

skin. Although the kits can remove a large portion of the residue, complete decontamination requires washing with water. An entire Army division—between 7,500 and 10,000 soldiers—would require about 200,000 gallons of water to completely wash down from a chemical attack. Fortunately, after all these necessary preparations, chemical warfare proved not to be a significant feature of the war in the Persian Gulf.

The first two levels of military medical care

To cope with the thousands of wounded troops that were originally expected to require treatment during the war, military medical planners relied upon the *Theater Combat Medical System*. In this system, military medical care is organized in four levels, or echelons, beginning with basic lifesaving measures in the field and progressing to increasingly sophisticated treatment as distance from the fighting increases. A key to the system is flexibility. Although each level is designed to offer a specific range of medical services, battle conditions and casualty rates may require that higher level facilities perform basic emergency care or move closer to the fighting. This system, in some form, is used in all four branches of the U.S. military services.

The first level consists of immediate first aid given by soldiers on the battlefield and care offered at *battalion aid stations*, where the wounded can be prepared for evacuation to more sophisticated medical facilities. Soldiers in Desert Storm paired up in "buddy" teams and used first-aid skills they learned in basic training to help each other if needed. Each platoon—about 25 to 27 soldiers—also had four combat lifesavers. Above the combat lifesaver is the traditional Army medic, generally one per platoon.

Medics evacuate the wounded from the front lines to a battalion aid station. Such stations, staffed by a doctor and six or seven medics, are equipped with minimal equipment such as bandages, splints, IV's, painkilling drugs, and blood plasma. The facility is most commonly a tent with cots. It has no hospital beds and is designed to hold patients no longer than the time it takes to perform the emergency care necessary to save a life or a limb. In heavy fighting, the number of wounded may limit battalion aid station doctors or medics to no more than 15 or 20 minutes per patient. Although doctors at these stations do not perform surgery, they can carry out immediate measures designed to prevent shock and bleeding—such as taking off and reapplying tourniquets, installing more permanent breathing passages, and renewing IV solutions. But the main duty of battalion aid station personnel is to separate out the most severely wounded and prepare them for evacuation.

The second level of care consists of *medical clearing companies*, which offer more advanced emergency care. Medical staff at these facilities also decide where soldiers should be taken for further treatment, based on the severity of their wounds. A medical clearing company is a temporary facility designed to treat the wounded from an entire division, usually between 7,500 and 10,000 troops. In Operation Desert Storm, clearing companies were set up in tents with 80 to 100 cots, three or four doctors, and basic medical equipment such as X-ray machines, a small laboratory, and a small pharmacy. In general, medical clearing companies are about 40 miles (65 kilometers) behind the lines, though this distance varies widely depending on the nature of the battle and the terrain.

As in the battalion aid station, no surgery is performed at a medical clearing company, but it can hold soldiers whose injuries require a recuperation time of no more than 72 hours. If needed, the medical clearing company staff can perform more extensive procedures than those at the battalion aid station, including reinflating lungs and administering antibiotics.

The third level of care

Level three facilities consist of mobile army surgical hospitals (MASH's), combat support hospitals (CSH's), evacuation hospitals, land-based fleet hospitals, and hospital ships at sea. According to Knisely, the Army had 8 MASH's, 9 CSH's, and 21 evacuation hospitals in the Persian Gulf.

Each of the MASH's in the Persian Gulf had a staff of about 115 medical workers, including such specialists as vascular surgeons to treat severe, complex battlefield wounds. A typical facility had 6 operating rooms and 60 beds, but was not intended to hold patients long after surgery. MASH's, housed in light, portable buildings that assemble and break down in sections, are designed to be taken down and set up quickly so they can stay close to the front lines.

MASH and CSH facilities are designed primarily to provide a wide range of lifesaving surgery. CSH's offer a level of care between that of a MASH and an evacuation hospital. The CSH's in the Persian Gulf had staffs of about 250 medical workers, 200 beds, and 4 operating rooms, according Knisely. CSH's have the capability for many types of surgery, and the extra beds in a CSH can hold recuperating patients as well. Although they have fewer operating rooms than a MASH unit, CSH's have more elaborate surgical facilities, including preoperative and postoperative rooms, intensive care areas, even air conditioning.

Fleet hospitals, evacuation hospitals, and hospital ships can provide the same range of surgery, but offer more specialized treatment as well, such as neurosurgery. Evacuation hospitals are large, full-scale hospitals of about 400 beds. They are designed to receive overflow patients from MASH or CSH facilities in heavy fighting or to provide follow-up surgery and more specialized treatment than is available in MASH's or CSH's. Evacuation hospitals in the Persian Gulf had staffs of about 420 medical workers, including a wider range of specialists—such as neurosurgeons, plastic surgeons, burn specialists, and kidney specialists—than are found in either CSH's or MASH's. Although evacuation hospitals can be set up in schools or other existing structures, those in the Persian Gulf were generally housed in the same type of portable building used for MASH's.

Evacuation hospitals can also provide space and care for recuperation of up to several weeks, if needed. Although they are generally at least 100 miles (160 kilometers) behind the front lines, these facilities were as much as 500 miles (800 kilometers) behind the lines in the Persian Gulf due to the great distances U.S. troops covered during Desert Storm, Knisely said.

The Navy operated three land-based, level-three fleet hospitals in Saudi Arabia. These 500-bed hospitals, which closely resembled evacuation hospitals in size and function, were set up to serve the 90,000 marines in the Persian Gulf, but were available for other members of the armed forces as well.

Transport for the wounded to these facilities ranges from stretchers to ambulances, and from helicopters to medical evacuation aircraft equipped with life-support systems. During the Vietnam War, from the mid-1960's to the early 1970's, the military used helicopters to transport the wounded from the front lines. Helicopters were necessary there because the enemy often occupied territory between the front lines and medical stations. Land vehicles did not work well because the country was mainly swamps and jungles. Because Vietnam is a small country, a helicopter could usually transport a severely wounded soldier to a hospital in about 20 minutes. This is within the "golden hour" trauma specialists agree is critical for patients going into shock from blood loss.

During Desert Storm, commanders feared that helicopters could be spotted too easily in the flat desert terrain and shot down with shoulder-held rockets. Instead, medics relied on ground transportation such as tanks and trucks to get to a battalion aid station. This initial trip could be a difficult one, covering several kilometers over rough terrain. Away from the front lines, however, transporting the wounded was far less difficult. The Air Force's Military Airlift Command (MAC) transported wounded soldiers from Saudi Arabia to Europe and from Europe to the United States. The MAC had special planes outfitted and staffed for the medical care of troops during transportation.

Medical care at sea

During the Gulf War, the U.S. Navy also supplied the first three levels of care at sea, depending on the size of the ship. The most complete care available at sea was on two hospital ships, the

The medical lessons of war

The challenge to military medicine has been to bring state-of-the-art civilian medicine to the battlefield. But the pressures of wartime have also led to advances in medical procedures.

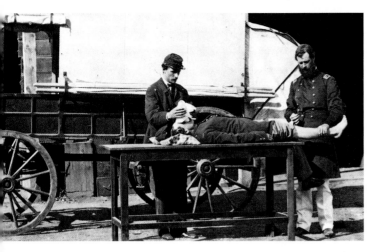

Field hospitals during the American Civil War consisted of little more than wooden tables, where amputation of a wounded limb was a common procedure. Doctors knew nothing about antiseptic surgery, and many soldiers died of infections. But an early version of the current *echelons*, or levels, of care was established.

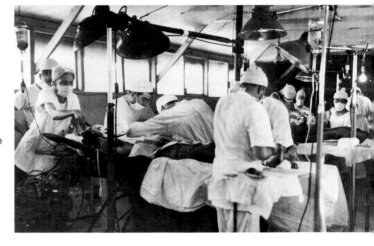

The Mobile Army Surgical Hospital (MASH), *right*, was developed during the Korean War in the 1950's. These field hospitals were equipped with the tools of modern medicine: powerful anesthetics, sterile operating conditions, and germ-killing antibiotics to ward off infections. Military doctors during this era also made improvements in vascular surgery (surgery on veins), and the use of dialysis.

Mercy and the *Comfort*, which provided third-level care. The *Mercy* and the *Comfort* offer the most sophisticated sea-based medical care, but all Navy ships can provide some care. Amphibious assault ships, which are designed to carry large numbers of troops, can be converted to hospital ships, offering second-level care. Aircraft carriers can also provide second-level care, according to the Navy. Smaller ships have a single corpsman whose job is to stabilize wounds and prepare patients for evacuation to a higher level of care, if needed.

The *Mercy* treated 6,700 patients during the conflict, and the *Comfort* treated 8,721, according to Navy spokesmen, though most treatment was for noncombat injuries. These ships were anchored about an hour's flight from most of the battle areas,

Treating chemical warfare wounds

Medical personnel in the Persian Gulf were prepared to treat wounds caused by chemical weapons in the form of nerve gas and mustard gas. These "gases" are actually liquids that form vapor when sprayed.

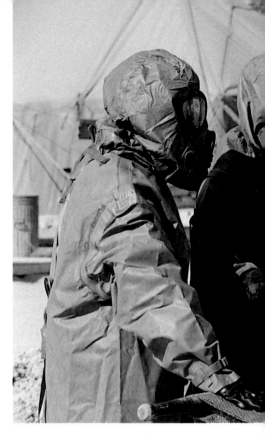

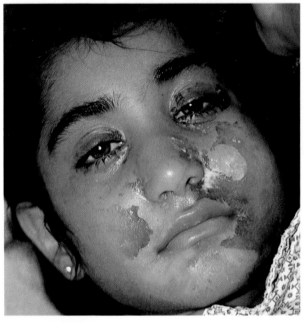

A Kurdish girl's face bears the painful chemical burns caused by contact with mustard gas, *above*. Mustard gas can also burn the lungs if inhaled.

and the wounded were brought to them by helicopter or boat.

These hospital ships are enormous converted oil supertankers about the length of three football fields. Each carries 1,000 beds and a crew of 800 medical workers. The sophisticated medical equipment on the *Mercy* and the *Comfort* includes computerized tomography (CT) scanners (an advanced type of imaging device that uses multiple X-ray exposures), a laboratory that can fabricate different parts of the human face for facial surgery, an optometry laboratory, and two oral surgery rooms. Each ship has the equivalent of 40 large hospital emergency rooms below deck, according to Knisely.

The best care available

Injured troops who required more than 14 days' care were usually transported to military hospitals in Europe for fourth-level care. In all, the military transported some 15,000 injured Desert Storm troops to Europe for treatment, most of whom had injuries unrelated to combat, according to Knisely. Except for the most complex and most difficult procedures—such as extended burn treatment and transplants, which would be performed in the United States—fourth-level hospitals offer the most sophis-

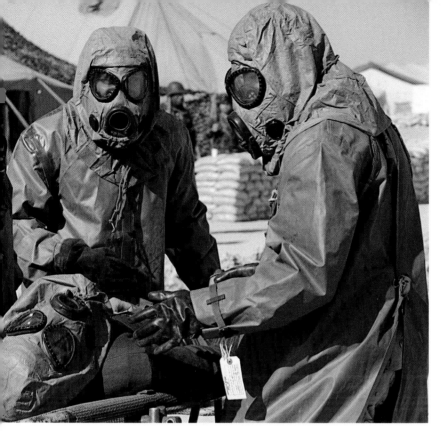

Military doctors and medics practice caring for a wounded soldier while wearing gear to protect against injury in the event of a chemical attack, *left*. During the Persian Gulf War, the military provided gas masks to prevent troops from inhaling chemicals, special clothing to protect them against chemical burns, and antidotes to nerve gas, which can be fatal if it is inhaled or comes in contact with the skin.

ticated medical care available. There were 11 Air Force and Army level-four military hospitals with approximately 10,000 beds equipped to receive wounded in Germany. More were available in Great Britain.

Many of the injured troops who were transported to European hospitals could have been treated in Saudi Arabia, on hospital ships, in fleet hospitals, and in evacuation hospitals, according to Knisely. The light number of casualties, the months that medical planners had to prepare, and the extensive military medical air transportation system allowed many of the wounded to make the trip to Europe. "It was a luxury for us to be able to treat that many in Europe," he said.

In addition to transporting the wounded to the best possible medical facilities, military medical planners must bring the best medical technologies to the battle zone. During the Gulf War, the military had available four CT scanners, two in Saudi Arabia and two on hospital ships. The large number of X rays employed by CT scanners provide detailed cross-sectional images of the body. This device can locate and help identify severe internal injuries much more accurately and quickly than can conventional X-ray machines.

Another sophisticated technology made available to military physicians was an advanced laser system that was designed to stop bleeding. A California medical equipment manufacturer donated two argon beam systems, which use lasers of argon gas to cauterize (burn) severed arteries in order to close them and stop wounds from bleeding.

Military doctors also had access to the latest in drug treatment. One such drug, called Centoxin, fights septic shock, a deadly infection of the bloodstream that is common on the battlefield. The drug was approved for military use on Feb. 14, 1991, just days before the allied ground offensive began.

Blood transfusions are often needed to save lives on the battlefield, so there must be an adequate blood supply close at hand. To move its blood supply closer to front-line troops during Operation Desert Storm, the Army installed refrigerators in medical facilities closer to the front than ever before. The refrigerators, powered by generators in field tents, allowed soldiers to receive blood within minutes rather than after a long trip across the desert to a medical unit far from the front.

Advanced identification techniques

In addition to new medical equipment and treatments, the armed forces used several new techniques to help identify unidentified human remains that resulted from the fighting—a difficult issue in past wars where there was a greater loss of life. The Armed Forces Institute of Pathology in Washington, D.C., used a new process called *antibody profiling* to scientifically determine which separated body parts came from the same body. According to Major Victor Weedn, chief of the institute's Armed Forces DNA Identification Laboratory, this process involves taking samples of *antibodies* (infection-fighting proteins) from blood in the tissue of one body part and comparing them with those from other body parts. The process produces an antibody pattern similar to the bar code on grocery packaging. Because everyone has unique antibody patterns, tissue samples that produce matching patterns should belong to the same body.

Military pathologists also used DNA (*deoxyribonucleic acid*, the molecule that genes are made of) to identify soldiers. Each person's DNA is unique—a kind of molecular fingerprint that is found in every cell of the body. If injuries disfigure a soldier so badly that identification is impossible from fingerprints and dental records, DNA samples from the body may provide the necessary information. For this process to work, however, previous samples of the soldier's DNA must exist for comparison.

Because the military had not yet collected DNA samples from soldiers, other tissue samples had to be found. In one case, according to Weedn, pathologists helped resolve an identity by comparing DNA in hair taken from a soldier's electric shaver with DNA in tissue from battlefield remains.

The U.S. military has begun plans to collect DNA from cells inside each soldier's mouth and from blood samples. The military will store the DNA samples, thus providing each soldier with a "DNA dog tag." If this method is successful, there may be no more "unknown soldiers."

The Gulf War did not produce the thousands of U.S. and allied casualties that were initially feared. The military had prepared for heavy losses—33,000 men and women, roughly 1 in 16 of all U.S. troops in the area. In actuality, there were 273 deaths among American forces during Operation Desert Storm, according to the Department of Defense. Of that total, 148 were combat deaths. The rest of the deaths resulted from illness or injury.

Surprisingly, the overall rate of death compared favorably with a peacetime population of roughly the same age and size. From August 1990 to the end of the war in March 1991, there were fewer than 70 deaths per 100,000 American military personnel stationed in the Persian Gulf, according to the Department of Defense. By contrast, there were more than 100 deaths per 100,000 men between the ages of 20 and 30 living in the United States during this same time period, according to the National Center for Health Statistics in Hyattsville, Md.

In the end, Desert Storm (as with many wars in history) produced a high ratio of noncombat-to-combat injuries. American lives were lost in accidents on sandswept highways crowded with camels and armored vehicles, by "friendly fire" (inadvertent loss of life caused by weapons fired by allied forces), and in aircraft that crashed due to noncombat causes. But when the shooting stopped, the death rate remained low for an active population of more than half a million.

When military historians look back on the Persian Gulf War, they may point to the conflict as the first example of air power and "smart weapons" substantially defeating an enemy's land force. Medical historians may similarly note that the low casualty rate was a testament to both superior military strategy and superior military medical care.

For further reading:

Hines, William. "Doctors at the Front." *MD*. April 1991.

The Journal of the American Medical Association. The News and Comments sections of *Journal* issues published between August 1990 and March 1991 provide accounts of the role of military medicine during the Persian Gulf War.

"Military Medicine." *American Heritage*. October/November 1984.

Rather than subject people
with incurable diseases to
often futile treatment, hospices
help make their final days
as comfortable as possible.

Caring for the Terminally Ill

By Paul Galloway

Jesse, a 56-year-old Chicago police officer, was lifting an air conditioner from a window in his home when he felt a sharp, jabbing pain in his back. He thought he had pulled a muscle—a common cause of back pain—but when he went to the doctor the news was much worse.

Jesse had prostate cancer. The likelihood of curing it was slim, because the cancer had been in his body for some time and had spread from the prostate to other areas, including the bones of his spine. The pain in his back was a sign of how far the disease had spread.

His physician referred Jesse to John Merrill, a cancer specialist, who began an aggressive plan of treatment to fight the cancer, including radiation and drugs. Jesse felt better for a while, but the improvement was only temporary.

The doctor sat down with Jesse and his wife, Beverly, to explain that conventional treatment would not defeat the cancer and to discuss what to do next. After thinking it over, Jesse chose to enter the hospice program at Northwestern Memorial Hospital, a 750-bed teaching and research institution affiliated with Northwestern University in Chicago.

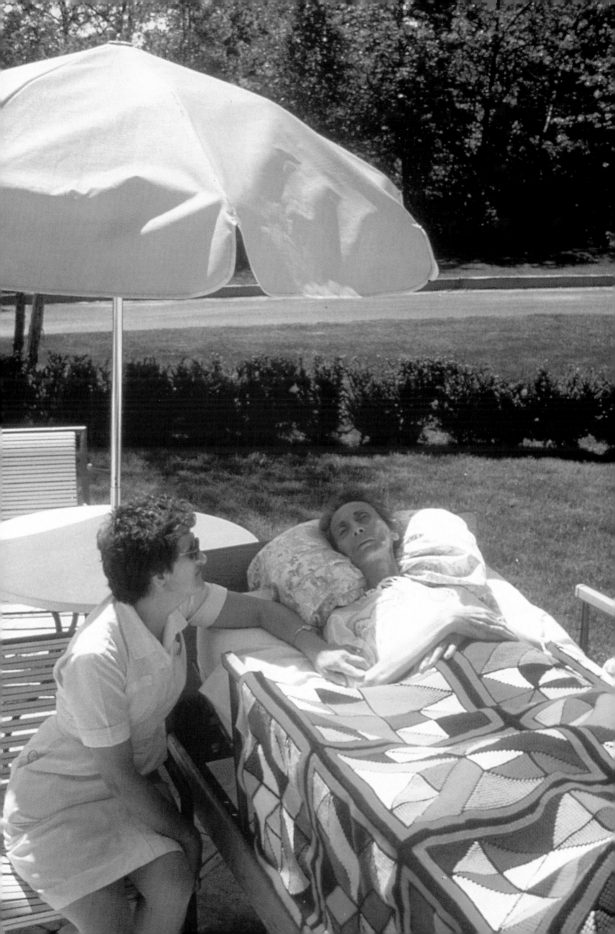

Hospices are programs designed specifically to help patients with terminal illnesses die with dignity and comfort. Instead of trying to cure the incurable, hospice treatment focuses on helping patients stay alert, communicative, and involved during the last stage of life.

"We want patients to be free from pain and to lead as normal a life as possible," says Janet Neigh, executive director of the Hospice Association of America (HAA), an organization based in Washington, D.C., and affiliated with the National Association for Home Care. "We want them to be able to say good-bye to their loved ones and tie up any loose ends with relationships or financial matters. Their final days can and should be positive and constructive for everyone."

The growth of hospice programs

Hospice programs have gained remarkably wide acceptance in a very short time. The first modern hospice was founded in London in 1967. The first American hospice opened in 1974 in Connecticut. Today, there are more than 1,700 hospices in the United States, according to the National Hospice Organization (NHO), another national association for hospice providers.

About 1.6 million patients die annually in American hospitals or long-term care facilities. Statistics from the NHO indicate that about 200,000 terminal patients were cared for in American hospices in 1990.

Hospice patients include nearly equal numbers of men and women. About two-thirds of them are age 65 or older, and about 85 per cent have incurable cancers. The rest have a variety of conditions, notably heart disease, lung disease, and—increasingly—AIDS.

The swift growth of hospice programs is all the more noteworthy because the concept revolves around an extremely unpleasant subject: death. "The hospice movement recognizes that we don't live forever," says Jeanne Martinez, a registered nurse and the clinical manager of Northwestern's hospice program. "Even with the best medical technology, we die."

A more humane approach to death

In fact, hospices arose in part as a reaction to medical technology—or more specifically, to technology's effects on treatment of the terminally ill. Leaders of the hospice movement observed that doctors, despite their best intentions, often became so involved in fighting patients' diseases that they overlooked the patients' human needs.

In particular, hospice advocates charged, physicians dedicated to prolonging life sometimes prescribed medicines that caused debilitating side effects and conducted procedures to sustain pa-

The author:

Paul Galloway is a writer for the *Chicago Tribune*.

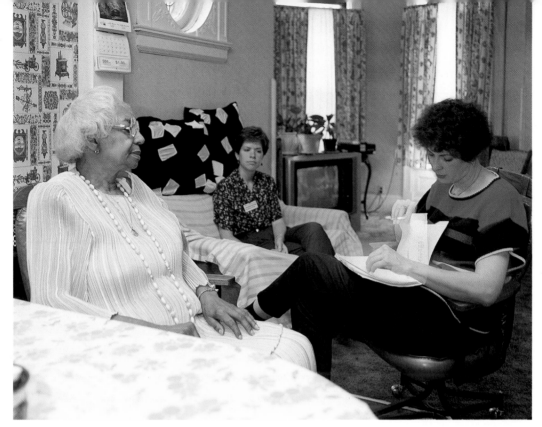

A patient (left) discusses her home care with an occupational therapist and a nurse from the hospice program at Northwestern Memorial Hospital in Chicago. Patients and their families often consult with hospice staff about how and where the patients will spend their last days.

tients' lives that prolonged their suffering. Often, these critics pointed out, death occurred while patients were attached to ventilators and monitoring machines—unable to talk to their families and friends or to have a say in their own course of care.

Hospice proponents said that in many cases, this approach offered no real hope. It only made the end of life more difficult for both patients and their families. A more humane alternative, they suggested, would be to quit battling the illness and to concentrate on improving the quality of the patients' last days. These ideas formed the basis of the hospice alternative.

Basic hospice concepts

As the hospice concept developed, it focused on several key points that hospice advocates believed traditional medical practice failed to address. These points now form the basis of hospice care.

First, hospices shift the primary emphasis of treatment from curing disease to alleviating pain—an approach called palliative care. The intent is not to reject traditional treatment, but rather to choose the option appropriate to the patient's condition. At times, this means that making the patient more comfortable makes more sense than administering aggressive treatment.

"Medically and ideally, we should focus on symptom management all the way through treatment," says Jamie Von Roenn,

Hospice: an ancient concept

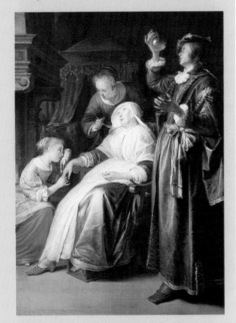

The tradition of caring for sick and dying patients is an ancient one. Care at home was the rule in earlier times, though by the 1100's, monasteries had established shelters called hospices to house sick people, along with weary pilgrims and travelers and orphaned children. The word *hospice* became synonymous with care for the dying in the late 1800's, when the Irish Sisters of Charity, a Roman Catholic order, opened such a hospice in Dublin.

The modern hospice movement grew out of the efforts of Cicely Saunders, an English physician. Saunders pioneered research in palliative care (treatment to control pain rather than cure disease). Her work led her to found the first modern hospice, St. Christopher's, in 1967 in London.

During a visit to the United States in the early 1960's, Saunders spoke at Yale University in New Haven, Conn., about her methods of caring for the terminally ill. Saunders' visit inspired the founding in New Haven of the first hospice in the United States.

medical director of Northwestern's hospice program. "But we don't. We focus on getting rid of problems." And some problems, she notes, simply cannot be cured.

Second, hospices insist that patients and their families participate in decisions about how and where patients spend the last weeks or months of their lives. In fact, as some hospice workers see it, a patient doesn't enter a hospice program alone—rather, a whole family enters together.

Third, hospices employ a *holistic* (all-encompassing) approach, addressing psychological, social, and spiritual issues as well as physical needs. Thus, hospices generally employ many kinds of experts—some full-time, some part-time or temporary—plus trained volunteers. In addition to physicians, a hospice might involve nurses, social workers, psychologists, psychiatric counselors, occupational therapists, clergy, home-care specialists, and legal or financial counselors.

Fourth, the focus of hospice care is the home. At least 90 per cent of hospice care takes place in the home, according to the NHO. For patients who are too ill to stay at home, some hospice programs offer inpatient facilities of their own, while others make arrangements with hospitals. But a "hospice" is not actually a particular place. "A hospice is a philosophy, a service, a concept, a program," says Neigh of the HAA.

Making the hospice choice

As reasonable as the hospice concept seems, many people do not find it immediately appealing—especially if they first hear of the idea as they face a terminal disease themselves. Thinking about death is never easy. "Denial is widespread," says Ira J. Bates, former vice president of the NHO and now a national consultant for hospice programs. "Death is inevitable. But lots of folks would rather ignore the subject."

That's true, he adds, even among doctors and other professionals who must deal frequently with death. Members of the hospice movement believe that some physicians resist

Volunteer and professional care

Hospice care for incurably ill patients involves a team of health-care professionals and volunteer workers who focus not on treating the disease but on easing pain and making the person's final days as comfortable as possible. Professional staff members supervise pain control and other medical concerns while family, friends, and hospice volunteers provide a variety of supportive services.

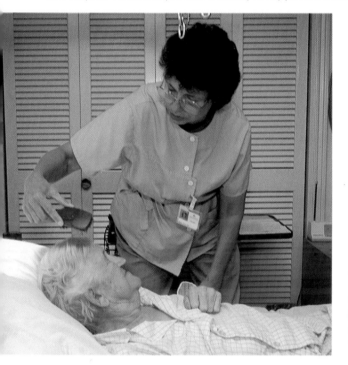

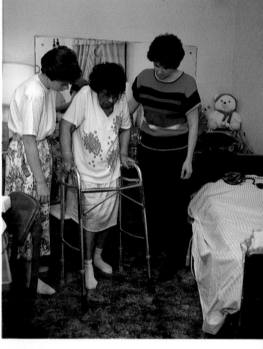

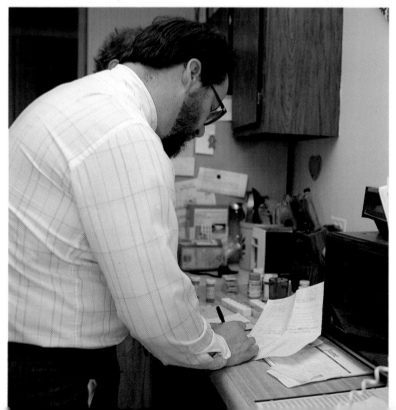

A hospice worker lifts a patient's spirits by brushing his hair, *above left,* while a nurse and occupational therapist help another patient learn how to use a walker, *above.* A nurse records information about pain control medication for his patient, *left,* as part of the effort to help the patient remain as pain-free as possible.

359

the hospice idea at first because they were trained never to surrender in the fight against disease. "Many physicians are given the idea that if they don't cure somebody, they've failed," says Northwestern's Von Roenn, a physician herself.

Still, with today's medical technology, it's more important than ever for doctors, patients, and families to discuss the process of death. Doctors often use machines or advanced procedures to sustain a hospital patient's life in a crisis—using ventilators, for example, to maintain breathing when lungs fail or administering electric shocks to revive a stopped heart. For a terminal patient, however, these so-called "heroic" measures can be viewed as simply prolonging the dying process.

Hospice patients generally decide—after discussion with doctors and family members—to decline such intervention in advance. And, by entering a hospice program, patients are in effect choosing to forgo continued attempts to cure their diseases.

These are hardly easy decisions. "People are resistant to hospice because it means they have to accept their mortality," says Von Roenn. "Most hospice programs require a consent form that says something like: 'I realize I have a disease for which there is no cure.' It's very hard to see these words in black and white."

Entering a hospice program

When prospective patients contact Northwestern, Von Roenn says, the hospice first consults the patient's physician to verify that the patient's condition is incurable. Typically, this means that life expectancy is six months or less—and that the physician agrees hospice treatment would be appropriate.

Often, the suggestion comes from the physicians themselves. For example, Chicago cancer specialist Merrill describes how he introduces the subject to his patients. First, he says, he usually reviews the course of the patient's disease. "When I talked with Jesse and Beverly, I explained what treatments he'd had and what these treatments accomplished and what trouble they caused. I then went over the options that remained and told them why I would or would not recommend them."

It's essential, he says, to explain that the disease is incurable. "You have to be honest with your patients. If you don't tell the truth about cancer, the disease will ultimately make you a liar."

Patients may ask about an experimental drug or procedure they've heard about. And while such measures may offer some hope, Merrill notes that patients also need to consider the often appreciable drawbacks—such as unpleasant or debilitating side effects—of experimental therapies. "Usually they've been through a lot already, and they know there's no such thing as saying 'It won't hurt to give it a try,'" explains Merrill. Then he introduces the alternative. "I tell them there is also the option of not treating the disease but entering a program that aims to keep them at home and in comfort by treating the symptoms. I tell them I would be happy to be their doctor for that phase," says Merrill.

He then tries to discuss questions about the patient's quality of life. "I can tell patients what it will be like if they use an experimental drug. I can tell them they wouldn't be spending much time at home and they'd probably go through a great deal of painful side effects."

Merrill continues working with patients who enter hospice programs. For such patients, he changes the emphasis from fighting the disease to controlling pain and treating the symptoms. "I consider that a high calling, one to which I have skills to contribute," explains Merrill.

The hospice family

Anywhere from 30 to 60 patients are enrolled in Northwestern's hospice program at any one time. Ninety per cent of them live at home, where a hospice doctor visits them regularly. After each visit, the doctor reports back to the patient's own physician, who must authorize any changes in treatment.

A nurse visits weekly, and nurses are on call 24 hours a day. "Sometimes when patients first enroll, the family will phone and ask for a nurse to come by," says Martinez. "Sometimes they just want to know that we really are available."

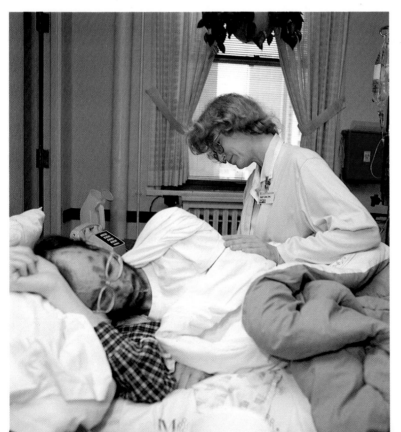

A volunteer comforts a terminally ill man at Northwestern Memorial Hospital's acute-care facility for hospice patients. Patients too ill for home care may spend time in a hospice's in-patient facility. Many hospices strive to make the setting more home-like than conventional hospital rooms, with plants, carpeting, and comfortable furnishings.

Hospices for children

"**A** child's death goes against nature," says Ann Armstrong-Dailey, a longtime hospice volunteer. "You can rationalize the death of an older person, but how do you rationalize the death of an 8-year-old child?"

Armstrong-Dailey realized that dying children and their families had special problems that most hospice programs were not addressing. So in 1983, she founded the nonprofit advocacy group Children's Hospice International to help families in which a child was dying.

"When we began," she says, "only four of 1,400 hospices were able to accept children, and none were exclusively for children. Today, more than 400 accept children, and four are programmed exclusively for them." Children's Hospice International is also working with officials in 18 countries interested in developing hospice programs for children.

In addition to encouraging the establishment of children's hospice programs, the Alexandria, Va.-based group acts as a clearinghouse for support groups, training programs, and research projects involving care of children with life-threatening conditions. The organization also offers publications on children's pain management, home care for seriously ill children, and related topics.

Many hospices do not accept children because they require specialized care as well as specially trained physicians. Furthermore, says Robert Milch, a hospice physician in Buffalo, N.Y., doctors are often hesitant to pronounce some children's diseases—especially cancer—incurable. Hospices typically accept only patients with no hope of a cure.

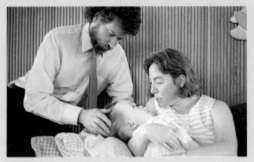

At the children's hospice at St. Mary's Hospital for Children in Bayside, N.Y., parents cuddle their terminally ill child.

"Children are incredibly resilient, much more so than adults," Milch explains. "So treatment can be much more aggressive. It's harder to know when to draw the line, and there's a tendency to go down with all guns firing."

Correspondingly, children's hospice programs do not automatically rule out treatment aimed at a cure. But instead of focusing only on the chance of a cure, they also help seriously ill children and their families deal with their fears and questions about death. "You can offer good holistic medicine and still potentially go for a cure in the context of a supportive program," Milch says.

Hospice staff members meet each week to discuss patients' needs, Von Roenn says. "We review the care plan for each patient: what's going on, who should see the patient, what kind of intervention should be made. Do we need a chaplain, nurses, more volunteer support? We consider not just medical issues but total support."

Volunteers form an essential core of hospice work. "Volunteers assist nurses in feeding, bathing, dressing, and turning patients," says John DeBerry, coordinator of volunteers and bereavement for Northwestern's hospice. "They hold a patient's hand. They take patients for walks or wheelchair rides."

Volunteers also help families by running errands, shopping, housekeeping, or simply listening when someone needs to talk. Another especially important job is respite care—sitting for a few hours at a dying patient's bedside to give family members a break from an emotionally draining vigil.

Patients too ill for home care may move temporarily to the hospice's acute-care facility at the hospital. The 10 single rooms look more like bedrooms than hospital rooms, with rose-colored carpets and elegant furniture. The family areas have kitchens and fold-out beds for relatives who don't want to leave a patient who is near death. About 40 per cent of Northwestern's hospice patients die in the facility. The rest die at home, often with a hospice staff member present.

After a patient's death, hospices stay in touch with the family, often for a year or more. "Bereavement support" may include grief counseling, support groups, memorial services, individual therapy, visits, and calls.

Many hospice advocates see a hospice death as a positive experience, because the hospice program encourages everyone involved to prepare for the event. "It is the sudden, unexpected death that leaves unfinished business and feelings that can be much more difficult to deal with," says Bates.

The cost of hospice care

Most medical insurance companies approve payments for hospice care, which generally is far less expensive than hospital care. The NHO says home-centered hospice programs generally reduce treatment costs by 20 to 40 per cent. People who qualify for benefits under Medicare (a federal program devoted mostly to health care for people over age 65) are entitled to hospice-care coverage in programs with Medicare certification. Some, but not all, states provide hospice benefits through Medicaid, a state-administered federal program that funds some health care for the uninsured poor. Many hospices also provide some care free of charge to patients who cannot pay.

The NHO says that, as of 1989, about 30 per cent of American hospices were both owned and operated by hospitals, 23 per cent were owned by home-health agencies, and 41 per cent were independent programs. The remaining few have other administrative arrangements, such as programs run entirely by volunteers. About 96 per cent of all hospice programs are nonprofit, depending on contributions for 25 per cent or more of their budgets.

Influence of the hospice movement

As the hospice community has expanded, so has its influence on the American health-care landscape. For example, Neigh of the HAA points to signs of growing awareness of the hospice alternative. "We've been concentrating on educating physicians about hospices," she says. "Increasingly longer stays at hospices indicate we're making progress."

Robert Milch, a hospice physician in Buffalo, N.Y., believes

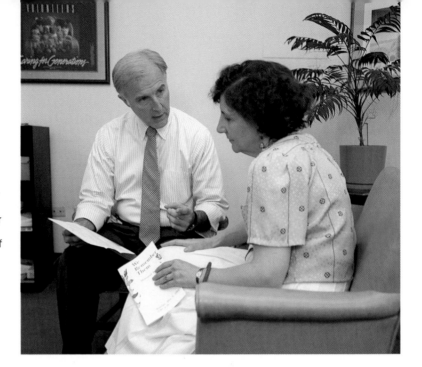

The coordinator of Northwestern Memorial Hospital's bereavement support program (left) confers with a volunteer about how to comfort the family and friends of a deceased hospice patient. Many hospice programs offer bereavement support after a patient's death. Such support may include grief counseling, support groups, and memorial services.

that hospices are having an impact on the health-care system in general. "Physicians historically haven't been well trained in palliative care and symptom management, but I've seen an increase in training in medical schools as well as in residencies," he says. At Northwestern's medical center, for example, residents may now take a course on palliative care that involves working with the hospice team and focusing on the care of patients who choose to die at home.

"We have a new generation of young physicians who have a decade of experience with the hospice concept, and that counts for a good deal," says Milch. "Hospices encourage the emergence of the best in human nature—caring, grace, dignity. I tell young medical students and physicians that working in hospices will make them better physicians and better human beings."

One hospice experience

Jesse, wearing a blue bathrobe, sat quiet and erect on his living room couch while Kathy Neely, one of the two staff physicians for Northwestern Memorial Hospital's hospice program, listened to his heart with a stethoscope. He told Neely that all morning he had been vomiting and could not keep any food or liquids down. She asked him to go to his bed for further examination. On a nearby end table sat a picture of Jesse, before his illness, looking healthy and robust—in sharp contrast to his present frailty.

A few minutes later, Jesse's brother, Nathaniel, also a Chicago police officer, arrived. "I'm going to take care of him to the end," said Nathaniel. "I work nights now so I can come in and stay with him during the day while Beverly's at work."

Nathaniel bathes his brother and takes him for drives. "I take him to see our mother. She's 81. He cries over there. I take him to see his friends. He's talked to my pastor. He has moments of depression, but I try to keep him cheered up."

Late in the 1960's, psychiatrist Elisabeth Kubler-Ross wrote in her landmark book, *On Death and Dying*, of the five stages people go through as they approach death. The first stage is denial; then come anger, bargaining (with God or fate), depression, and finally acceptance.

"People misunderstand these stages," Martinez says. "You don't necessarily start at denial and end up at acceptance. It's not that neat. It's more like a seesaw. Patients go back and forth. Some days they are accepting and want to talk about death and some days they don't."

On this day, Jesse was concerned with his nausea. He did not talk about what he was going through or what lay ahead. There would be opportunities, if he wished, to talk about death later, with family members, with good friends, or with a sympathetic hospice volunteer. Jesse's decision to enter a hospice program has given him more flexibility to choose how and where he will spend the time he has left.

For now, he talked with the hospice physician about managing his symptoms and his pain. And when Neely got up to leave for her next house call to see another hospice patient, he used his walker to see her to the door.

"Thank you," he said. "Thank you for coming."

For more information:

For answers to questions about hospice care, information on hospices, or free brochures, contact:

Hospice Education Institute, P.O. Box 713, Essex, CT 06426, or call HOSPICELINK toll-free at (800) 331-1620.

National Hospice Organization, 1901 N. Moore St., Suite 901, Arlington, VA 22209, or call toll-free at (800) 658-8898.

Foundation for Hospice and Homecare, 519 C St., NE, Washington, DC 20002, or call the publications department at (202) 547-6586. A free brochure, "Consumer's Guide to Hospice Care," is available.

For materials on the care of seriously ill children or referrals to hospice programs that admit children, contact:

Children's Hospice International, 700 Princess St., Suite 3, Alexandria, VA 22314, or call toll-free at (800) 242-4453.

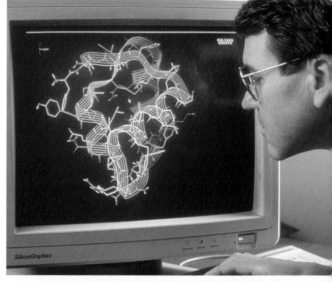

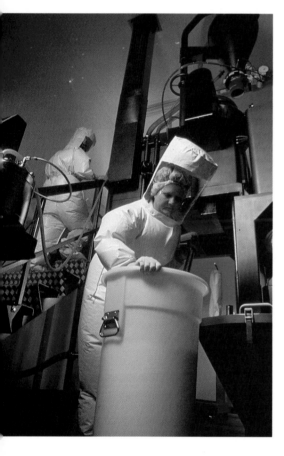

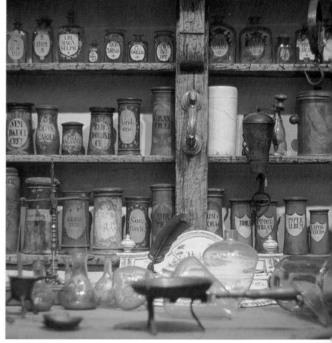

Health Studies

The World Book Health & Medical Annual takes a wide-ranging, in-depth look at an important aspect of health care today.

Prescription Drugs and Human Health
by Ricki Lewis

Medicinal drugs have helped millions of people live longer, healthier lives. The most powerful of these drugs require a prescription from a physician. This report reviews the basic classes of drugs and gives a brief history of drugs through the ages. It also explains how drugs are administered and how they work in the body. In addition, it describes how new drugs are developed and provides a glimpse of drugs of the future.

How drugs have improved human life   368

Classes of drugs   369

The history of drugs   370

How drugs are administered   372

How drugs work   373

How new drugs are developed   376

Drugs of the future: genetic medicine   384

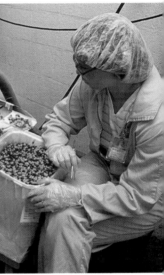

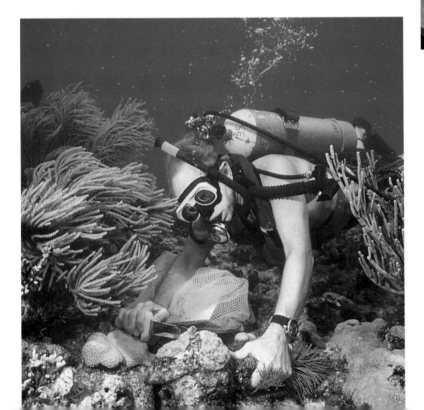

Prescription Drugs and Human Health

By Ricki Lewis

In our century, medicinal drugs have helped millions of people live longer, healthier lives and have vanquished some diseases completely. The most powerful of these drugs require a prescription from a physician. More than 1.5 billion bottles, vials, and other containers of prescription medicines are dispensed each year in the United States for the treatment of a staggering variety of disorders. But prescription drugs also have the potential for doing harm. They often have side effects that must be weighed against their benefits. And, if taken incorrectly or when not needed, these drugs can be more dangerous than helpful.

bring TB under control. The death rate from TB dropped from about 33 per 100,000 population in 1947, when streptomycin became available, to 0.5 per 100,000 by the mid-1980's.

The ability to cure TB and other infectious diseases is just one of many benefits that drugs have brought us. Other drugs that have markedly transformed the practice of medicine and improved people's lives in this century include medications for heart ailments, drugs that fight cancer, oral contraceptives, drugs for the treatment of mental disorders, and a great many others.

Drugs now save lives from the moment of birth. For example, 50,000 of the 250,000 babies born prematurely in the United States each year develop a condition called *respiratory distress syndrome*, in which the lungs cannot inflate because their air sacs lack an essential substance. About 5,000 infants died every year from the disorder. But since mid-1990, a new drug, Exosurf, has been available for the treatment of respiratory distress syndrome. The drug proved so effective in hospital tests that the U.S. Food and Drug Administration (FDA) took just five months to issue its final approval.

How drugs have improved human health

The success story of prescription drugs can be chronicled by noting the diseases that took the greatest number of lives at an earlier time and how those diseases were brought under control. At the beginning of the 1900's, before the discovery of *sulfa drugs* and *antibiotics*—drugs that fight bacteria as well as other disease-causing microorganisms—infectious diseases were a major cause of death. In fact, pneumonia, tuberculosis, and intestinal infections were the top three killers in the United States. Today, thanks to modern medications, deaths from infectious diseases are much less common here and in other developed countries.

The decline of tuberculosis (TB) as a health threat was one of the major medical victories of the 1900's. TB is a chronic and often fatal lung infection caused by *mycobacteria*, a type of *microbe* (a tiny organism that can be seen only with the aid of a microscope). The first successful TB treatment came from the soil. In 1943, Selman A. Waksman, a bacteriologist at Rutgers The State University of New Jersey, discovered that a certain soil bacterium manufactures a chemical called streptomycin that halts the growth and activity of mycobacteria. Streptomycin, together with other drugs developed in the 1950's, helped

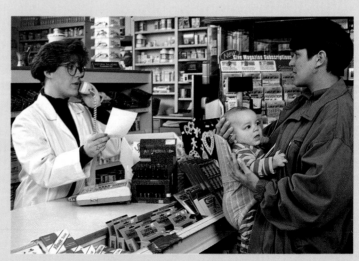

A pharmacist checks on a patient's prescription. A modern pharmacy carries more than a thousand prescription drugs.

Few success stories in the history of drugs are as dramatic as the conquest of bacterial infections. The record of deaths in the United States from influenza complicated by bacterial pneumonia shows that in the early 1900's, influenza combined with pneumonia caused nearly 200 deaths per 100,000 population annually. In the late 1930's, sulfa drugs greatly reduced deaths from this illness, and the widespread introduction of penicillin in the 1940's lowered the influenza-pneumonia death rate even further.

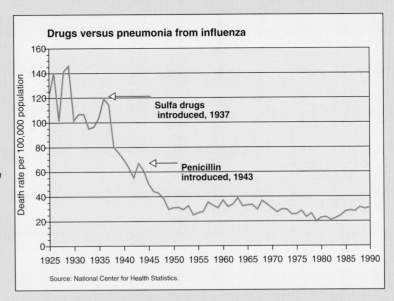

Drugs versus pneumonia from influenza

Sulfa drugs introduced, 1937

Penicillin introduced, 1943

Source: National Center for Health Statistics.

Classes of drugs

Drugs are chemicals, either produced synthetically or derived from biological sources, that are designed to produce a specific effect in the body. *Pharmacologists*, the scientists who study drugs, classify prescription drugs into 83 broad groups, 16 of which account for about 85 per cent of all drugs prescribed in the United States. According to the FDA, the top 6 categories of those 16, representing some 55 per cent of all drugs prescribed are: (1) *cardiovascular drugs*, for the treatment of heart and blood-vessel disorders; (2) antibiotics and sulfa drugs; (3) *psychotherapeutic drugs*, used to treat mental disorders; (4) *analgesics* (pain relievers); (5) *hormones,* natural and synthetic versions of chemicals made by the body's glands; and (6) *diuretics*, drugs that cause increased urine production.

Cardiovascular drugs account for 15 per cent of all prescribed drugs in the United States, with approximately 250 million prescriptions written each year. There are several kinds of cardiovascular medications, including drugs to strengthen and regulate the heartbeat, drugs that widen narrow

blood vessels to improve blood flow, medicines that control high blood pressure, and drugs that are given during a heart attack to break up blood clots and limit damage to heart muscle.

The second most prescribed class of drugs—antibiotics and sulfa drugs—represents about 13 per cent of all U.S. prescriptions. These drugs are used to treat a great variety of infections caused by bacteria or other organisms, such as fungi. They work by killing the microorganisms, preventing them from multiplying, or slowing their reproduction so that the patient's immune system can mount an effective attack against the infection. (Antibiotics and sulfa drugs cannot fight infections caused by viruses. The most effective defense against viral infections is prevention with *vaccines*, preparations that are usually made with killed or weakened viruses. In addition, there are a growing number of *antiviral drugs* that fight infections by viruses.)

Psychotherapeutic drugs, which alter mood or behavior, account for about 8 per cent of U.S. prescriptions. This class of drugs includes stimulants, antidepressant medications, tranquilizers, and sedatives.

Analgesics include narcotic drugs, the most common of which are morphine and other *opiates* (drugs derived from the opium poppy). The analgesics make up approximately 7 per cent of all U.S. prescriptions. The analgesics also include several widely used nonprescription pain relievers—mainly aspirin, acetaminophen (Tylenol), and ibuprofen.

Hormones, substances ordinarily produced in the body by glands, represent about 6 per cent of the drugs prescribed for Americans. In some cases, these drugs are administered to people whose bodies do not produce enough of a certain hormone. For example, many people with *diabetes*, in which the body cannot use sugar normally, take supplemental doses of the hormone insulin. Doctors may also prescribe a hormone to treat some disorders, such as rheumatoid arthritis, that do not stem from a deficiency of that hormone. Birth control pills also contain hormones, which prevent pregnancy by interfering with a woman's normal reproductive cycle.

Diuretics relieve the build-up of water and salt in the body that occurs when a disorder hinders the functioning of the kidneys. Be-

369

cause removing fluids from the body can bring down high blood pressure, diuretics may also be prescribed for that condition. Diuretics account for about 6 per cent of the prescriptions written in the United States each year.

The history of drugs

The discovery of "natural" medicines—chemicals extracted from plants or other living organisms—probably began thousands of years ago in prehistoric times. By the start of recorded history, some 5,000 years ago, many drugs were apparently already in use. Physicians in Sumer, an early civilization in Mesopotamia, inscribed the first known *pharmacopoeia*, or catalog of drugs, on clay tablets in about 2100 B.C. At around the same time, the ancient Egyptians were also increasing their medical knowledge. According to an Egyptian scroll dating from about 1550 B.C., the healers of the Nile Valley had at least 700 drugs at their disposal. Historians and archaeologists have discovered other lengthy pharmacopoeias in records left by the early Chinese, Greeks, and Romans. But how well most of those ancient drugs worked against disease is unknown.

Works of ancient literature also include many mentions of drugs. In the Old Testament book of Psalms, King David says, "Purge me with hyssop [a plant in the mint family] and I shall be made clean." The Roman philosopher Pliny the Elder, writing sometime after A.D. 50, commented, "If remedies were sought in the kitchen garden, none of the arts would become cheaper than the art of medicine." Dating from about 100 years later, the writings of the Greek physician Galen, one of the towering figures in the early history of medicine, include many drug "recipes"—instructions for making a variety of medications.

Over the centuries, people continued to seek out healing substances in nature. Beginning in the 1500's, European colonists in the New World encountered new species of plants, some of which were used by Native Americans for medicinal purposes. In addition, the Europeans brought their own knowledge of drugs to the Americas. In colonial North America, physicians also served as *apothecaries* (druggists), a carry-over from English tradition. Benjamin Franklin separated the two fields, appointing an apothecary to a Pennsylvania hospital in 1752—thereby creating the division between doctor and pharmacist that has persisted to this day.

Painless surgery
By the mid-1800's, scientists in Europe and the United States were making a systematic study of drugs and their potential uses. In the 1840's, two Americans—Georgia physician Crawford W. Long and Boston dentist William T. G. Morton—made a momentous discovery that opened up a new era of surgery. Working independently, Long and Morton found that breathing gaseous ether causes *general anesthesia*, a state of unconsciousness in which the patient is insensitive to pain. Up to that time, surgeons had prepared patients for the ordeal of an operation by getting them drunk or rendering them unconscious by strangulation or a blow to the head. In later decades, researchers discovered other anesthetic drugs, including ones that could be used to numb the part of the body being operated on without causing the patient to lose consciousness.

By the end of the 1800's, other new pain drugs were also coming into use. In 1899, Heinrich Dreser, a German scientist, wrote about

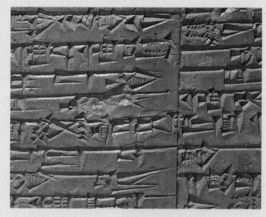

A Sumerian clay tablet from about 2000 B.C. contains the oldest known drug prescription. Physicians in Sumeria, China, Egypt, Rome, and other civilizations of the ancient world compiled long lists of drugs for a variety of human illnesses.

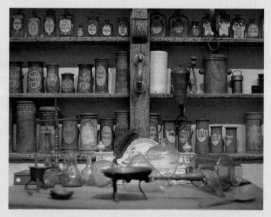

Containers that once held drugs line the shelves of a replica of an old German pharmacy. The exhibit, typical of many European pharmacies of the 1600's, also includes some of the implements druggists used to compound prescriptions.

the effectiveness of aspirin in easing pain and reducing inflammation and fever. Although a related compound extracted from willow bark had long been used for those purposes, Dreser's report led to the widespread use of synthetic aspirin. Many addictive drugs that are now available only by prescription were also in general use in those days. One of the most common was opium, which was taken by many people in an alcohol-water mixture called laudanum for the relief of pain and mental stress.

Conquering infection

The conquest of pain was a major triumph, but medicine still had another formidable menace to contend with: infection. Historians note that during the American Civil War (1861-1865), many more soldiers died of infections than were killed on the battlefield. In hospitals in the North and South, men died by the thousands from infected wounds, typhoid, pneumonia, dysentery, and malaria.

In the late 1800's, the *germ theory* of disease (the recognition of microbes as the cause of many illnesses), a scientific advance pioneered by the French scientist Louis Pasteur and the German physician Robert Koch, led to the next revolution in medicine. Although doctors still had no way to cure an infection once it had taken hold in a patient's body, they learned to prevent many infections by using *antiseptics* (agents that kill bacteria or inhibit their growth) to wash infected wounds and sterilize operating rooms and surgical instruments.

The first major advance in controlling bacterial infections in the body came in the 1930's with the development of sulfa drugs. In 1935, Gerhard Domagk, a German pathologist, reported that a dye called Prontosil cleared up streptococcal infections in mice. Subsequent research showed that the dye was broken down to a sulfur compound called sulfanilamide in the mice's bodies. Sulfanilamide prevented the streptococcal bacteria from multiplying, making it possible for the body's natural immune defenses to destroy them. Researchers soon found several related compounds that also were effective against bacteria.

The sulfa drugs saved many lives that would have been lost to such infectious diseases as pneumonia, dysentery, and urinary tract infections. But the drugs were far from ideal. They were useless against some kinds of infections, and they could cause serious side effects, including damage to the blood and kidneys.

The wonder drugs

In the mid-1940's, sulfa drugs were eclipsed by a far more important drug: penicillin. Penicillin was the first of the so-called wonder drugs that, virtually overnight, swept away many diseases that had been leading causes of death throughout history.

The discovery of penicillin happened by chance. In the late 1920's, a British bacteriologist in London, Alexander Fleming, was examining various kinds of bacteria for substances that might be taken orally to treat infections. At the time—this was before the introduction of sulfa drugs—most scientists thought that any substance potent enough to stop an internal infection would also kill the patient. So no one was very optimistic about Fleming's work.

One day in autumn 1928, Fleming noticed with some annoyance a dark green blob in one of his laboratory dishes of staphylococcus bacteria, caused by some sort of contaminating organism. As he was about to discard the ruined culture, he noticed a clear area around the green where no bacteria were growing.

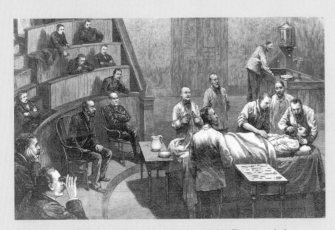

Physicians at Massachusetts General Hospital in Boston administer ether to a surgical patient in the late 1880's. Ether was the first of the general anesthetics, *drugs that put patients into an unconscious state. By enabling doctors to operate without causing patients pain, anesthetics revolutionized surgery.*

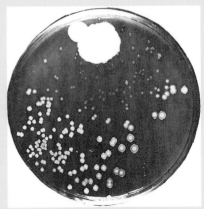

A Penicillium *mold (large blob) kills nearby bacteria in a laboratory dish. From this discovery, made by British scientist Alexander Fleming in 1928, came the first antibiotic, penicillin.*

Suspecting that something from the green splotch was killing the bacteria, Fleming analyzed the contaminant and discovered that it was a soil mold called *Penicillium*. He named the bacteria-killing substance produced by the mold penicillin.

Subsequent studies showed that penicillin not only killed many kinds of bacteria but also did no harm to laboratory animals or human cells grown in culture. And in 1941, a hospital test of penicillin proved that the drug was safe and effective for use against internal infections. Penicillin temporarily relieved the symptoms of an English policeman suffering from a severe bacterial infection. The man then relapsed and died, but only because there was insufficient penicillin available to completely destroy the infection.

Penicillin was in short supply because it was hard to purify or to produce in large amounts. Thus, despite the drug's apparent effectiveness against bacterial infections, most medical researchers had only limited interest in it.

All that changed in the early 1940's, when World War II was raging. Hoping to save wounded troops from fatal infections, researchers in the United States and Great Britain began looking for a way to mass-produce penicillin. The answer was found by way of another fortunate accident. A U.S. Department of Agriculture scientist browsing at a vegetable stand in Peoria, Ill., noticed a cantaloupe with an interesting mold on it. The mold proved to be a strain of *Penicillium* that produced much greater quantities of penicillin than the strain that had been isolated by Fleming. By mid-1943, a growing number of U.S. pharmaceutical companies were culturing the newly found mold, making penicillin for military hospitals around the world.

That same year, streptomycin was discovered. In the years that followed, scientists added one antibiotic drug after another—and many other kinds of drugs as well—to the arsenal against disease. The terms wonder drug or miracle drug, which were originally applied just to antibiotics, are now used in a more general sense to mean any drugs that offer seemingly miraculous cures for once-dreaded afflictions.

How drugs are administered

Drugs come in many forms and can be taken in various ways. Drugs meant to be taken orally are produced in capsule, tablet, powder, or liquid form. Other drugs must be inhaled, injected into a muscle or vein, or administered as an intravenous solution that is slowly dripped through a needle in the patient's arm.

Some drugs are applied locally—that is, just to the place where they are needed. Eye drops, nasal inhalants, and ointments and lotions that are rubbed into the skin are examples of drugs that go directly to the affected area of the body. Most drugs, however, are carried throughout the body in the bloodstream.

The way a drug is administered depends in part on the patient. Whereas an adult might take a particular medication in capsule form, the drug would probably be mixed with a pleasant-tasting liquid for an infant. A person lying semiconscious in a hospital bed would most likely be given a drug intravenously.

Other factors determining how a drug is administered include the nature of the drug and where in the body it is needed. Many synthetic chemicals, for instance, can be taken orally, but that is not the

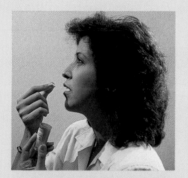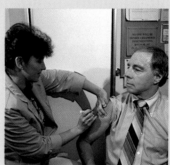
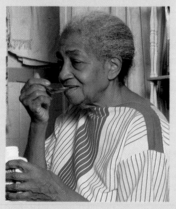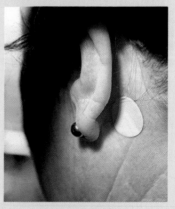

Drugs come in many forms and are administered in a variety of ways. Some drugs are available in pill or capsule form, top left, *while others are liquids that are taken orally,* above left, *or injected,* top right. *An adhesive patch,* above right, *releases a drug slowly through the skin.*

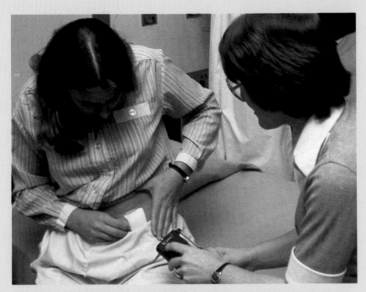

A portable pump that injects small doses of insulin is a recent option in drug delivery systems for some people with diabetes.

case with drugs that are proteins, such as insulin and many other hormones. That is because digestive juices in the stomach break down protein-based drugs just as they do the proteins in food. Thus, protein drugs must usually be injected into the bloodstream.

Delivering drugs to the brain is particularly difficult. Many drugs are blocked from entering the brain by the *blood-brain barrier*, a physical and biochemical "barricade" of tightly packed cells lining the blood vessels in the brain. The purpose of the barrier is to prevent chemical fluctuations that might disrupt the brain's delicately balanced internal chemistry. Fortunately, researchers have succeeded in developing a number of chemicals that can cross the barrier. Drugs linked to such chemicals are carried into the brain.

Another approach to overcoming the blood-brain barrier is to develop chemical *precursors* of drugs. A precursor is an inactive molecule that is converted by the body to an active drug. The kinds of precursors researchers are seeking are ones that would cross the blood-brain barrier and be transformed within the brain to functioning drugs. One such

chemical is administered to many people with *Parkinson's disease*, a brain disorder marked by muscle tremors and rigidity. Parkinson's disease develops when the brain produces an insufficient amount of *dopamine*. Dopamine is a *neurotransmitter*, a chemical that conveys signals between brain cells. Parkinson's patients cannot be given dopamine itself because the chemical cannot cross the blood-brain barrier. Instead, patients take a drug called L-dopa, a precursor of dopamine that is not stopped by the barrier. Within the brain, L-dopa is converted to dopamine.

Other ways of administering drugs include timed-release capsules that slowly empty their contents into the small intestine for absorption into the bloodstream and skin patches that deliver hormones, heart drugs, and other medicines through the skin. Yet another approach, being tested for the treatment of diabetes, uses a tiny pump that is implanted under the skin of the patient's abdomen. The pump releases precise amounts of insulin into the bloodstream throughout the day.

Scientists are working on other delivery systems, including im-

plants made of various kinds of *polymers* (giant molecules) that enclose drugs. In most cases, these slowly break down to release small, steady doses of medication. A polymer device named Ocusert is now being used for the treatment of glaucoma, a condition that causes a build-up of fluid in the eye. A new contraceptive for women, Norplant, releases its contents over a five-year period from a polymer implant placed under the skin of the arm.

Researchers are also looking for ways to release drugs at precise moments when the body most needs them. One approach uses polymer-based systems that respond to chemical changes in the body. For example, scientists at Enzytech, a company in Cambridge, Mass., have developed a polymer that swells when exposed to a higher-than-normal level of sugar in the blood. They suggest that this polymer, impregnated with insulin and implanted into the body, might provide a way to treat diabetes. With a rise in blood sugar, which normally signals the body to release insulin into the blood, the polymer would expand and allow insulin to escape. When blood-sugar levels returned to normal, the polymer would contract, shutting off the release of insulin.

How drugs work

Most drugs work by altering or interfering with biochemical reactions in cells. By so doing, drugs can boost the level of a deficient chemical, decrease the amount of a chemical that is present in excess, or prevent some chemicals from being produced at all.

Most drugs act by way of *cell receptors*, protein molecules on the surface of a cell that serve as highly selective gateways into the cell. A drug that can *bind* (make a molecular connection) to receptors normally involved in controlling a particular biochemical reaction can enhance or prevent that reaction. Some drugs, rather than acting at the cell surface, use receptors to pass into the interior of a cell. Once inside, they affect the cell's inner workings.

Among the drugs that operate at the cell surface are many psychotherapeutic drugs. These drugs bind to brain-cell receptors for neurotransmitters. Some brain cells, for instance, have receptors that are shaped to receive a neurotransmitter called *norepinephrine*, which is deficient in the brains of many depressed patients. Molecules of *imipramine*, a drug used to treat depression, can also bind to those receptors. The drug thereby prevents norepinephrine from being absorbed at those receptors and broken down by the nerve cells. This action results in a build-up of norepinephrine between cells, making more of the chemical available for the transmission of nerve signals.

A class of drugs known as *antihistamines*, taken by many people with allergies, works by plugging receptors on cells called mast cells, which when stimulated release substances that cause allergic symptoms. The antihistamine molecules thus prevent allergy-provoking molecules from pollen or other substances from binding to the mast-cell receptors and stimulating an allergic attack.

Not all drugs work by attaching to receptors on the body's cells. An antibiotic, for example, fastens onto and penetrates an invading microbe. The cholesterol-lowering drug Lovastatin works by attaching to molecules of an *enzyme* (a protein that speeds chemical reactions in cells) that the liver requires to manufacture cholesterol. With the needed enzyme inactivated by the drug, cholesterol levels in the blood drop.

Side effects and dosage

Because most drugs circulate throughout the body via the bloodstream, they often cause undesirable side effects. Most antihistamines, for instance, cause

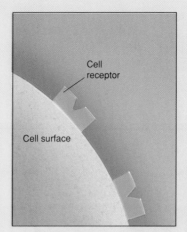 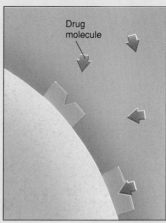

How drugs work in the body
Almost all drugs work by a kind of "lock and key" effect. They do so by attaching to cell receptors, molecules on the cell surface that serve as entrances to the cell, above left. Ordinarily, cell receptors take in nutrients or other molecules that affect the cell's activities. A drug molecule with the proper shape, above right, can attach to a receptor and alter chemical activity in the cell.

drowsiness in many people, and the antibiotic tetracycline can make users more sensitive to the sun, increasing the risk of sunburn. In many cases, a drug produces side effects that are very troublesome to patients. The antidepressant imipramine, to name just one example, can cause a variety of unpleasant effects, including constipation, dizziness, heart palpitations, and blurred vision. With some drugs that work in the brain, such as morphine, patients can become addicted if they take the drug over a period of weeks. In this state, the patient has developed a physical dependency on the drug and feels ill or agitated when deprived of it.

Occasionally, a patient has a severe—and sometimes even fatal—reaction to a drug. Some patients lapse into a coma, suffer serious organ damage, or die of respiratory failure after taking a particular drug. Serious effects of this sort occur when too large a dose of a drug is administered; when the drug reacts with other medications the patient is taking; or when the patient has a health condition, unrelated to the one for which the drug has been prescribed, that is aggravated by the

drug. A serious reaction can also result if the patient is allergic to a given drug, though such allergies cannot always be predicted. Because of the potential hazards involved with many drugs, it is vital for the physician to know a patient's health history before prescribing a drug for that patient.

Even when the physician is armed with that knowledge, prescribing the right dosage of a drug can be difficult. Some drugs are effective only over a very specific range of concentrations. If the patient takes too little of the drug, the condition being treated is not eliminated or effectively controlled. If he or she takes too much, symptoms of poisoning or some other severe reaction may occur. To be sure the patient receives just the right amount of a medication with such a narrow "safety margin," the doctor may find it necessary to periodically measure the drug's concentration in the patient's blood. Such blood tests are available for only a few drugs, however.

The age of the patient is another important consideration. Physicians must be especially careful when prescribing drugs for children and the elderly. Children are at a higher risk for many serious reactions or side effects than the general population because their physical development is not complete. For example, tetracycline can cause permanent discoloration of children's teeth.

The elderly are similarly at increased risk of experiencing reactions to many drugs. The changes brought on by aging, such as declining liver and kidney function, cause drugs to be retained in the body for a longer time. In addition, an older patient is more likely than a younger person to be suffering from more than one ailment and thus to be taking other medications that could interact with the drug.

When a patient stops taking a drug, its amount in the body begins to drop, and sooner or later the body eliminates the drug completely. Many drugs are broken down by the liver into smaller, inactive molecules that travel in the bloodstream to the kidneys and are excreted in the urine. Some drugs, such as penicillin, go directly to the kidneys for rapid excretion, bypassing the liver. Because the body gets rid of penicillin so quickly, large doses of the drug must be used against an infection to destroy the microbe.

Not all medications exit the body in the urine. Drugs may also be expelled in solid body wastes, sweat, tears, and even exhaled breath.

Factors that influence a drug's effectiveness

There are many variables that determine a drug's effectiveness in treating a particular condition. A drug's effects are never identical in all patients taking it, and even one person taking the same drug at different times may experience different results. In some cases, this could no doubt be attributed to subtle differences in body chemistry. But dosage is another important factor. A dose of a medication that would be adequate for a thin person might be too small for a heavier individual, simply because the drug would

be more diluted in the larger person's body.

Taking drugs at the proper time is also important. Doctors advise patients to take some medications at least one hour before or two hours after meals, when the stomach and upper small intestine are relatively empty. That is because food in the digestive tract can decrease the amount of drug absorbed into the bloodstream and thus lessen the drug's effectiveness. Other drugs, however, such as the antibiotic *amoxicillin*, are not affected by food and can be taken anytime. And some drugs should be taken with food to avoid irritating the stomach lining. That is the case with many drugs that fight inflammation, including aspirin and ibuprofen.

To complicate matters, certain drugs should not be taken with particular foods. For example, milk and other foods that contain appreciable amounts of calcium should not be consumed while the antibiotic tetracycline is being taken, because the calcium may reduce the drug's absorption and effectiveness.

Drug-resistant bacteria

An antibiotic's effectiveness can also be diminished when the microorganisms it attacks become resistant to it. When an antibiotic is given to many patients, it might kill billions of bacteria but leave unharmed a few that possess a natural immunity to the drug. In other cases, bacteria that are initially susceptible to an antibiotic are able to adapt in such a way that they acquire an immunity to the drug. After widespread and prolonged use of a particular antibiotic to treat an infection, the bacteria that are resistant to the drug become the most common strains that people encounter. When that happens, physicians must prescribe other antibiotics to quell the infection.

The widespread use of penicillin has led to the emergence of such drug-resistant bacterial strains. During World War II, 300,000 units of penicillin were

sufficient to cure many infections. (A unit of penicillin is 0.6 millionths of a gram.) Then, following years of worldwide use of the drug, 600,000 units were often needed —and then 1.2 million units, or even larger doses.

During the Vietnam War in the 1960's and early 1970's, many U.S. troops stationed in Southeast Asia contracted a form of *gonorrhea* (a sexually transmitted bacterial infection) that was unaffected by penicillin. Biologists speculate that the strain of bacteria causing the disease took hold in the brothels of the Philippines and other parts of the Far East. Prostitutes in those areas of the world commonly take regular low doses of antibiotics as a preventive measure against infection, a practice that encourages the growth of any drug-resistant strains of bacteria the women encounter. Carried back to the United States by infected military personnel, the penicillin-resistant bacteria spread through the general population. As a result, doctors must now prescribe other antibiotics to treat many cases of gonorrhea.

How new drugs are developed

The process of bringing a new drug to market is long and expensive. According to the Pharmaceutical Manufacturers Association (PMA), a trade association in Washington, D.C., it takes an average of nearly 10 years and costs at least $125 million for a pharmaceutical company to develop a drug, demonstrate its safety and effectiveness, and get approval to market it from the FDA.

This lengthy process begins with the identification of a new compound that shows promise as a drug. Every year, pharmaceutical researchers conduct laboratory tests on hundreds of such compounds, the vast majority of which are not developed further because they turn out to be less effective than had been hoped, because they are too toxic, or for other reasons. The PMA estimates that of every 10,000 potential drugs examined, only 1 eventually becomes a commercially available drug.

Some new compounds are found by accident, as happened with penicillin. In other cases, a new use is found for an existing drug. Minoxidil, approved in 1988 to treat baldness in men, was originally developed to treat high blood pressure. When researchers noticed hair growth in 80 per cent of the patients taking the drug, they decided to investigate the drug as a baldness remedy.

In the case of protein drugs, including many hormones, scientists often set out to find a way of producing a known protein in large quantities. Because genes, which carry the basic "blueprint" of life, code for all proteins, researchers are increasingly using the techniques of genetic engineering to make protein-based drugs. This entails taking a gene from one organism and inserting it into the genetic material of another organism. In this way, a human gene that carries the code for making a certain protein, such as insulin, can be spliced into a bacterium or yeast cell. The rapidly multiplying microorganism carries out the instructions in the spliced-in gene, producing large quantities of the protein coded for by that gene. The protein is then isolated and purified to be used as a drug.

Many drugs, particularly ones other than proteins, have come from nature. Following up on the discoveries of folk healers over the centuries, scientists have long explored the natural world for compounds with possible medical uses. One rich source of potential drugs is the sea. Many soft marine animals, lacking the protection of a shell or the ability to fight back, have evolved chemical defenses against their predators. Although such chemicals are used by the animals as poisons or repellents, in some cases they also have healing properties. A compound produced by sponges, for example, became the anticancer drug *cytarabine,* and a chemical called *didemnin-B,* derived from the sea squirt, is used to treat some kinds of herpesvirus infections as well as yellow fever and cancer.

An even greater source of drugs is the plant kingdom. Plants, too, have evolved legions of chemicals for self-defense, and many of those compounds have been adapted to human uses. Among them are the heart stimulant *digitalis; quinine,* used in the treatment of malaria; *ephedrine,* a drug used to treat respiratory conditions; and *scopolamine,* an antinausea drug.

Today, scientists are scouring the world's tropical rain forests to find new plants of potential importance to medical science. Because the rain forests are being destroyed at an alarming rate, the investigators are in a race against time. They must find those still-

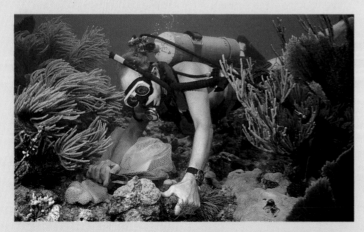
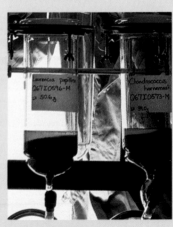

A diver, above left, *harvests organisms that may contain medically useful chemicals. Many modern drugs were derived from oceanic organisms or* dry-land plants. The chemicals are extracted in the laboratory, *above right.* Scientists may then try to make synthetic versions of the natural drugs.

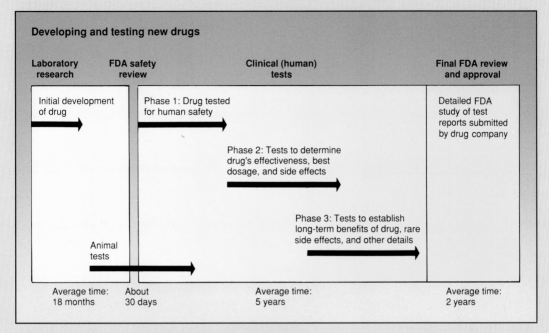

Developing and testing new drugs

Laboratory research	FDA safety review	Clinical (human) tests	Final FDA review and approval
Initial development of drug ⟶	Phase 1: Drug tested for human safety ⟶	Phase 2: Tests to determine drug's effectiveness, best dosage, and side effects ⟶ Phase 3: Tests to establish long-term benefits of drug, rare side effects, and other details ⟶	Detailed FDA study of test reports submitted by drug company
Animal tests ⟶			
Average time: 18 months	About 30 days	Average time: 5 years	Average time: 2 years

It takes several years for a pharmaceutical company to develop a new drug, test its safety and effectiveness in animals and human patients, and obtain approval to market it from the U.S. Food and Drug Administration.

unknown species before the plants—and the beneficial drugs that might be made from them—are lost to humanity for all time.

When researchers discover a promising new compound, they analyze it in the laboratory to learn its chemical structure. They then try to duplicate the compound synthetically so that supplies of the organism it came from will not be necessary for further development and production of the drug. Most mass-produced drugs are synthetic.

But waiting for a stroke of luck

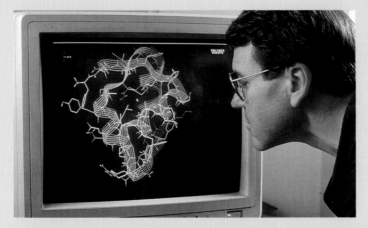

A researcher scrutinizes the structure of a drug molecule on a computer monitor. Experimental drugs that will fit specific points on other molecules are being designed with the aid of computers.

The history of a drug

Discovering and developing a drug can take many years, as the chronology of tretinoin (Retin-A), a drug applied to the skin to treat severe acne, illustrates:

1946—Tretinoin, a vitamin A derivative, is first synthesized.

1962—Tretinoin is tested as a treatment for certain types of skin damage resulting from overexposure to the sun.

1968—Ortho Pharmaceutical Corporation requests permission from the U.S. Food and Drug Administration to test tretinoin as a treatment for severe acne.

1971—Retin-A is marketed to treat severe acne. Although animal tests have indicated that the drug presents little risk (unlike the more hazardous acne drug isotretinoin, approved in 1983), pregnant women are advised to use Retin-A only if they are suffering from a serious acne problem.

1984—Ortho begins studies on using lower doses of Retin-A.

1988—A low-dose formulation of Retin-A is approved. It is just as effective against severe acne as the original higher-dose drug but is less irritating to the skin.

and painstakingly screening nature's medicine chest are not the most efficient ways to get started on the development of a new drug. A more direct route is *rational drug design,* an approach to drug production that makes extensive use of computers.

In rational drug design, scientists first use X-ray analysis to determine the three-dimensional structure of a specific portion of a cell receptor or other molecule that would be a target for the drug. They look for a *binding site,* the point on the target molecule where the drug molecule would attach itself to carry out its activity. The researchers then use a high-powered computer and a computer-graphics program to custom-design a drug that would fit perfectly with the binding site.

Next, they analyze protein molecules on the body's vital organs in the same way to ensure that the newly designed drug would not be able to attach to any cell receptors on the body's vital organs and thereby cause harmful side effects. If everything looks good, chemists and biologists can then get down to the business of actually synthesizing the drug. A new drug can in many cases be "assembled" from basic chemicals, but scientists usually find it easier to make it by modifying existing compounds.

Testing a new drug

Once pharmaceutical researchers have developed a new drug, they conduct exhaustive tests to ensure that it is both safe and effective. The compound is first tested in laboratory animals—a necessary step that saves many human lives. After animal testing, physicians administer the drug to selected groups of patients in carefully monitored clinical trials. If the drug lives up to expectations, the FDA approves it for mass production and general use.

The animals most often used in drug testing include rats, mice, rabbits, guinea pigs, and monkeys. Animal experiments can be done in a number of ways, de-

pending on the nature of the drug being tested. If, for example, the drug is meant to help people control their weight, the researchers might use a strain of mice that tend to get fat and see whether the drug makes them lose weight. If the compound is an antibiotic, the investigators would give the animals an infection and then see whether the drug helps the animals recover.

Scientists usually test a new compound on two or more kinds of animals, because a drug may affect different species in different ways. For example, a toxic effect that would make the drug unusable for human patients might

show up in monkeys but not in rats. The researchers also use animal studies to "fine-tune" a drug. If they find, for instance, that a drug promises to work as hoped but is not absorbed readily into the bloodstream, they may be able to modify it or add other ingredients to increase its absorption rate.

Animal tests typically go on for one to three years. If the drug does what it is supposed to and does not cause unacceptable side effects, it is ready for human trials, pending FDA permission. The agency reviews the data from the animal experiments, and, if it sees no danger, gives its approval

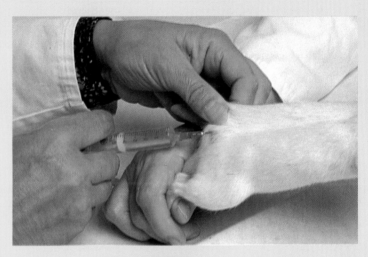

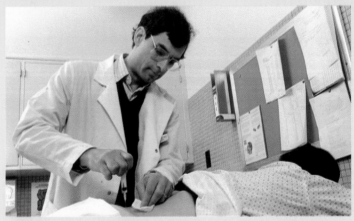

To test a newly developed drug, a scientist injects a dose of the experimental compound into a laboratory rat, top. *Once animal tests have shown that a new drug is safe and works as intended, the drug is administered to human patients,* above, *in a series of clinical trials.*

378

for clinical testing of the drug.

The clinical studies consist of three phases. Phase I, which lasts from six months to a year, tests the safety of the new drug on healthy volunteers. The volunteers, typically 20 to 100 people, are recruited for the study and are usually paid for their participation. The Phase I trials examine how the drug is absorbed, used by the body, and excreted, and assess its effects on specific tissues and organs. As the trials progress, the researchers gradually increase the dose to determine the drug's side effects and the dosage level at which they start to appear. One of the main reasons potential drugs fail during human testing is that they cause side effects at dosage levels lower than would be required to produce any beneficial result.

About 70 per cent of drugs tested go on to Phase II, which lasts from several months to two years. This stage, aimed at testing the drug's effectiveness as well as its risks, involves hundreds of patients who have the condition the drug is meant to treat. The patients are assigned at random to receive the experimental drug; a drug—if there is one—conventionally used to treat the condition; or a *placebo* (an inactive substance). This system enables the testers to learn whether the experimental drug has any more effect than an existing medicine or, in the case of the placebo group, no treatment at all.

In most cases, the pharmaceutical company or research organization involved assigns code numbers to supplies of the drugs and placebo. This ensures that neither the patients participating in the test nor the physicians administering it know who is getting what. This technique, called a *double-blind study,* guarantees that the conclusions reached by the testers will be completely without bias.

Less than 50 per cent of Phase II drugs proceed to Phase III. By now, researchers know that the drug is effective, and they have

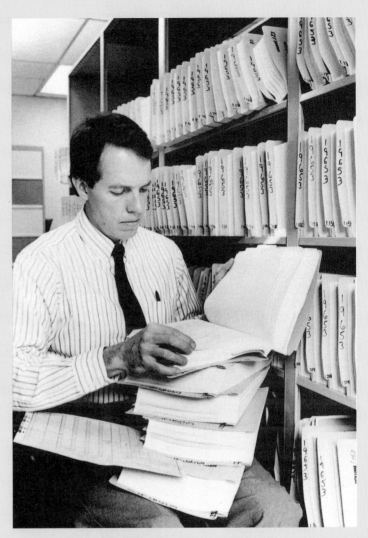

At the Food and Drug Administration (FDA), which approves new drugs, an official examines study results submitted by a drug firm.

determined its optimum dosage and side effects. In Phase III, the final stage of testing, they administer the drug to thousands of patients over a period of three to four years, and sometimes longer. These trials clarify all of the information needed to market the drug—its long-term beneficial effects, rare side effects, interactions with foods and other medications, and various other details. About 90 per cent of drugs that make it through Phase II also survive Phase III. Thus, of every 100 drugs that are approved for the first phase of human testing, 25 to 30 are ultimately considered worthy of being marketed.

Once all tests are completed, the drug's sponsor sends detailed records to the FDA as part of an application for permission to market the new drug. Experts at the FDA, including chemists, microbiologists, physicians, pharmacologists, and statisticians, then pore over the reams of documents to evaluate every aspect of the drug and the results of the clinical trials. If they are persuaded that the drug is both effective and safe, the agency approves the drug for production. This final approval process is painstaking and thorough and can take as long as seven years, though the average is two years. Of the 25 to 30 drugs out of 100 that make it to the end of Phase III testing, about 20 will finally receive FDA sanction and be manufactured.

Manufacturing and long-term monitoring

With the testing and approval process at last at an end, full-scale manufacture of a new drug begins. Pharmaceutical companies use mass-production methods to turn out millions of doses of any given drug each year.

The formulation of a drug, such as a tablet or capsule, generally contains a number of substances, called the *active* and *inactive* ingredients. The chemical causing the desired effect in the body is the active ingredient. Commonly used inactive ingredients include materials that provide bulk and chemicals that are added to a drug to prevent it from breaking down and losing its potency. Finally, drug manufacturers typically add flavors, colors, fragrances, thickeners, and other ingredients to make their products more appealing to patients.

Whether it is a synthetic chemical or a genetically engineered protein, a drug is produced in large batches under precisely controlled conditions. Automated equipment processes the completed drug into its final form, such as tablets, capsules, or bottled liquid, and then packages it for shipment to hospitals and pharmacies.

But even with full production of a new drug underway, the FDA's role is not ended. The FDA sends agents to examine and evaluate the equipment and production methods used in making the drug, just as it checks regularly on the manufacture of other, long-established medications.

The agency also requires the maker of a new drug to supply reports from physicians of any adverse patient reactions to the drug. If FDA computers uncover

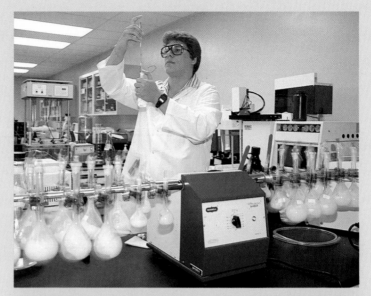

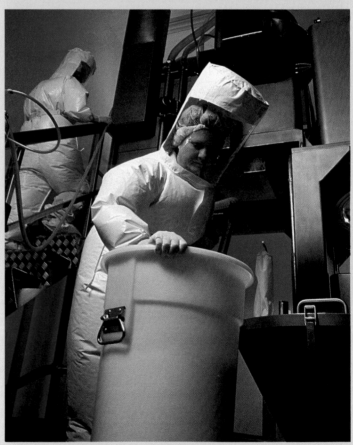

In a laboratory at a pharmaceutical plant, a chemist conducts tests on samples of drugs being manufactured, top. The production of drugs requires adherence to extremely high manufacturing standards. Formulating a compound, technicians at a plant wear special suits designed to prevent contamination of the drugs, above.

Understanding prescription information

There are many things people should know about drugs their doctor has prescribed for them. Sources of information include:

The prescribing physician. Before leaving the doctor's office, a patient should ask for an explanation of the drug that has been prescribed—what it does and when and how to take it. The physician can also explain when the patient should expect to feel better, what side effects might arise from the medication, and what the patient should do in the event of missing a scheduled dose. Patients should mention other medications they are taking or conditions they have that might cause a reaction with the drug.

Pharmacists. Pharmacists spend 5 years in training learning about drugs. A survey by the FDA found that pharmacists spend nearly one-fourth of their working day counseling patients on prescription drugs and how to take them. Nearly all pharmacists now use computers to keep track of patients' prescriptions. A pharmacist who is advised of all the medications a patient is taking can warn against harmful interactions between different drugs.

Drug-company handouts. Many pharmaceutical companies send drug information sheets or pamphlets to physicians and pharmacists. These materials are written with the patient in mind, so the language is not technical, and they often contain illustrations that can be quite helpful.

Package information. Health experts recommend that patients read every sticker and label on the medicine container and follow the instructions to the letter. Such instructions may warn, for example, against driving a motor vehicle or using heavy equipment while taking the drug. Directions concerning food warrant special attention because drug reactions with food are a frequent complication with prescription drugs.

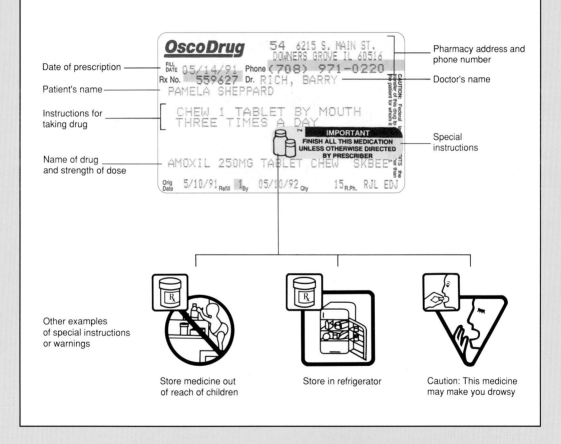

Date of prescription

Patient's name

Instructions for taking drug

Name of drug and strength of dose

Pharmacy address and phone number

Doctor's name

Special instructions

Other examples of special instructions or warnings

Store medicine out of reach of children

Store in refrigerator

Caution: This medicine may make you drowsy

any pattern of reactions in the reports, the drug company is directed to take action. The FDA orders the company either to change the written directions for using the medication or to add a warning for those people—for example, individuals with high blood pressure—who are considered to be at risk in taking the drug. In cases where serious reactions are occurring, the FDA may order the drug to be taken off the market if the manufacturer does not withdraw it voluntarily.

One drug that proved to have a tragic side effect after going on the market was *isotretinoin* (Accutane), a vitamin A derivative used to treat a severe form of acne. Less than one year after Accutane received FDA approval in 1982, some women who had been using the drug during pregnancy gave birth to babies with misshapen heads, heart problems, and other serious defects. The potential hazards of Accutane had been known from animal studies, but the warnings provided on the instructions accompanying the drug were apparently not forceful enough to prevent its use by pregnant women.

Because Accutane was far more effective against disfiguring acne than any other medication, the FDA did not order its removal from the market. Instead the agency worked with the manufacturer, Hoffmann-La Roche, Inc., of Nutley, N.J., to hammer out even more prominent and strongly worded cautions to both physicians and prospective users of the drug. The new warnings included a prohibition against prescribing Accutane for a woman unless she undergoes a laboratory test to ensure that she is not pregnant.

Fluoxetine (Prozac) is another drug that has been surrounded by controversy. More than 50 lawsuits have been filed against the manufacturer of this antidepressant drug, Eli Lilly and Company of Indianapolis, claiming that the medication produces suicidal tendencies in some users. But because suicidal thoughts are common in people suffering from depression, it may be hard to determine if the drug has caused any Prozac users to take their life.

Sometimes, a majority of physicians feel that a prescription drug is safe enough for patients to take without undue restrictions. In such cases, the FDA, after extensive review of the medication and its side effects, may change the drug's status to *over-the-counter* (OTC)—available without a prescription. A recent example is *ibuprofen,* a drug for the relief of pain and inflammation. Ibuprofen was introduced as Motrin in 1974, and received OTC status—though only for use by adults and in lower dosages—in 1984.

Speeding up drug approval

Sometimes there is such pressing need for a particular new drug that the normal process by which medications are tested and approved can seem intolerably slow.

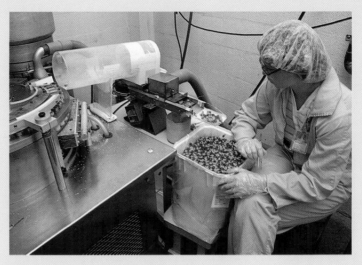

A worker checks drug capsules as they emerge from a capsulating machine. The drug will next be packaged and shipped to buyers.

During the 8 to 10 years that it takes the typical drug to reach the marketplace, many sufferers of the disease the drug is meant to treat may die.

That problem became a major issue in the 1980's with the AIDS epidemic. With AIDS deaths in the United States mounting each year and patients clamoring for any experimental drug that showed promise against the disease, the FDA was forced to reconsider its drug-approval policy. In late 1986,

the agency approved the drug *AZT* (also called zidovudine) for AIDS patients in the last stages of the disease. AZT was so effective at prolonging some patients' lives that the FDA in May 1987 established a *treatment investigational new drug* (treatment IND) program. The program allows people with AIDS or other life-threatening illnesses to obtain an experimental drug after the drug has successfully passed Phase II safety testing. By 1990, more than 10,000

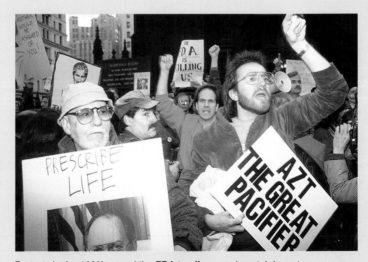

Protests in the 1980's urged the FDA to offer experimental drugs to AIDS patients. As a result, the FDA liberalized drug-testing policies.

AIDS patients were taking a drug called *dideoxyinosine* (DDI) that had been made available under the treatment IND policy. The FDA is considering a *parallel track* drug testing program that would make some experimental drugs available to seriously ill patients at the end of Phase I trials.

In October 1988, the FDA implemented another reform, aimed at shortening the time required for human trials of drugs for serious illnesses. The new regulation enables drug developers to eliminate Phase III testing if Phase I and Phase II trials provide strong evidence that a drug is safe and effective. That measure was expected to bring many needed drugs to market in record time.

Generic drugs

A pharmaceutical company that develops a new drug receives a 17-year patent on the drug and may renew the patent for up to 5 more years. The patent period begins when the drug receives FDA approval. During that time, the firm has the exclusive right to manufacture and distribute the drug. The manufacturer usually chooses to market the drug only under the company's own *trade name* (brand name).

After the patent on a drug has expired, other manufacturers are free to produce the drug and sell it under their own trade names. To increase their sales of the drug, companies may also decide to make it available to buyers at a lower price under its generic, or chemical, name.

The FDA requires that a generic drug match the original drug in active ingredients and strength and that it be *therapeutically equivalent,* meaning that it must produce the same effect as the original when administered in the same way. A generic drug may, however, differ in shape from the original drug and may have different inactive ingredients, such as flavor and color.

In the 1980's, the number of generic drugs available in the United States exploded from a few hundred to several thousand. A major impetus for this consumer windfall was the Drug Price Competition and Patent Term Restoration Act, which Congress passed in 1984. The act permits companies to receive FDA approval to begin marketing generic versions of a brand-name medication on which the patent has expired without having to repeat the lengthy testing process. The company need only conduct limited trials with patients to show that its generic product works as well as the brand-name drug. This abbreviated testing process also holds if a company plans to market a previously patented drug under a trade name. Such drugs are sometimes referred to as "branded generics."

Orphan drugs

Most familiar prescription drugs are taken by millions of people with common afflictions. But there are at least 5,000 diseases, such as leprosy and hemophilia, whose sufferers number in the thousands—or in some cases even the dozens—rather than the millions. For a great many of these less common illnesses, no drugs are available. Pharmaceutical companies are hesitant to invest the huge amounts of money necessary to develop new drugs to treat such illnesses, because the market for the drugs is relatively small and therefore unprofitable.

In 1983, Congress provided a financial incentive for the production of these so-called orphan drugs with the passage of the Orphan Drug Act. The act provides grants, federal tax credits, and a seven-year monopoly to developers of orphan drugs. An orphan drug was defined as one that would benefit fewer than 200,000 people in the United States. By 1991, the FDA had approved more than 40 orphan drugs and was evaluating more than 130 others.

In some instances, the FDA grants more than one company orphan-drug protection for the same drug. This occurs when the drug is marketed in different forms or when it is intended for the treatment of separate diseases. For example, both Genentech, Incorporated, of South San Francisco, Calif., and Eli Lilly and Company have received orphan-drug designation for slightly different forms of genetically engineered human growth hormone for children suffering from one form of dwarfism.

The Orphan Drug Act has aroused a considerable amount of controversy. Although the legislation has increased the number of drugs being developed for uncommon diseases, it has also in several instances brought windfall profits to companies, which—in the absence of competition—can charge what they like for an orphan drug. The example of Eli Lilly and Genentech demonstrates that even when some degree of market competition is preserved, it is not sufficient to hold down the price of a drug. The two companies charge from $10,000 to $30,000 for a year's worth of human growth hormone for a single patient. Although there are only about 12,000 children in the United States afflicted with the kind of dwarfism that responds to human growth hormone, the companies' combined sales of growth hormone amount to more than $150-million a year. That is about three times the combined total that Lilly and Genentech spent to develop the drug, a ratio that critics say is too high.

Occasionally, a company's sales for an orphan drug increase spectacularly when another use is found for the drug. The orphan drug law forbids a company to promote an orphan drug for any condition other than the one for which it was originally intended, but nothing prevents physicians from prescribing it for different conditions. That is precisely what occurred with *erythropoietin,* a drug developed by Amgen Incorporated of Thousand Oaks, Calif., to treat anemia in patients with kidney failure. Doctors soon began prescribing erythropoietin for other kinds of anemia as well, and annual sales of the drug soared to $200 million. Human growth hormone, too, is expected to bring in additional millions in profits. Recent research has shown that the protein is useful for treating burns and that it seems to reverse some of the effects of aging.

Because the Orphan Drug Act was never intended to produce financial bonanzas for drug companies, Congress decided some fine-tuning of the law was called for. In 1990, Representative Henry A. Waxman (D., Calif.) introduced a bill calling for a drug's orphan status to be revoked when the number of patients using the drug exceeds 200,000. The bill would also have allowed more than one company to market identical versions of an orphan drug if the companies began their work at about the same time. The bill was passed by Congress but vetoed by President George Bush, who argued that the legislation would "endanger the success of the [orphan drug] program."

Drugs of the future: genetic medicine

On Sept. 14, 1990, shortly after noon, a 4-year-old girl made medical history as she sat in her hospital bed at the National Institutes of Health (NIH) in Bethesda, Md. Because her body lacked a vital enzyme, the girl was threatened by infections that would not bother a healthy person. That afternoon, the child received an intravenous infusion of her own white blood cells, which had been extracted from her earlier. With the aid of a harmless virus, NIH scientists had added to the white blood cells a human gene instructing the cells to manufacture the needed enzyme. This FDA-sanctioned experiment, which seems to have improved the girl's immunity, was the first federally approved attempt at gene therapy—treating disease by giving people new genes or altering their existing genes.

This foray into gene therapy marked the beginning of a new era for medical science—and for the drug industry. Although drug makers will undoubtedly continue to benefit from screening nature's bounty and from the occasional lucky find, our rapidly expanding knowledge of how the human body works at the molecular level may someday make those traditional avenues of development increasingly less important.

As researchers learn more about genes and their role in disease, experts believe that computer drug design will be applied to the challenge of creating new drugs that can compensate for the effects of faulty genes. We can only guess what sorts of drugs will result, but the future for human health looks promising.

For further reading:

Long, James W. *The Essential Guide to Prescription Drugs.* Harper & Row, 1991.

United States Pharmacopeial Convention. *Drug Information for the Consumer.* Consumer Reports Books, 1990.

For more information:

The U.S. Food and Drug Administration
Office of Consumer Affairs
HFE-88
5600 Fishers Lane
Rockville, MD 20857

The U.S. Pharmacopeial Convention
Drug Information Division
12601 Twinbrook Parkway
Rockville, MD 20852

The author:

Ricki Lewis teaches biology at the State University of New York in Albany and is a genetic counselor. She has published many magazine articles on scientific topics and is the author of two biology textbooks, *Beginnings of Life* and *Life.*

Index

How to use the index
This index covers the contents of the 1990, 1991, and 1992
editions of *The World Book Health & Medical Annual.*

D-fenfluramine, 92: 131-132
Dairy products, 91: 221, 274
Dalkon Shield, 92: 243-244
Daminozide, see **Alar**
Deafness, see **Ear and hearing**
Deaths
  accidental, **92:** 319
  blacks, **92:** 297
  drug and alcohol abuse, **92:** 234-235
  exercise level, **91:** 277-278
  health-care facility, **91:** 292
  hospice care, **92:** 354-365
  Persian Gulf War, **92:** 353
  plague, **92:** 168, 172, 176
  smoking, **92:** 326-328, **91:** 255, 328, **90:** 316, 328
  see also specific diseases and **Infant mortality; Right to die**
Debridement, 90: 219-221
Defibrillation, 91: 355, **90:** 273-274
Delayed sleep phase syndrome (DSPS), 91: 307
Delusions, 92: 154, 156, 157
Dendritic cells, 92: 232
DENTISTRY, 92: 262-263, **91:** 260-262, **90:** 261-262
  AIDS risk, **92:** 230, 297-298
  artificial joint risks, **92:** 248
Deoxyribonucleic acid, see **DNA**
Department of Agriculture, U.S. (USDA), 91: 222
Deprenyl, 92: 149-150
Depressants, 92: 117
Depression
  chronic fatigue syndrome, **92:** 238
  drug abuse, **92:** 116-117
  drug treatment, **92:** 309-311
  elderly, **90:** 229
  L-tryptophan, **91:** 237, 310
  smoking, **92:** 327-328
  women, **92:** 125-137, 308
DES, see **Diethylstilbestrol**
Desensitization
  anxiety disorders, **90:** 24
  immunotherapy, **90:** 194-195
Detoxification, see **Withdrawal**
DIABETES, 92: 263-265, **91:** 262-264, **90:** 262-264
  animals, **90:** 332
  carpal tunnel syndrome, **91:** 49
  obesity, **91:** 133
  protein intake, **92:** 307
  stroke risk, **90:** 65
  women, **92:** 98, 108-109, **91:** 297, 314
Diabetic retinopathy, 92: 264, 280 (il.), **90:** 357
Dialysis, 92: 306-307, **91:** 303-304
Diarrhea, 91: 115, 119, 126

Each index entry gives the edition year
and the page number or numbers—for example, **Dalkon Shield, 92:** 243-244. This
means that information on the Dalkon
Shield may be found on pages 243 to 244
of the 1992 *Health & Medical Annual.*

When there are many references to a topic,
they are grouped alphabetically by clue
words under the main topic. For example,
the clue words under **Deaths** group the
references to that topic under nine
subtopics.

When a topic such as **DENTISTRY** appears in all capital letters, this means that
there is a Health & Medical News Update
article entitled Dentistry in at least one of
the three volumes covered by this index.
References to the topic in other articles
may also appear after the topic name.

When only the first letter of a topic such as
Depression is capitalized, this means that
there is no Health & Medical News Update
article entitled Depression, but that information on this topic may be found in the
edition and on the pages listed.

The "see" and "see also" cross references
are to other entries in the index—for example, **Detoxification,** see **Withdrawal.**

The indication (il.) means that the reference is to an illustration only, as in the
Diabetic retinopathy entry on page 280
of the 1992 edition.

A

Abortion
birth control drug, **90:** 243
fetal brain tissue, **92:** 150, **91:** 382
laws, **92:** 244, 298, **91:** 294
Soviet Union, **90:** 94
Accidents, see **Emergency medicine;
Injuries; Safety**
Accutane, see **Isotretinoin**
Acetaminophen, 91: 185, 195, **90:**
303-304
Acetylcholine, 92: 147, 240, **90:** 228
Acne, 92: 381-382
**Acquired immune deficiency syn-
drome,** see **AIDS**
Acupuncture, 92: 120 (il.), **90:** 209
Acyclovir, 92: 221
Addiction, see **Alcohol and drug
abuse**
Additives, Food, 91: 216-220
Adenoids, 91: 272
**Adenomatous polyposis coli (APC),
92:** 265-266, 289
**Adenosine deaminase (ADA) defi-
ciency, 92:** 286-287, **91:** 284-285
Adipsin, 90: 335
Adrenal glands, 92: 150, **91:** 382
**Adrenocorticotropic hormone
(ACTH), 92:** 236
Aerobic exercise, 92: 271-272
Aflatoxin B1, 92: 255
Agent Orange, 90: 275
Aggressive behavior, 90: 48, 49, 258,
307-308
AGING, 92: 228-229, **91:** 228-230, **90:**
228-229
aspirin and strokes, **91:** 331
bone disorders, **92:** 246-247, **91:**
246-247, 287-289
books, **92:** 248, **91:** 247, **90:** 248
Down syndrome births, **92:** 100
drug dosage, **92:** 375
influenza risk, **91:** 301
prostate disorders, **92:** 70, 78
weight guidelines, **92:** 336
see also **Alzheimer's disease; Bone
disorders; Menopause**
Agoraphobia, 90: 12, 13, 20, 25
Agranulocytosis, 91: 270
AIDS, 92: 13-27, 230-232, **91:** 230-233,
90: 230-233
AZT treatment, **92:** 14, 23-24, 231,
382, **91:** 231, 233, 245, 266-267,
90: 230-231
blood supply safety, **92:** 18, 244-245,
91: 233, 341-350
books, **92:** 248, **90:** 248
condoms, **92:** 18, 27, **91:** 323-324
costs, **92:** 16-17, **91:** 284, **90:** 294
drug approval, **92:** 382-383
Epstein-Barr virus, **90:** 137
erythropoietin treatment, **92:** 23-24,
231, **91:** 245
ethical issues, **92:** 297-298, **90:** 112-
125
free needle distribution, **90:** 295
joint inflammation, **91:** 242
kidney disease, **91:** 303
other sexually transmitted diseases,
link with, **92:** 212, 213, 222-224,
323
Soviet Union, **90:** 92

testing, **92:** 18-20, 22, 297-298, **90:**
232, 239
tissue transplants, **92:** 230-231
tuberculosis, **90:** 153
see also *Pneumocystis carinii*
pneumonia; Vaccines
Air pollution
asthma trigger, **90:** 189
global, **90:** 276-277
lead poisoning, **90:** 173-176
Legionnaires' disease, **90:** 167
lung damage, **92:** 274-275
Airbags, Automobile, 92: 320
Airlines
emergencies, **90:** 274
safety, **91:** 317, 318, **90:** 321-323
smoking, **91:** 330
Alar, 90: 320
Alcohol, Consumption of
cancer risk, **91:** 255, **90:** 30
coffee and drunkenness, **91:** 13
epilepsy and withdrawal, **91:** 150
pregnancy, **92:** 105, 107
ulcers, **90:** 76
Alcohol abuse
genetic tendency, **92:** 66-67, 235, **91:**
251-252, 285-286, 305, **90:** 233-
234
Soviet Union, **90:** 86, 97
see also **Alcohol and drug abuse**
ALCOHOL AND DRUG ABUSE, 92:
233-236, **91:** 233-236, **90:** 233-236
books, **91:** 247-248
parenting style, **91:** 259
sudden infant death syndrome, **91:**
62
truckers, **91:** 318
see also **Alcohol abuse; Drug
abuse**
Alcoholics Anonymous (AA), 92: 122
Alcoholism, see **Alcohol and drug
abuse**
All-terrain vehicles, 91: 274
ALLERGIES AND IMMUNOLOGY, 92:
236-240, **91:** 237-239, **90:** 236-240
see also **Antihistamines; Asthma;
Immune system**
Allografts, 90: 222
Alpha blockers, 92: 332
Alpha interferon, 92: 24, 269, **90:** 232
Alphafetoprotein (AFP), 92: 100-101,
91: 109
Alprazolam, 92: 115, 195
ALS-PD, 92: 144-145
Altretamine, 92: 268
Alveoli, 92: 84-88
Alzheimer's disease
book, **92:** 248
brain grafts, **92:** 150, **91:** 382
causes, **92:** 250-251
Down syndrome patients, **91:** 107
drug, **92:** 228-229
families, research on, **91:** 250
heart attacks, **91:** 230
nose, changes in, **90:** 250-251
suicide case, **91:** 293
Amantadine, 92: 147, **91:** 240-241
American Red Cross, 92: 244
Amino acids, in diet, 90: 106
Amniocentesis, 92: 101-102, 316, **91:**
107-108
Amoxicillin, 92: 271
Amphetamines, 92: 114-116, 233
Amygdala, 92: 191
Amyotrophic lateral sclerosis (ALS),

92: 144, 253-254, 289-290
Anabolic steroids, 90: 43-55
Analgesics, 92: 369, **90:** 53
Anemia
AIDS, **92:** 23-24, 231, **91:** 245
aplastic, and tanning, **92:** 325
Fanconi's, **91:** 245
iron-deficiency, **90:** 108
sickle-cell, **91:** 244
sudden infant death syndrome, **91:**
62
Anencephaly, 91: 314-315, **90:** 379
Anesthesia, 92: 370
Aneurysm, 90: 59-61, 270
Angel dust, see **PCP (drug)**
Angina, 92: 312
Angiography, 91: 298
Angioplasty, 90: 331
see also **Plaque, Arterial**
Animals
drug tests, **92:** 378
organ transplants, **91:** 379-380
see also **Veterinary medicine**
Ankylosing spondylitis (AS), 92: 241-
242, **91:** 29, 35
Anorexia nervosa, 91: 24, 253
Antacids, 91: 80, **90:** 79
Antibiotics, 92: 369, 371-372
burns, **90:** 219
drug-resistant bacteria, **92:** 375
pneumonia, **92:** 90-91, 94
rheumatoid arthritis, **91:** 241
tuberculosis, **90:** 149-150
Antibodies
AIDS, **92:** 14
donated blood, **91:** 349
Epstein-Barr virus, **92:** 238, **90:** 132
pneumonia, **92:** 85, 94-95
pregnancy failure, **91:** 290
rheumatoid arthritis, **91:** 30-31, 36
soldier identification, **92:** 352
transplant rejection, **92:** 239, **91:** 370
Anticholinergic drugs, 92: 147, 149
Anticoagulant drugs, 90: 62
Anticonvulsant drugs, 91: 148, 151,
153-154
Antidepressant drugs
anxiety disorders, **90:** 20-22
deaths, **92:** 234
depression, **92:** 309-311
obsessive-compulsive disorders, **91:**
270
premenstrual syndrome, **92:** 137
shyness, **92:** 195
tricyclic, for drug abuse, **92:** 117
Antigens, 91: 30, 342-343
Antihistamines, 92: 374, **90:** 270-271
Anti-inflammatory drugs, 92: 236-237
see also **Nonsteroidal anti-inflam-
matory drugs**
Antilymphocyte serum, 91: 370
Antipsychotic drugs, 91: 96-98
Antitoxin, 92: 199
Antiviral drugs, 91: 240-241
Anxiety, 92: 116, 184
Anxiety disorders, 91: 20-23, **90:** 11-
25
Aphasia, 90: 58, 63
Appendicitis, 90: 266
Appetite, see **Eating disorders;
Weight control**
Armadillo, and leprosy, 91: 207-208
Arteriography, 90: 62

ARTHRITIS AND CONNECTIVE TIS-SUE DISORDERS, 92: 240-242, **91:** 240-242, **90:** 240-242
  book, **92:** 248
  repetitive strain injuries, **91:** 43-55
  running injuries, **91:** 278
  see also **Bone disorders; Ligaments; Osteoarthritis; Rheumatoid arthritis;**
Arthrodesis, 91: 40
Asbestos, 91: 64, 275-276, 317, **90:** 277
Aspiration pneumonia, 92: 84
Aspirin
  arthritis, **91:** 36, **90:** 74
  asthma trigger, **90:** 189
  fever, **91:** 185, 194-195
  heart attacks, **92:** 300-302, **91:** 245
  origins, **92:** 371
  pregnancy, **92:** 106
  repetitive strain injuries, **91:** 52
  stroke, **91:** 331, **90:** 62
Asthma, 90: 183-197
  book, **91:** 247
  caffeine, **91:** 23-25
  childhood, **92:** 237
  deaths, **92:** 236 (il.), 316-317, **90:** 316
  drugs, **92:** 236-237, 317, **91:** 269
  guidelines, **92:** 317
  smoking risk, **91:** 238 (il.)
Asymptomatic infection, 92: 213
Atherosclerosis
  endothelial cells, **91:** 298-299
  fat in diet, **91:** 133-137, **90:** 101-104
  plaque removal devices, **90:** 296-297
  stroke, **91:** 331, **90:** 58
  see also **Heart disease**
Athletics
  anabolic steroid abuse, **90:** 42-55
  eye injuries, **92:** 282
  repetitive strain injuries, **91:** 45-46
  see also **Exercise and fitness**
Atlantoaxial instability, 91: 106-107
Atrial fibrillation, 92: 291, 301, 331, **91:** 331, **90:** 67
Atropine, 92: 343
Attention deficit disorder, 92: 308, **91:** 88
Autism, 90: 305 (il.)
Autograft, 91: 367-368, **90:** 221
  see also **Skin grafting**
Autoimmune diseases
  arthritis, **92:** 240
  Graves' disease, **92:** 291
  myasthenia gravis, **92:** 240
  vaccines, **91:** 238-239
  see also **AIDS; Multiple sclerosis**
Autoimmune reaction, 91: 31
Autologous blood donation, 91: 351, **90:** 246
Automobile accidents, 92: 320, **90:** 319-322, 342, 352
  see also **Safety**
Ayala, Anissa, 91: 379
Azathioprine, 92: 265
AZT, see AIDS

B

B cells
adenosine deaminase deficiency, **91:** 284-285

Epstein-Barr virus, 90: 136
  immune response, **90:** 370
  myasthenia gravis, **92:** 240
  rheumatoid arthritis, **91:** 30-31
  transplanted immunity, **90:** 240
Back pain, 90: 199-211
Bacteremia, 92: 303, **91:** 191
Bacteria
  ankylosing spondylitis, **92:** 241-242
  blood poisoning, **92:** 303
  botulism, **92:** 198-209
  cholera, **92:** 304
  contact lenses, **90:** 283
  drug development, **92:** 371-372
  food poisoning, **92:** 204
  Legionnaires' disease, **90:** 164 (il.), 166-167
  Lyme disease, **92:** 332-333
  Parkinson's disease, **92:** 143
  plague, **92:** 168-172, 176-181
  pneumonia, **92:** 83-84, 90-94
  reactive arthritis, **90:** 241-242
  sexually transmitted diseases, **92:** 213-218, 223
  stomach cancer, **92:** 305
  vaccines, **90:** 369-370
  see also **Infection; Streptococcus**
Baldness, 92: 324 (il.), **91:** 327, **90:** 270 (il.)
Balloon dilation, 91: 296
Barbiturates, 92: 112, 114, 115
Basal ganglia, 92: 142
Battalion aid stations, 92: 346
Bed-wetting, 91: 290 (il.), 332
Behavior, see Child development; Mental health
Behavioral inhibition, 92: 186-187
  see also **Shyness**
Behavioral therapy, 92: 121
Bellybutton surgery, see Laparoscopic surgery
Benign prostatic hyperplasia (BHP), 92: 78-79
Benzodiazepines, 92: 115, 117, **90:** 20
Bergalis, Kimberly, 92: 230, 297
Beta amyloid, 92: 250-251
Beta-blockers, 92: 195, **90:** 22, 53
Beta cells, 92: 265
Beta-endorphin, 92: 132
Bias, in science, 91: 61-62
Bilateral orchiectomy, 92: 76-80
Bile, 92: 42, 43
Bilirubin, 92: 42, 43, 45
Biobehavioral problems, 92: 126
Biofeedback, 91: 33 (il.), 40, **90:** 196, 209, 264
Biological clock, 91: 66-68, 307
Biopsy
  cancer, **92:** 73, **91:** 81-82, **90:** 36, 37
  ulcers, **90:** 78
Bipolar disorder, see Manic-depressive disorder
BIRTH CONTROL, 92: 243-244, **91:** 242-244, **90:** 243-244
  cancer risk, **91:** 75, **90:** 30
  rheumatoid arthritis, **90:** 241
  sexually transmitted diseases, **92:** 323-324
  Soviet Union, **90:** 94
  toxic shock syndrome, **91:** 125
  vaccine, **90:** 383
  see also **Condoms; Norplant contraceptive**
Birth defects
  aortic valve obstruction, **91:** 296

  caffeine, **91:** 20, 22
  drugs, **92:** 106
  epilepsy, **91:** 149
  fetal surgery, **91:** 296, 312-313
  fetal tissue for organ transplants, **91:** 379
  folic acid, **92:** 315-316, **91:** 314-315
  testing, **91:** 100-102, 316
  video terminal use, **92:** 314-315
Birth weight, 92: 102, **91:** 61, 313-314
Birthmarks, 90: 327
Bisexuality, see Homosexuality, and AIDS
Black Death, see Plague
Blacks
  death rates, **92:** 297
  diabetes, **90:** 263 (il.)
  organ transplants, **91:** 378, 380
  sickle-cell anemia, **91:** 244
Bladder cancer, 92: 254-255
Bleeding
  digestive system, **92:** 266-267
  small blood vessels, **92:** 273
  vaginal, **92:** 109
Blinded studies, 92: 65 (il.)
Blindness, see Eye and vision
BLOOD, 92: 244-246, **91:** 244-245, **90:** 244-246
  sudden infant death syndrome, **91:** 68
  see also **Bleeding; Leukemia; White blood cells**
Blood banks, 91: 343
  see also **Blood transfusions**
Blood-brain barrier, 92: 149, 373
Blood clots
  blood types discovery, **91:** 343
  heart attack, **92:** 301, 302, **91:** 245, 269
  Norplant side effects, **91:** 243
  stroke, **91:** 330, **90:** 58-59, 62
  see also **Hemophilia**
Blood donation, 91: 345-348
  see also **Blood transfusions**
Blood doping, 90: 53
Blood poisoning, 92: 303
Blood pressure, 92: 278-279, **90:** 249
  see also **Hypertension**
Blood sugar, see Glucose, Blood
Blood testing
  AIDS, **92:** 18-20, 22, **90:** 116-118
  alcoholism, **90:** 234
  botulism, **92:** 199
  cancer, **92:** 73, 74, **90:** 318
  cholesterol, **91:** 135
  diabetes, **92:** 264
  Down syndrome, **91:** 109, **90:** 314-315
  hepatitis, **91:** 265, **90:** 301
  lead poisoning, **90:** 179-180
  mononucleosis, **90:** 138-139
  pregnancy, **92:** 98-100
  stroke, **90:** 330-331
Blood transfusions
  AIDS, **92:** 18-20, 244-245, **91:** 233, 341-351, **90:** 116-118
  blood supply safety, **91:** 341-351
  hepatitis, **91:** 265, 302
  Persian Gulf War, **92:** 352
Blood types, 91: 342-343, **90:** 76
Body building, 90: 229
  see also **Anabolic steroids**

BONE DISORDERS, 92: 246-248, **91:** 246-247, **90:** 246-247
  back pain, **90:** 199-211
  elderly, **92:** 246-247, **90:** 228, 229
  healing method, **90:** 247
  menstrual cycle, **92:** 290
  prednisone, **92:** 242
  see also **Arthritis and connective tissue disorders; Osteoporosis**
Bone infusion needle, 91: 273-274
Bone marrow transplants
  AIDS and lymphoma, **91:** 232
  bone healing method, **90:** 247
  ethical issues, **91:** 379
  Fanconi's anemia, **91:** 245
  Hodgkin's disease, **90:** 244-245
  infection risk, **92:** 268-269
  procedure, **91:** 374-376
  rejection problem, **91:** 372
  statistics, **91:** 369
Bone spurs, 91: 37
Bone transplants, 91: 366, 367
BOOKS OF HEALTH AND MEDICINE, 92: 248-250, **91:** 247-249, **90:** 248-250
Borrelia burgdorferi (bacteria), **92:** 306, 332-333
Botox, 92: 208
Botulism, 92: 197-209
Bradykinesia, 92: 140, 141
BRAIN AND NERVOUS SYSTEM, 92: 250-254, **91:** 249-253, **90:** 250-253
  anxiety disorders, **90:** 18
  birth defects, **92:** 100-102, 315-316, **91:** 314-315
  blood-brain barrier, **92:** 149, 373
  books, **91:** 249, **90:** 248, 249
  caffeine, **91:** 24
  emotional development, **91:** 257
  epilepsy, **91:** 143-155
  hyperactivity, **92:** 308
  imaging of arteries, **91:** 298
  lead poisoning, **90:** 177-179
  menstrual cycle, **92:** 128, 134
  schizophrenia, **92:** 155 (il.), 156, 158-160, **91:** 304-305
  shyness, **92:** 191
  stress and aging, **92:** 229
  sudden infant death syndrome, **91:** 64-66
  Tourette syndrome, **91:** 88, 93-99
  see also **Alzheimer's disease; Neurons; Parkinson's disease; Spinal cord injuries**
Brain damage
  epilepsy, **91:** 149-150
  fever, **91:** 191
  nerve tissue regrowth, **91:** 249-250, **90:** 228
  stroke, **90:** 57-62
Brain death, 91: 376, 377
Brain tissue implants, 92: 150-151, **91:** 382, **90:** 228
Breast
  augmentation, **90:** 33
  examinations, **91:** 254, **90:** 38-39
  fibrocystic changes, **92:** 135
  reconstruction, **90:** 37
Breast cancer, 90: 26-41
  age differences, **92:** 256 (il.)
  books, **92:** 248-249, **91:** 249
  estrogen replacement therapy, **91:** 288-289
  fat in diet, **91:** 137-140
  medical study design, **92:** 58-59
  screening, **92:** 254
Breast-feeding, 91: 236
Bromocriptine, 92: 130
Bronchi, 92: 85, 86 (il.), 316
Bronchial pneumonia, 92: 88
Bronchioles, 92: 85, 86 (il.)
Bronchodilators, 92: 236, 316-317, **90:** 193
Bronchopulmonary dysplasia, 92: 318
Bronchoscope, 92: 84, 88, 92 (il.)
Buboes, 92: 171-172
Bubonic plague, 92: 171-172
Bulimia, 90: 235
Burns, 92: 213-225
  epidermal growth factor, **90:** 326
  pressure garments, **90:** 223 (il.), 224, 327 (il.)
Bush, George and Barbara, 92: 291

C

CAD-CAM, see **Computers**
Caesarean section, 92: 109, **90:** 313-314
Caffeine, 92: 269 (il.), **91:** 11-25, 255
Calcium, 91: 220, 288, 311, **90:** 108-110, 251-252
Calcium antagonists, see **Calcium channel blockers**
Calcium channel blockers, 90: 62-63, 252, 269-270
Calcium disodium edetate, 90: 180
CANCER, 92: 254-258, **91:** 253-257, **90:** 254-257
  airline flight radiation, **91:** 318
  back pain, **90:** 204
  books, **92:** 248-249
  caffeine, **91:** 23, 255
  electromagnetic fields, **92:** 273-274, 322
  Epstein-Barr virus, **90:** 136-137
  estrogen replacement therapy, **92:** 290-292, **91:** 288-289
  fever as symptom, **91:** 191
  fluoridation, **91:** 319
  food labeling claims, **91:** 213
  gene therapy, **92:** 256-257, 286-287, **91:** 253, 285, **90:** 254-255, 286-287
  genetic basis, **92:** 254-257, 265-266, 287-288, **90:** 255
  grade, **92:** 74, 77 (il.)
  hospice care, **92:** 354, 360
  medical study design, **92:** 58-61
  new drugs, **92:** 268, 270, **91:** 271
  organ transplants, **91:** 370
  rain forest drugs, **91:** 164-168
  smoking, **92:** 258, 317, 327, **91:** 74, 328, **90:** 328-329
  stage, **92:** 74, 77 (il.)
  see also **Chemotherapy** and specific cancer types
Candidiasis, 92: 24
Canthaxanthin, 92: 325-326
Carbidopa, 92: 149
Carbohydrates, 92: 131-132, **91:** 220
Carcinogens, see **Cancer**
Cardiac arrhythmia, 91: 22, 24
Cardiac monitors, 91: 355
Cardiopulmonary resuscitation (CPR), 92: 273
Cardiovascular disease, see **Heart disease**
Cardiovascular drugs, 92: 369
Carotid endarterectomy, 92: 329-330
Carpal tunnel syndrome, 92: 247-248, **91:** 44-55
Cartilage, 91: 29-33, 37, 367
CAT scan, see **Computerized tomography**
Cataracts, 92: 281-282, **91:** 106, 330, **90:** 283-284, 357
Catatonic schizophrenia, 92: 157
Cauterization, 91: 82-83
Ceftriaxone, 92: 216
Cell receptors, 92: 373-374, 378
Centoxin, 92: 352
Cerebral cortex, 92: 142
Cerebral embolism, 90: 58-59
Cerebral hemorrhage, 90: 58-62
Cerebral thrombosis, 90: 58, 62
Cervical cancer, 91: 71-85
  passive smoking, **90:** 328-329
  screening, **92:** 254
  venereal warts, **92:** 221, **91:** 332
  viruses, **91:** 257
Chamorro, 92: 144-145
Chancre, 92: 217-218
Chancroid, 92: 212, 213, 223-224
Chemical Abuse and Addiction Treatment Outcome Registry (CATOR), 92: 122
Chemical weapons, 92: 342-346, 350 (il.)
Chemotherapy
  breast cancer, **90:** 35 (il.), 40
  cervical cancer, **91:** 85
  colon cancer, **90:** 257
  infections, **92:** 246, 268-269
  prostate cancer, **92:** 80
  rectal cancer, **92:** 257-258
Chenodiol, 92: 48
Chicken pox vaccine, 90: 383
CHILD DEVELOPMENT, 92: 258-261, **91:** 257-260, **90:** 257-260
  abuse, **92:** 311, **90:** 306-307
  food choices, **92:** 313-314
  growth hormone, **90:** 290
  hyperactivity, **92:** 308
  mental disorders, **90:** 305-306
  obesity, **92:** 335
  shyness, **92:** 186-194, **90:** 19-20, 260
  see also **Birth defects; Children; Pregnancy and childbirth**
Children
  AIDS, **92:** 15, 19, 20, 23
  asthma, **92:** 237
  bed-wetting, **91:** 290 (il.)
  books, **91:** 247
  caffeine addiction, **91:** 15
  cancer and sunburn, **91:** 254-255
  drug dosage, **92:** 374-375
  drug infusions, **91:** 273-274
  fever, **91:** 188-191, 195
  hospice care, **92:** 362
  immunization, **92:** 34-39, 303-305, **91:** 301, **90:** 382-383
  lead poisoning, **92:** 275-276, **90:** 170-181
  lice infestations, **91:** 325
  passive smoking, **92:** 327
  pediatric trauma centers, **90:** 341-353
  plague victims, **92:** 176

radiation exposure, **91:** 274
see also **Child development; Down syndrome; Infants; Safety**
Chiropractors, 90: 208-209
Chlamydia, 92: 92, 212-215, 225
Chlorpromazine, 92: 160
Chocolate, 92: 334
Cholecystectomy, 92: 46 (il.), 50-53
Cholecystitis, 92: 43
Cholera, 92: 304
Cholesterol
anabolic steroids, **90:** 47-48
caffeine, **91:** 16, 19
fat in diet, **91:** 129-141
food labeling, **91:** 212-216, 221-222
gallstones, **92:** 42, 43, 47
"good" and "bad," **90:** 298-299
heart disease, **92:** 300, **91:** 296-297, **90:** 289-290
oat bran, **92:** 64-66, **91:** 224-225, 308-309, **90:** 309
stroke, **90:** 65-67
vegetarian diet, **90:** 101-104
vitamin E, **92:** 312
weight loss, **90:** 279-280
see also **Heart disease; High-density lipoproteins; Low-density lipoproteins; Plaque, Arterial**
Chorionic villus sampling (CVS), 92: 102, 316, **91:** 108, **90:** 289
Chromosomes
amyotrophic lateral sclerosis, **92:** 253, 290
fragile X syndrome, **92:** 285-287
schizophrenia, **92:** 157-158
translocation, **91:** 103
Chronic fatigue syndrome (CFS), 92: 238-239, 240-241, **90:** 137
Chronic granulomatous disease (CGT), 91: 239
Chronic motor tics, 91: 91
Cigarette smoking, see **Smoking**
Ciguatera, 92: 204
Cimetidine, 91: 22
Circadian rhythms, 91: 66-68
see also **Biological clock**
Circumcision, 90: 315
Clinical ecology, 90: 239
Clinical trials, 92: 58
Clostridium botulinum (bacteria), **92:** 198-209
Clotrimazole, 92: 270
Clozapine, 92: 161
Cocaine, 92: 105-106, 112-119, 234
see also **Crack**
Cockroaches, 92: 237
Codeine, 92: 114, 115
Coffee, see **Caffeine**
Cognitive therapy, 92: 121
Colds, 91: 189, **90:** 238-239, 300-301
Collagen, 90: 177, 223
Colon cancer
diet, **92:** 255 (il.), 311, **91:** 23, 137, 140
drug treatment, **91:** 253-254, 271
gene, **92:** 256, 265-266, 289, **90:** 255-256
screening, **92:** 254
Colony stimulating factors, 92: 268-269
Colposcopy, 91: 81-82
Combat lifesavers, 92: 343, 346

Combat support hospitals (CSH's), 92: 347-348
Comfort (hospital ship), **92:** 345 (il.), 349
Compound Q, 92: 25
Computerized tomography (CT)
back problems, **92:** 206
hearing loss studies, **90:** 272
pediatric trauma units, **90:** 351-353
Persian Gulf War, **92:** 350, 351
stroke diagnosis, **90:** 61-62
Computers
communication by disabled, **90:** 252 (il.)
dentistry, **90:** 261
drug design, **92:** 378, 384
health effects, **92:** 314-315, **91:** 43-46, 53-55
psychotherapy, **91:** 307-308
skull surgery, **92:** 247 (il.)
Condoms
AIDS prevention, **92:** 18, 27
cervical cancer prevention, **91:** 76
sexually transmitted diseases, **92:** 225, 324
teen-age use, **91:** 323-324
Conization, 91: 83, 84
Conjunctivitis, 92: 31, 215
Constipation, 92: 107
Contact lenses, 91: 281, **90:** 281-283
Contingency contracting, 92: 121
Contraception, see **Birth control**
Control groups, 92: 61, 63 (il.)
Coprolalia, 91: 91-93
Cornea, 92: 281, **91:** 279-280, **90:** 357
Cornea transplants, 91: 366, 367, 369, 373 (il.), 376
Coronary artery bypass surgery, 92: 299-300
Coronary artery disease, see **Atherosclerosis; Heart disease**
Corpus callosum, 91: 148 (il.)
Corticosteroids
AIDS, **92:** 24, 232
asthma, **92:** 236, **90:** 193, 195
organ transplants, **91:** 368
repetitive strain injuries, **91:** 51-52
rheumatoid arthritis, **91:** 36-38
Cortisol, 90: 234
Cosmetic surgery, 90: 37, 224
Costs, Medical and health-care, see **Financing medical care**
Cough, Chronic, 90: 317-318
Crack (cocaine), 92: 106, 114-116, 119, **91:** 235
Creatine kinase, 91: 174
Cruzan, Nancy Beth, 92: 296
Cryosurgery, 91: 82-83
Cryptococcal meningitis, 92: 21, **91:** 231-232, 267
CT scan, see **Computerized tomography**
Cumulative trauma disorders, see **Repetitive strain injuries**
Curare, 91: 160
Cutaneous T-cell lymphoma, 90: 326-327
Cyclosporine, 91: 303, 326-327, 370-371, **90:** 222
Cyst, 90: 36
Cystic fibrosis, 91: 285 (il.), 315
Cystoscopy, 92: 74
Cytokines, 92: 239
Cytomegalovirus (CMV), 92: 21, **91:** 267, 272, 350, **90:** 232

D

D-fenfluramine, 92: 131-132
Dairy products, 91: 221, 274
Dalkon Shield, 92: 243-244
Daminozide, see **Alar**
Deafness, see **Ear and hearing**
Deaths
accidental, **92:** 319
blacks, **92:** 297
drug and alcohol abuse, **92:** 234-235
exercise level, **91:** 277-278
health-care facility, **91:** 292
hospice care, **92:** 354-365
Persian Gulf War, **92:** 353
plague, **92:** 168, 172, 176
smoking, **92:** 326-328, **91:** 255, 328, **90:** 316, 328
see also specific diseases and **Infant mortality; Right to die**
Debridement, 90: 219-221
Defibrillation, 91: 355, **90:** 273-274
Delayed sleep phase syndrome (DSPS), 91: 307
Delusions, 92: 154, 156, 157
Dendritic cells, 92: 232
DENTISTRY, 92: 262-263, **91:** 260-262, **90:** 261-262
AIDS risk, **92:** 230, 297-298
artificial joint risks, **92:** 248
Deoxyribonucleic acid, see **DNA**
Department of Agriculture, U.S. (USDA), 91: 222
Deprenyl, 92: 149-150
Depressants, 92: 117
Depression
chronic fatigue syndrome, **92:** 238
drug abuse, **92:** 116-117
drug treatment, **92:** 309-311
elderly, **90:** 229
L-tryptophan, **91:** 237, 310
smoking, **92:** 327-328
women, **92:** 125-137, 308
DES, see **Diethylstilbestrol**
Desensitization
anxiety disorders, **90:** 24
immunotherapy, **90:** 194-195
Detoxification, see **Withdrawal**
DIABETES, 92: 263-265, **91:** 262-264, **90:** 262-264
animals, **90:** 332
carpal tunnel syndrome, **91:** 49
obesity, **91:** 133
protein intake, **92:** 307
stroke risk, **90:** 65
women, **92:** 98, 108-109, **91:** 297, 314
Diabetic retinopathy, 92: 264, 280 (il.), **90:** 357
Dialysis, 92: 306-307, **91:** 303-304
Diarrhea, 91: 115, 119, 126
Diazepam, 92: 115
Dideoxycytidine (DDC), 92: 25
Dideoxyinosine (DDI), 92: 23, 383
Diet
liquid, **90:** 336
premenstrual syndrome, **92:** 131-132, 136-137
ulcers, **90:** 74 (il.), 78
weight guidelines, **92:** 336
see also **Fat, Dietary; Nutrition and food; Recommended Dietary Al-**

lowances; Vegetarianism; Weight control
Diet pills, 92: 335-337, 91: 24
Diethylstilbestrol (DES), 91: 74, 90: 32
DIGESTIVE SYSTEM, 92: 265-267, 91: 264-266, 90: 264-267
see also Gall bladder disorders; Intestines; Ulcers
Digital rectal examination, 92: 70-73
Digitoxin, 91: 158
Dioxin, 90: 275
Disabled, 90: 252 (il.)
Disease, see specific diseases
Diskogram, 90: 206
Disorganized schizophrenia, 92: 157
Diuretics, 92: 137, 369-370, 90: 53
Divorce, 92: 261
DNA
  alcoholism gene, 91: 286
  human genome project, 90: 288
  schizophrenia gene, 90: 287
  soldier identification, 92: 352
  see also Chromosomes; Genes
Donor organs, see Transplantation surgery
Dopamine
  alcoholism, 92: 235, 91: 286, 305
  Parkinson's disease, 92: 142-150, 91: 250, 382, 90: 251 (il.)
  schizophrenia, 92: 160
  Tourette syndrome, 91: 93
Double pneumonia, 92: 88
Doulas, 92: 109
Down syndrome, 91: 101-113
  prenatal screening, 92: 100-102, 91: 107-109, 90: 314-315
Drowning by infants, 91: 322
Drug abuse, 92: 111-123
  AIDS transmission, 92: 14, 16-21, 26, 90: 118-121, 295
  pregnancy, 92: 105-106
  sexually transmitted diseases, 92: 212, 91: 322-323
  testing, 90: 53-55, 324
  see also Alcohol and drug abuse
Drug Price Competition and Patent Term Restoration Act, 92: 383
DRUGS, 92: 267-270, 91: 266-271, 90: 267-271
  books, 90: 248
  generic, 92: 383, 91: 268-269
  new drug approval, 90: 123 (il.), 295-296
  organ transplants, 91: 368-372, 376, 382
  orphan, 92: 383-384
  over-the-counter, 92: 269 (il.), 382
  Persian Gulf War, 92: 352
  pregnancy, 92: 106
  prescription, 92: 368-384
  rain forest plants, 91: 157-169
  resistance, 90: 268-269
  terminal illness, 92: 360-361
  see also Chemotherapy; Drug abuse; and specific drugs and disorders
Drunken driving, 92: 233
Duchenne muscular dystrophy, 91: 170-183
Ducts (gall bladder), 92: 42
Duodenal ulcers, 90: 72-74
Dyskinesia, 92: 149
Dysmenorrhea, 92: 135

Dysplasia, 91: 82-83, 333-334
Dystonias, 92: 208
Dystrophin, 91: 181-183

E

EAR AND HEARING, 92: 271-272, 91: 271-272, 90: 271-273
  infants and language, 92: 258-259, 91: 260
Eating disorders, 91: 24, 252-253, 90: 235-236
EBV, see Epstein-Barr virus
ECG, see Electrocardiography
Eclampsia, 92: 108
Ectopic pregnancy, 92: 214, 323
EEG, see Electroencephalogram
Elderly, see Aging
Electrocardiogram, see Electrocardiography
Electrocardiography, 92: 279, 90: 273-274
Electroencephalogram, 91: 143, 146 (il.), 152-154, 90: 63
Electromagnetic fields (EMF's), 92: 273-274, 314-315, 322
Electromyography, 91: 51
Elephant man's disease, see Neurofibromatosis
EMERGENCY MEDICINE, 92: 272-273, 91: 273-274, 90: 273-274
  pediatric trauma units, 90: 341-353
  Persian Gulf War, 92: 341-353
  Soviet Union, 90: 91-93
Emphysema, 92: 275, 91: 315
EMS, see Eosinophilia-myalgia syndrome
Encephalitis, 92: 31, 33, 90: 177-179
Endometrial cancer, 91: 288
Endometriosis, 92: 135
Endoscopy, 90: 77-78, 264-265
Enrichment (food), 91: 219-220
ENVIRONMENTAL HEALTH, 92: 273-276, 91: 274-276, 90: 275-277
  see also Air pollution; Water
Environmental medicine, 90: 239
Enzyme, Diabetes, 92: 264-265
Enzyme-linked immunosorbent assay (ELISA), 92: 20, 91: 349-350
Eosinophilia-myalgia syndrome, 91: 310-311
Epidemic, see specific diseases
Epidemiologic studies, 92: 56-58, 199-200
Epilepsy, 91: 143-155, 269
EPO, see Erythropoietin
Epstein-Barr virus (EBV), 92: 238, 90: 127-139
Ergot, 91: 164
ERT, see Estrogen replacement therapy
Erythromycin, 92: 91, 92
Erythropoietin (EPO), 92: 24, 231, 384, 91: 245, 90: 245-246
Esophagus, 92: 267, 91: 264-265
Estrogen, 92: 80, 129, 290
Estrogen replacement therapy, 92: 228, 290-292, 91: 288-289, 297, 90: 289-290
Ether, 92: 370
Ethical issues
  AIDS, 92: 297-298, 90: 113-125
  books, 92: 250, 91: 247-248
  organ transplants, 91: 377-381

right to die, 92: 296, 91: 294-295
Etidronate, 91: 247
Euthanasia, 91: 293
Evacuation hospitals, 92: 347-348
EXERCISE AND FITNESS, 92: 276-279, 91: 277-279, 90: 277-281
  asthma, 90: 316 (il.)
  books, 92: 249
  diabetes, 92: 264
  ear damage, 92: 271-272
  elderly, 92: 229 (il.), 90: 229
  heart disease, 92: 276-278, 91: 298
  joint diseases, 91: 37, 39-40, 90: 242
  low-impact, 90: 278
  women, 92: 104-105, 136, 278-279, 290
  see also Body building
Exosurf Neonatal, 92: 269, 368
Experimental studies, 92: 58, 379
External beam radiation, 92: 76
Extracorporeal shock-wave lithotripsy (ESWL), 90: 266-267
EYE AND VISION, 92: 279-282, 91: 279-282, 90: 281-284
  AIDS drug treatment, 90: 232
  Project Orbis, 90: 354-365
  retinitis pigmentosa, 91: 281-282
  see also Cataracts; Contact lenses; Cornea; Diabetic retinopathy
Eye bank, 90: 365
Eye chart, 90: 283 (il.)
Eye surgery
  nearsightedness, 91: 279-280
  Project Orbis, 90: 356, 360 (il.), 363-365
  Soviet Union, 90: 84-85
  see also Cornea transplants

F

Factor VIII, 92: 246
Fallopian tubes, 92: 214
Familial adenomatous polyposis (FAP), 92: 256, 265
Family therapy, and drug abuse, 92: 118, 122
Fanconi's anemia, 91: 245
Fasting, 90: 336
Fat, Body
  abdominal, risk of, 92: 336, 337, 90: 299
  genetic influence, 91: 286-287
  smoking redistribution, 90: 330
  see also Weight control
Fat, Dietary, 91: 129-141
  atherosclerosis, 91: 133-134, 299
  cancer, 91: 256-257, 90: 32
  food labeling, 91: 212-217, 222-225
  guidelines, 92: 336
  substitute, 91: 311-312
  vegetarian diet, 90: 101-104, 111
Fatigue, see Chronic fatigue syndrome
Fear, see Anxiety disorders
Fel D1 (protein), 91: 239
Fetal alcohol syndrome, 92: 105, 91: 247, 90: 234
Fetal surgery, 91: 296, 312-313
Fetal tissue transplants, 92: 150, 91: 250-251, 379, 90: 251 (il.), 294-295
Fever, 91: 185-195
  febrile seizures, 91: 150-151

measles, **92:** 30-32
toxic shock syndrome, **91:** 115-116, 119
Fiber, Dietary, 91: 213, 224-225, **90:** 104, 309
Fibroadenoma, 90: 36
Fibrocystic breast changes, 92: 135, **90:** 32
Fibromyalgia, 92: 240-241
Filgrastim, see **Granulocyte colony stimulating factor**
FINANCING MEDICAL CARE, 92: 283-285, **91:** 282-284, **90:** 284-286
AIDS, **92:** 16-18, **90:** 124
books, **90:** 248
drug addiction, **92:** 115
hospices, **92:** 363
schizophrenia, **92:** 165
see also **Health care facilities; Medicaid; Medicare**
Fingerprint forecasts, 90: 287 (il.)
Fish, Raw, 90: 312 (il.)
Fitness, see **Exercise and fitness**
5-fluorouracil, 92: 257-258
FK506 (drug), 92: 267, **91:** 303
Flashbacks, 90: 14-16
Fleas, and plague, 92: 168-171, 176, 179-181
Flu, see **Influenza**
Fluconazole, 92: 24
Fluoridated water, 92: 262, **91:** 260, 319
Fluoxetine, see **Prozac**
Folate, 92: 104
Folic acid, 92: 315-316, **91:** 314-315
Follicular phase, 92: 128-129
Food, see **Diet; Nutrition and food**
Food and Drug Administration, U.S. (FDA)
blood supply safety, **92:** 244
drug testing, **92:** 378-383, **91:** 268-269
food labeling, **91:** 212-225
reform plan, **92:** 267-268
Fortification (food), 91: 219-220
Fragile X syndrome, 92: 285-287
Fungal infection, of nervous system, 91: 267

G

Gall bladder disorders, 92: 42-45
see also **Gallstones**
Gallo, Robert, 92: 232
Gallstones, 92: 40-53
dietary fat, **91:** 140
overweight patients, **91:** 335-336
treatments, **90:** 265-267, 271
Ganciclovir, 92: 24, **90:** 232
Gastric ulcers, 90: 72
Gene splicing, see **Genetic engineering**
Gene therapy, 92: 285, 384
adenosine deaminase deficiency, **92:** 286-287, **91:** 284-285
cancer, **92:** 256-257, 286-287, **91:** 253, **90:** 254-255, 286-287
immune system disorder, **91:** 239
Gene transfer, see **Gene therapy**
Generally recognized as safe (GRAS), 91: 219

Genes
alcoholism, **92:** 66-67, 235, **91:** 251-252, 285-286, 305, **90:** 233-234
Alzheimer's disease, **92:** 250-251
amyotrophic lateral sclerosis, **92:** 253-254, 289-290
anxiety disorders, **90:** 19
arthritis, **92:** 241, 242, **91:** 246, **90:** 240
cancer, **92:** 254-257, 265-266, 287-288, **90:** 255
cancer-suppressing, **92:** 81, 254-256, 286-288
diabetes, **92:** 263-264
Down syndrome, **91:** 102-103
drug abuse, **91:** 234-235
eating disorders, **90:** 235-236
eye disorder, **91:** 281-282
leprosy, **91:** 199
long life, **91:** 228-229
muscular dystrophy, **91:** 170-183
Parkinson's disease, **92:** 147
schizophrenia, **92:** 157-158
shyness, **92:** 188, 191
Tourette syndrome, **91:** 93-94
see also **Gene therapy; Genetic engineering; Genetics; Hereditary disorders**
Genetic counseling, 92: 98, **91:** 103, 109, 181
Genetic engineering
Alzheimer's disease, **92:** 251
artificial insulin, **91:** 264
drug design, **92:** 376
hemoglobin production, **92:** 245-246
hemophilia, **90:** 245
Parkinson's disease, **92:** 150-151
wound healing, **90:** 326
GENETICS, 92: 285-289, **91:** 284-287, **90:** 286-289
see also **Gene therapy; Genetic engineering; Genes**
Genital herpes, 92: 212, 213, 220-222
Genital warts, 91: 76, 257, 332
Germ theory of disease, 92: 371
German measles, see **Rubella**
Gerstmann-Sträussler-Scheinker syndrome (GSS), 92: 251-253
Gingivitis, 91: 260
GLANDS AND HORMONES, 92: 290-292, **91:** 287-290, **90:** 289-291
drug types, **92:** 369
Graves' disease, **92:** 291
premenstrual syndrome, **92:** 128-130, 134
see also **Sex hormones**
Glaucoma, 92: 279-281, **91:** 280-281
Gleason score, 92: 74-75
Glucose, Blood, 91: 263, 343
see also **Diabetes**
Glutamic acid decarboxylase (GAD), 92: 265
Gold salts, 91: 38
Gonorrhea, 92: 212-216, 225, 375, **91:** 323
Gout, 91: 29
Graft-versus-host disease, 91: 372
Gram-negative bacteremia, 92: 303
Granulocyte colony stimulating factor (G-CSF), 92: 246, 268
Graves' disease, 92: 291
Group A streptococcus, 92: 83-84
Group therapy, for drug abusers, 92: 118, 122
Growth hormone, 91: 289-290

see also **Human growth hormone**
Gum disease, 92: 263, **91:** 260, **90:** 261-262

H

HA-1A (protein), 92: 303
Hair cells, of inner ear, 91: 272
Hair loss, see **Baldness**
Hallucinations, 92: 154, 156, 157
Hallucinogens, 92: 115
Hand injuries, 92: 247-248, **91:** 43-44
Hansen's disease, see **Leprosy**
Hashish, 92: 114
Head injuries, 92: 321, **91:** 149, **90:** 321
Headache, 92: 125, 137, 253, **91:** 13-15
HEALTH-CARE FACILITIES, 92: 293-295, **91:** 290-293, **90:** 291-294
drug addiction, **92:** 115
hospices, **92:** 354-365
see also **Health maintenance organizations; Hospitals; Nursing homes**
Health maintenance organizations (HMO's), 90: 293-294
HEALTH POLICY, 92: 295-298, **91:** 293-295, **90:** 294-296
AIDS, **92:** 26-27, **90:** 116-124
books, **90:** 248-249
Soviet Union, **90:** 83-97
HealthAmerica plan, 92: 295-297
Heart, Artificial, 91: 367
HEART AND BLOOD VESSELS, 92: 299-302, **91:** 296-299, **90:** 296-300
alcohol abuse, **91:** 236
caffeine, **91:** 24
drugs, **91:** 269-270
Heart attacks
Alzheimer's disease, **91:** 230
aspirin, **92:** 300-302, **91:** 245
clot-dissolving drugs, **92:** 302
emergency treatment, **90:** 273-274
exercise, **92:** 277-278
fever as symptom, **91:** 191
hypertension, **92:** 229
platelet count, **91:** 244
Heart defects
Down syndrome, **91:** 106
stroke risk, **90:** 67
sudden infant death syndrome, **91:** 63-64
valves, **92:** 302, **90:** 67
Heart disease
anabolic steroids, **90:** 45, 47-48
book, **91:** 249
caffeine, **91:** 17-19
cholesterol, **92:** 300
estrogen replacement therapy, **91:** 288, 289
exercise, **92:** 276-278, **91:** 298
fat in diet, **91:** 133-137, **90:** 104
Norplant side effects, **91:** 243
smoking, **92:** 327, **91:** 255-256
Vitamin E, **92:** 311-312
weight changes, **92:** 312-313, 335
women, **92:** 64, 299-300, **91:** 296-297, 336, **90:** 289-290
see also **Atherosclerosis; Cholesterol; Heart and blood vessels; Heart attacks**

Heart-lung transplants, **91:** 369, 370, 381
Heart murmur, **91:** 106
Heart rate, and exercise, **92:** 278
Heart transplants
  development, **91:** 366-370, 381-382
  ethical issues, **91:** 377, 380
  portable pump, **92:** 299
  procedure, **91:** 373-377
  statistics, **91:** 369
Heartburn, **92:** 107, **91:** 264-265
Helicobacter pylori (bacteria), **92:** 305
Helper T cells, see T-helper cells
Hemodialysis, see Dialysis
Hemoglobin, **92:** 245-246, **91:** 244
Hemophilia, **92:** 18, 246, **90:** 245
Hemorrhagic stroke, **90:** 59-61
Henson, Jim, **92:** 83, 94
Hepatitis, **92:** 303-305
  cancer risk, **92:** 255
  infections in U.S., **91:** 302, **90:** 301
  tests, **91:** 265, **90:** 265, 301
  toxic, **90:** 47
  treatments, **92:** 269, **91:** 157, 265-266
Hereditary disorders
  anxiety disorders, **90:** 19
  asthma, **90:** 185
  cancer, **92:** 80, **90:** 30-31
  epilepsy, **91:** 150
  pregnancy planning, **92:** 98
  rheumatoid arthritis, **91:** 34
  schizophrenia, **92:** 157-158
  shyness, **92:** 188-191
  see also Genes; Genetics
Herniated disks, **90:** 202-203, 209
Heroin, **92:** 112-114, 117
  deaths, **92:** 234
  pregnancy, **92:** 105-106
  strokes, **92:** 233
  synthetic, **92:** 143-144
Herpes, Genital, see Genital herpes
Herpesvirus, **92:** 220-221, **90:** 132-133, 136
High blood pressure, see Hypertension
High-density lipoproteins (HDL's), **91:** 134-136, **90:** 47-48, 280-281, 335-337
Hip dysplasia in dogs, **91:** 333-334
Hip fractures, **92:** 246-247, **91:** 287-289
Histoplasmosis, **92:** 279
HIV, see AIDS
HMO's, see Health maintenance organizations
Hodgkin's disease, **91:** 165, **90:** 244-245
Homelessness, **92:** 165
Homosexuality, and AIDS, **92:** 14, 18-21, 26-27, **90:** 123, 230
Hormone replacement therapy (HRT), see Estrogen replacement therapy
Hormones, see Glands and hormones; Sex hormones
Hospices, **92:** 354-365
Hospitals
  critical care nursing, **91:** 352-363
  Persian Gulf War, **92:** 347-352
  Soviet Union, **90:** 90-96
  see also Financing medical care; Health-care facilities
Human growth hormone (HGH), **92:**

384, **91:** 228, **90:** 53
Human immunodeficiency virus (HIV), see AIDS
Human papillomavirus (HPV), **92:** 221-222, 323, **91:** 76, 257
Humidifiers, Ultrasonic, **90:** 237
Hyperactivity, **92:** 308
Hypertension
  books, **92:** 249-250, **90:** 249
  caffeine, **91:** 19
  exercise, **92:** 278-279
  heart attacks, **92:** 229
  hormone as cause, **92:** 292
  obesity, **91:** 133
  sodium, **91:** 212
  stroke, **92:** 229, **90:** 65
  women, **92:** 278-279, **91:** 297, 314
Hyperthermia, **91:** 189
Hypoglycemia, **91:** 263-264, **90:** 263
Hypothalamus, **92:** 128
Hypothyroidism, **91:** 106
Hysterectomy, **91:** 83-84
Hytrin, **92:** 332

I

Ibuprofen, **92:** 137, 382, **91:** 304 (il.)
Imaginal flooding, **90:** 24
Imipramine, **92:** 310, 374
Immune globulin, **92:** 32
Immune system
  adenosine deaminase deficiency, **92:** 286-287, **91:** 284-285
  breast cancer, **90:** 28
  fever, **91:** 186
  nervous system link, **90:** 252-253
  organ transplants, **91:** 368-373
  pneumonia, **92:** 85-87, 90, 94-95
  rheumatoid arthritis, **91:** 30-31
  tuberculosis, **90:** 146
  vitamin E, **90:** 311
  see also Allergies and immunology; Antibodies; Immunosuppressant drugs
Immunization
  guidelines, **92:** 303
  measles, **92:** 34-39
  trends, **90:** 381-383
  see also Vaccines
Immunology, see Allergies and Immunology; Antibodies; Vaccines
Immunosuppressant drugs
  arthritis, **92:** 240, **91:** 38-39
  burns, **90:** 222
  organ transplants, **92:** 307, **91:** 368-373
Immunotherapy, **90:** 194-195
Implants, Surgical, **90:** 241 (il.), 251 (il.)
  see also Transplantation surgery
Impotence, **92:** 76, 79-80
In vivo exposure, **90:** 24
Incontinence, **90:** 332
Indians, American, **91:** 59
  see also Jívaro Indians
Infant mortality, **92:** 108, 298
  airline crashes, **91:** 317
  Soviet Union, **90:** 86-87
  sudden infant death syndrome, **91:** 57-69
  suffocation, **91:** 317-318
Infants
  AIDS, **92:** 19
  botulism, **92:** 206

deaf, and language, **92:** 258-259
drug abuse, **92:** 119, **91:** 233
lung disease, **92:** 318
measles immunization, **92:** 37, 39
premature, **92:** 269
safety, **92:** 293 (il.), **91:** 317-322
shyness, **92:** 189-192
sugar water effect, **92:** 261
see also Child development
Infection
  cancer patients, **92:** 268-269
  drug conquest, **92:** 371-372
  ear, **92:** 271, **91:** 272, **90:** 272
  fever, **91:** 186
  toxic shock syndrome, **91:** 125
  vaginal yeast, **92:** 270
INFECTIOUS DISEASES, **92:** 303-306, **91:** 300-303, **90:** 300-302
  see also specific diseases
Infertility, **91:** 19-20, 248, 290
Influenza, **91:** 300, 301
  drugs, **92:** 369 (il.), **91:** 240-241
  fever, **91:** 185
  vaccine, **90:** 378
Inhalers, **90:** 193
Inhibition, **92:** 186
  see also Shyness
Injuries
  back pain, **90:** 201-203
  exercise, **92:** 279 (il.)
  job, **90:** 323
  repetitive strain, **91:** 43-55
  see also Bone disorders; Head injuries; Occupational hazards; Safety; Spinal cord injuries
Insect stings, **92:** 240
Insecticides, **91:** 274-275
Insulin, **92:** 373, **91:** 262, 264, 367
Insulin pump, **92:** 373, **91:** 125, 262-263
Insulinlike growth factor 1, **91:** 228
Insurance, see Financing medical care; Health policy
Intelligence, **90:** 258-259
Intensive care units (ICU's), **91:** 352-363
Interferon, **92:** 269, **91:** 193, 239, 265-266
Interleukin-2 (IL-2), **91:** 238-239, 253, **90:** 255 (il.)
Intermediate care units (IMCU's), **91:** 354
Interposed abdominal compressions CPR (IAC-CPR), **92:** 273
Intestines
  bleeding, **92:** 266
  cholera, **92:** 304
  gall bladder problems, **92:** 42-44
  irritable bowel syndrome, **91:** 266 (il.)
  transplants, **92:** 267, **91:** 370, 381
Intrauterine devices (IUD's), **92:** 243-244, 324, **91:** 242
Intron A, see Alpha interferon
Introversion, **92:** 186
Iron, in diet, **92:** 104, **91:** 193, 220, 311, **90:** 108
Ischemic heart disease, **92:** 312, 328-329
Ischemic strokes, **90:** 58-59
Islet cell transplantation, **91:** 262
Isotretinoin, **92:** 106, 381-382
IUD's, see Intrauterine devices

J

Jaundice, 92: 44, 45, **90:** 134
Jívaro Indians, 91: 157, 160-164
Jogging, see **Running**
Joints, see **Arthritis and connective tissue disorders; Bone disorders**
Juvenile rheumatoid arthritis (JRA), 91: 29, 35, **90:** 240-241

K

Kaposi's sarcoma, 92: 14, 21, 24, **90:** 232
Kevorkian, Jack, 91: 293
KIDNEY, 92: 306-307, **91:** 303-304, **90:** 303-304
  caffeine, **91:** 12
  renal cell cancer, **90:** 254
Kidney stones, 90: 290-291
Kidney transplants
  rejection problem, **91:** 303, 368
  sources, **91:** 375
  statistics, **91:** 369, 376-377, 381
Knee, 91: 240 (il.)
Koop, C. Everett, 90: 352
Koplik's spots, 92: 30, 33 (il.)
Korean War veterans, 92: 308-309
Kosher foods, 91: 223

L

L-dopa, 92: 149, 373, **91:** 250
L-tryptophan, 91: 237-238, 310-311
Labor, see **Pregnancy and childbirth**
Lactose intolerance, 91: 217, 223, **90:** 310-311
Lamaze childbirth, 92: 106 (il.)
Laminectomy, 90: 209
Language development, 92: 258-259, **91:** 260
Laparoscopic surgery, 92: 50-53
Laser surgery
  birthmark removal, **90:** 327
  cervical cancer, **91:** 82-83
  coronary artery, **90:** 297
  eyes, **92:** 279-281
  inner-ear, **92:** 272
  tattoo removal, **92:** 324-325
Late luteal phase dysphoric disorder (LLPD), 92: 132-134
Latin America
  AIDS cases, **92:** 16
  cholera, **92:** 304
Lead exposure, 91: 275
Lead poisoning, 90: 169-181
  children, **92:** 275-276
  drug, **92:** 269
  epilepsy, **91:** 149
  lead crystal glasses, **92:** 321
  swans, **90:** 334
Lecithin, 92: 265 (il.)
Left ventricular assist device, 92: 299
Legionella pneumophila, see **Legionnaires' disease**
Legionnaires' disease, 92: 91-92, **91:** 320, **90:** 155-167
Leprosy, 91: 196-209
Leukemia, 92: 273-274, **91:** 165, 350
  see also **Bone marrow transplants**

Levamisole, 91: 253-254, **90:** 257
Levonorgestrel, see **Norplant contraceptive**
Li-Fraumeni syndrome, 92: 255-256, 287-288
Lice infestation, 91: 325
Licensed Practical Nurses (LPN's), 91: 362
Life expectancy
  mortality decrease, **92:** 228
  Soviet Union, **90:** 87
Life support systems, see **Right to die**
Ligaments, 91: 29-30, **90:** 200-203
Ligation, 92: 267
Limbic system, 92: 190
Lipoproteins, 91: 337, **90:** 47-48, 279-281
  see also **High-density lipoproteins; Low-density lipoproteins**
Listeriosis, 92: 204
Lithium, 92: 310-311
Lithotripsy, 92: 48-49
Liver
  breast cancer, **90:** 28-29
  caffeine, **91:** 12
  cirrhosis, **92:** 265 (il.)
  esophageal bleeding, **92:** 267
  mononucleosis, **90:** 134
  Norplant side effects, **91:** 243
  Parkinson's disease, **92:** 146-147
  see also **Hepatitis**
Liver cancer, 92: 255, **91:** 370, **90:** 29, 45
Liver transplants
  development, **91:** 367-371, 381-382
  ethical issues, **91:** 377-381
  procedure, **91:** 374-377
  statistics, **91:** 369
Living wills, 92: 293, 296, **91:** 295
Lobar pneumonia, 92: 88
Lobes (lung), 92: 86
Lou Gehrig's disease, see **Amyotrophic lateral sclerosis**
Lovastatin, 92: 374
Low-density lipoproteins (LDL's), 91: 16, 134-136, **90:** 19, 47-48
LSD, 92: 114, 115
Lumpectomy, 90: 37, 40
Lung cancer
  asbestos exposure, **91:** 317
  diagnosis, **91:** 315-317, **90:** 318
  screening, **92:** 254
  smoking, **92:** 317, **91:** 328
Lung transplants
  development, **91:** 315, 367, 370, 381
  donors, **91:** 377
  statistics, **91:** 369
Lungs, 92: 86 (il.)
  air pollution damage, **92:** 274-275
  surfactant product, **92:** 269, 318
  see also **Asthma; Pneumonia; Respiratory system**
Luteal phase, 92: 129, 132
Lyme disease, 92: 305-306, 332-333, **91:** 240, 300
Lymph nodes, see **Lymphatic system**
Lymphatic system
  cancer, **92:** 71, 75, **90:** 28, 37, 40-41
  mononucleosis, **90:** 129
  plague infection, **92:** 171-172
  see also **Hodgkin's disease**
Lymphocytes, see **White blood cells**
Lymphoma, 92: 24, **91:** 232, **90:** 326-327

M

Macrobiotics, 90: 101
Macrophages, 91: 193
Macular degeneration, 92: 279
Magnesium, 91: 126-127
Magnetic resonance imaging (MRI)
  arteries, **91:** 298
  back pain, **90:** 206
  blood sugar, in diabetes, **91:** 263
  exercise injuries, **91:** 279 (il.)
  stroke, **90:** 61-62
Malaria, 92: 305 (il.)
Malathion, 91: 274-275
Mammography, 92: 257, **90:** 27 (il.), 33
Manic-depressive disorder, 92: 132-134, 310-311, **90:** 305
Manipulation, for back pain, 90: 208
Marijuana, 92: 105-106, 113-115, 234, **90:** 233
Mastectomy, 90: 31, 34 (il.), 37-40
MCC gene, 92: 289
MDphone, 90: 273-274
Measles, 92: 28-39, 95, **91:** 300, **90:** 301
Measurement, 92: 62
Meat
  cancer, **92:** 255 (il.), 258, 311
  decision to eat, **90:** 99-111
  labeling, **91:** 222
Medicaid
  anniversary, **91:** 293
  health care costs, **92:** 284-285, 297, **91:** 282, 293-294
  hospital finances, **92:** 294
  organ transplant coverage, **91:** 381
  right to sue, **91:** 291-292
Medical clearing companies, 92: 346-347
Medical studies, 92: 55-67
Medical waste, 90: 292 (il.)
Medicare
  anniversary, **91:** 293
  book, **90:** 250
  dialysis length, **92:** 306
  health care costs, **92:** 283-284, **91:** 282
  health care quality, **91:** 292
  hospital finances, **92:** 294
  organ transplant coverage, **91:** 381
Medics, Army, 92: 343, 346
Melanoma
  gene therapy, **92:** 256, 286-287, **91:** 253, 285, **90:** 254-255
  sun exposure risk, **91:** 254-255
  vaccine, **90:** 383
Meningitis
  bacterial, **92:** 303
  cryptococcal, **91:** 231-232, 267
Menopause
  breast cancer risk, **90:** 31
  estrogen replacement therapy, **91:** 288-289, **90:** 331
  heart disease, **91:** 296-297, **90:** 289-290
Menstrual cycle, 92: 128-129, 131 (il.)
  see also **Premenstrual syndrome**
Menstruation
  breast cancer, **90:** 31
  exercise, **92:** 290
  premenstrual syndrome, **92:** 125-137
  see also **Toxic shock syndrome**

MENTAL HEALTH, 92: 308-311, **91:** 304-308, **90:** 304-308
anabolic steroids, **90:** 48
caffeine, **91:** 20-23
Clomipramine, **91:** 270-271
drug abuse, **92:** 115, 116
premenstrual syndrome, **92:** 125-137
Soviet Union, **90:** 94-96
see also **Anxiety disorders; Brain and nervous system; Psychotherapy; Schizophrenia; Shyness**
Mental retardation, **92:** 285
Mercury poisoning, **92:** 262, **91:** 318-320
Mercy (hospital ship), **92:** 349
Metabolism, **91:** 187
Metastasis, of breast cancer, **90:** 28-29, 37, 40-41
Methadone, **92:** 105-106, 115, 117, 120 (il.), **90:** 234
Methyl-CCNU, **92:** 257-258
Methyl-tertiary-butyl ether, **92:** 48
Methylphenidate, **92:** 233
Metronidazole, **92:** 219
Microcatheter embolization, **92:** 273
Microwave prostate treatment, **92:** 331-332
Midwives, **92:** 98
Mifepristone, **92:** 132
Milk, see **Dairy products**
Mind and body, **92:** 250, **91:** 249
Minnesota model for drug rehabilitation, **92:** 118
Minocycline, **91:** 241
Minoxidil, **92:** 376, **90:** 271
Miscarriage
exercise risk, **91:** 278-279
immune system disorder, **91:** 241
mother's age, **91:** 314
pregnancy testing, **92:** 102, 316
video terminal use, **92:** 314-315
Mitochondria, **92:** 146
Mobile army surgical hospitals (MASH's), **92:** 347-348
Monoclonal antibodies, **91:** 238, 372-373, **90:** 318
Mononucleosis, **92:** 238, **90:** 127-139
Monospot test, **90:** 138
Morphine, **92:** 114, 115, 234, **91:** 158
Mortality rate, **92:** 228
see also **Infant mortality**
Mosaicism, **91:** 103
Motorcycle injuries, **92:** 272-273
Motrin, see **Ibuprofen**
MPTP, **92:** 144, 146
MRI, see **Magnetic resonance imaging**
Multiple sclerosis, **91:** 238, 252
Muscles
back pain, **90:** 202
L-tryptophan, **91:** 310
myasthenia gravis, **92:** 240
Parkinson's disease, **92:** 140-141
relaxant drugs, **91:** 160
Muscular dystrophy, see **Duchenne muscular dystrophy**
Mustard gas, **92:** 343, 350 (il.)
Mutation of genes, **92:** 287-288
Myasthenia gravis, **92:** 240
Mycobacterium leprae (bacteria), **91:** 198-200, 206-209

Mycoplasmal pneumonia, **92:** 91
Myelograms, **90:** 206

N

Naloxone, **92:** 132
National Alliance for the Mentally Ill (NAMI), **92:** 163-164
Natural childbirth, **92:** 98
Natural gas explosions, **91:** 322
Nausea, in pregnancy, **92:** 107
Needle aspiration, **90:** 36
Nerve cells, see **Neurons**
Nerve conduction velocity tests, **91:** 49 (il.), 51
Nerve gas, **92:** 343
Nervous system, see **Brain and nervous system**
Neupogen, see **Granulocyte colony stimulating factor**
Neural tube defects, **92:** 100-102, 104, 315
Neuralgia, **91:** 249
Neurofibrillary tangles, **90:** 251
Neurofibromatosis, **91:** 285
Neuroleptic drugs, **92:** 160-161, 164 (il.)
Neurological problems, see **Brain and nervous system**
Neurons
food poisoning, **92:** 198-199, 208
nerve growth factors, **90:** 228
nerve growth inhibitors, **91:** 249
Parkinson's disease, **92:** 142-149
Neurotoxins, **92:** 144-147
Neurotransmitters
botulism, **92:** 198-199
drug craving, **90:** 235
dystonias, **92:** 208
Tourette syndrome, **91:** 93
see also **Dopamine; Serotonin**
Neutering of pets, **92:** 334
Neutrophils, **90:** 257
NF, see **Neurofibromatosis**
Nicardipine, **92:** 269
Nicotine, see **Smoking**
Nimodipine, **90:** 251-252, 269-270
Nocardia (bacteria), **92:** 143
Noise pollution, **91:** 271-272, **90:** 272-273
Non-Hodgkin's lymphoma, **92:** 24
Nonsteroidal anti-inflammatory drugs (NSAID's), **91:** 36, 52, **90:** 267-269
Norepinephrine, **92:** 374
Norplant contraceptive, **92:** 243 (il.), 269-270, 373, **91:** 243-244
Northwestern Memorial Hospital hospice program, **92:** 354, 361-364
Nose, and Alzheimer's disease, **90:** 250-251
Novello, Antonia C., **91:** 295
Nuclear scan, **92:** 47
Nurses
intensive-care unit, **91:** 352-363
shortage, **92:** 294-295
Nursing homes
books, **92:** 248, **91:** 247
care quality, **92:** 295, **91:** 292, **90:** 292-293
statistics, **92:** 295, **91:** 292
NUTRITION AND FOOD, 92: 311-314, **91:** 308-312, **90:** 308-312
allergies, **92:** 239-240

books, **92:** 249, **91:** 247, **90:** 249
botulism, **92:** 197-209
epilepsy, **91:** 149
eye injuries, **92:** 282
labeling of foods, **91:** 210-225
leprosy, **91:** 199, 202
pregnancy, **92:** 102-104
radiation in milk, **91:** 274
seafood safety, **92:** 321, **90:** 312
see also **Diet; Fat, Dietary; Meat; Pesticides; Vegetarianism**

O

Oat bran, **92:** 64-66, **91:** 224-225, 308-309, **90:** 309
Obesity, **92:** 335, 337, **91:** 132-133, 297-298
see also **Weight control**
Obsessive-compulsive disorder (OCD), **91:** 92, 270, 306
Obstetrics, see **Pregnancy and Childbirth**
Occupational hazards
AIDS and health care workers, **90:** 121-122
asthma, **90:** 190
job injuries, **90:** 323
osteoarthritis, **91:** 37
repetitive strain injuries, **91:** 43-55
Ocean, and drugs, **92:** 376
Omnibus Budget Reconciliation Act, **92:** 293
Oncogenes, **92:** 287
Ondansetron, **92:** 268
Operation Desert Storm, **92:** 341-353
Operations, see **Surgery**
Opiates, **92:** 115, 117
Opioids, **92:** 132, **90:** 236
Opportunistic infections, **92:** 14
Oral cancer, **91:** 261-262, **90:** 308-309
Oral cholecystogram, **92:** 46-47
Organ transplants, see **Transplantation surgery**
Organically grown food, **91:** 220
Orphan Drug Act, **92:** 383-384
Osteoarthritis, **92:** 242, **91:** 133, 246, **90:** 203-204
Osteopathy, **90:** 208
Osteoporosis, **92:** 247
back pain, **90:** 203
book, **90:** 249
caffeine, **91:** 22
calcium, **91:** 225
diagnosis, **91:** 246 (il.)
electric currents, **90:** 246-247
estrogen replacement therapy, **91:** 288-289
thiazide diuretic, **91:** 287-288
Otosclerosis, **92:** 272
Ouabain, **92:** 292
Ovarian cancer, **92:** 254
Ovaries, **92:** 128-129
Overuse syndrome, see **Repetitive strain injuries**
Ovulation, **92:** 129

P

p53 (gene), **92:** 254-257, 288-289
Pacemaker, **90:** 298 (il.)

Paget's disease, **90:** 38
Pain
   drugs, **92:** 370-371
   hospices, **92:** 357, 359 (il.)
   smoker tolerance, **92:** 328-329
Palliative care, 92: 357
Pancreas
   artificial, **91:** 262, 367, **90:** 263-264
   cancer, **90:** 264
   transplants, **91:** 369, 375-379, 381
Pandemic, 92: 15
Panic disorders, 91: 20-23, 306-307, **90:** 12, 13, 18-25
Pannus, 91: 29 (il.)
Pap test, 91: 71-72, 76-80
Papule, 92: 217-218
Paranoid schizophrenia, 92: 157
Parasites, 90: 370
Parkinson's disease, 92: 139-151
   brain tissue implants, **92:** 150-151, **91:** 250-251, 379
   neuroleptic drugs, **92:** 160
Paroxysmal supraventricular tachycardia (PSVT), 91: 269
Pasteur, Louis, 90: 374
Patient "dumping," 92: 293
Patient rights, 92: 293
Patient Self-Determination Act (1990), 92: 296
PCP (disease), see *Pneumocystis carinii* pneumonia
PCP (drug), 92: 105-106, 114, 115, 233
Pediatric trauma centers, 90: 342-353
Pelvic infections, 92: 243-244
Pelvic inflammatory disease (PID), 92: 212, 214, 216, 323
Pelvic tilt exercise, 92: 105
Penicillin
   development, **92:** 371-372
   dosage, **92:** 375
   drug-resistant bacteria, **92:** 375
   gonorrhea, **92:** 216, **91:** 323
   syphilis, **92:** 218
Pentamidine, 92: 24, 93, **90:** 232
Peptic ulcers, see **Ulcers**
Percutaneous cholecystolithotomy, 92: 49
Percutaneous diskectomy, 90: 211
Perilymphatic fistula, 90: 271
Periodontal disease, see **Gum disease**
Peristalsis, 92: 266
Peritonitis, 92: 43
Persian Gulf War, 92: 341-353
Pertussis vaccine, 91: 237, **90:** 377, 380, 383
Pesticides, 91: 220, 274-275, **90:** 320-321
Phagocytes, 91: 239
Phalen's test, 91: 49 (il.), 50-51
Pharmacists, 92: 368 (il.), 381
Phencyclidine, see **PCP (drug)**
Phenelzine, 92: 195
Phenylpropanolamine (PPA), 92: 335-337
Phobia, 90: 11-25, 306
Phoenix House, 92: 123
Photorefractive keratectomy (PRK), 91: 279-280
Physical fitness, see **Exercise and fitness**
Physical therapy
   back pain, **90:** 207-208

burns, **90:** 224
repetitive strain injuries, **91:** 44
rheumatoid arthritis, **91:** 39
stroke, **90:** 63-64
Physicians
   AIDS transmission, **92:** 230, 297-298
   drug prescriptions, **92:** 381
   hospices, **92:** 356-357, 363-364
   Medicare payments, **92:** 284
Pituitary gland, 92: 128, 130
Placebos, 92: 61-62, 130-132, 379
Plague, 92: 167-181
Plants, and pollution, 92: 275
   see also **Nutrition and food; Rain forest drugs; Vegetarianism**
Plaque, Arterial, 91: 133-134, **90:** 296-298
Plaque, Dental, 92: 263
Plaques, Brain, 92: 251, **90:** 251
Plasma (blood), 91: 348
Plastic surgery, see **Cosmetic surgery**
Platelets, 92: 301, **91:** 244-245, 348
PMS, see **Premenstrual syndrome**
Pneumococcus, 92: 83-84, 91, 95
Pneumocystis carinii **pneumonia, 92:** 14, 93, 231-232, **91:** 231, 267-269, **90:** 230
Pneumonia, 92: 83-95
   drug success, **92:** 369 (il.)
   plague, **92:** 172, 181
   pneumococcal, **90:** 378
   see also *Pneumocystis carinii* pneumonia
Pneumonic plague, 92: 171-172
Poisoning
   Agent Orange, **90:** 275
   botulism, **92:** 197-209
   cyanide in grapes, **90:** 321
   mercury, **92:** 262, **91:** 318-320
   see also **Asbestos; Lead poisoning; Pesticides; Toxins**
Polio vaccine, 92: 250, **90:** 368, 372, 375, 377-381
Pollution, see **Air pollution; Environmental health; Toxins; Water**
Polycythemia, 90: 67
Polymers, 92: 373
Polysaccharide vaccines, 90: 376
Positron emission tomography, 92: 308
Post-traumatic stress disorder (PTSD), 92: 308-309, **90:** 12, 14-16, 18, 20, 25
Postpartum depression, 92: 127
Poultry, 92: 311, 312, **91:** 222
Pralidoxime, 92: 343
Precursors (drug), 92: 373
Prednisone, 92: 242, 271
Preeclampsia, 92: 107-108
PREGNANCY AND CHILDBIRTH, 92: 314-316, **91:** 312-315, **90:** 313-315
   airline radiation, **91:** 318
   asthma, **91:** 238 (il.)
   book, **90:** 248
   caffeine, **91:** 20
   carpal tunnel syndrome, **91:** 49
   Down syndrome, **91:** 103
   exercise, **91:** 278-279
   fetal surgery, **91:** 296, 312-313
   fever, **91:** 191
   herpes, **90:** 324-325
   measles, **92:** 32, 33
   Medicaid coverage, **91:** 284

premenstrual syndrome, **91:** 237, 310
prenatal care, **92:** 97-109
sexually transmitted diseases, **92:** 214-215, 217, 221
Soviet Union, **90:** 93-94
substance abuse, **92:** 119, **91:** 236, **90:** 234
sudden infant death syndrome, **91:** 60-63
see also **Birth defects; Child development; Miscarriage; Premenstrual syndrome; Prenatal diagnosis**
Premenstrual syndrome, 92: 125-137, **91:** 237, 310
Premenstrual tension, 92: 126
Prenatal diagnosis
   Down syndrome, **91:** 107-109, **90:** 314-315
   risks, **92:** 316
   see also **Alphafetoprotein; Amniocentesis; Chorionic villus sampling**
Prenatal surgery, see **Fetal surgery**
Pressure garments for burns, 90: 223 (il.), 224, 327 (il.)
Prions, 92: 251-253
Prisoners of war (POW's), 92: 308-309
Progesterone, 92: 129-130, 290
Project MotherCare, 92: 108
Project Orbis, 90: 354-365
Prolactin, 92: 130
Proscar, 92: 79, 332
Prostaglandins, 90: 74
Prostate gland, 92: 70
   cancer, **92:** 69-81, 254, **91:** 331-332
   enlarged, **92:** 69-70, 78-79, 331-332, **91:** 332, **90:** 331-332
Prostate-specific antigen (PSA), 92: 73, 74
Prostatectomy, Radical, 92: 76
Prostatic acid phosphatase (PAP), 92: 74
Prostatic balloon dilation, 92: 79
Prostatitis, 92: 70
Prostratron, 92: 331-332
Protein
   brain disease, **92:** 252-253
   food labeling, **91:** 220, 222
   kidney failure, **92:** 307
   vegetarian diet, **90:** 106-108
Protein drugs, 92: 376
Protozoa, 92: 84, 93, 218-219
Prozac, 92: 137, 382
Psittacosis, 92: 92-93, **90:** 163
Psoriasis, 91: 326-327, **90:** 327
Psychiatry, see **Mental health**
Psychological disorders, see **Mental health; Psychotherapy; Stress**
Psychosis, 92: 156
Psychotherapeutic drugs, 92: 369, 374
Psychotherapy
   burn victims, **90:** 225
   computer, **91:** 307-308
   depression, **92:** 310
   drug abuse, **92:** 118-121
   schizophrenia, **92:** 161
   shyness, **92:** 193-195
Public health, see **Health policy**
Pulmonary function tests, 90: 190-192
Pyridostigmine, 92: 343

Q

Quinine, 91: 159-160

R

Rabies, 92: 306, 333-334, 91: 335
Radial keratotomy, 91: 279
Radiation
 airline travel, 91: 275 (il.), 318
 breast cancer, 90: 32, 33
 nuclear weapons plant, 91: 274
 see also Ultraviolet (UV) radiation
Radiation therapy, 92: 76, 257-258,
 91: 84
Radioactive waste, 92: 273
Radionuclear bone scan, 92: 74
Radon, 90: 275-276
Rain forest drugs, 92: 376-377, 91:
 157-169
Rape, 92: 309
Rapid eye movement (REM) sleep,
 91: 66
Rash
 measles, 92: 30-32
 toxic shock syndrome, 91: 115-116,
 119, 127
Rational drug design, 92: 378
RDA's, see Recommended Dietary Al-
 lowances
Reactive arthritis, 92: 241, 91: 241-
 242
Receptors (brain), 92: 160
Recombigen HIV-1 Latex Aggluntina-
 tion Test, 90: 232
Recombinant DNA technology, see
 Genetic engineering
Recommended Dietary Allowances
 (RDA's), 91: 220-221, 309-311, 90:
 106-111
Reconstructive surgery, see Cosmet-
 ic surgery
Rectal cancer, 92: 257-258
Red blood cells, 91: 349 (il.)
Reflux esophagitis, 91: 264-265
Registered Nurses (RN's), 91: 362
Reiter's syndrome, see Reactive
 arthritis
Relaxation techniques
 anxiety disorders, 90: 24-25
 asthma, 90: 196
 back pain, 90: 209
 diabetes, 90: 264
 drug abuse, 92: 118
 premenstrual syndrome, 92: 136
 rheumatoid arthritis, 91: 33 (il.), 40
Reliability, 92: 62
Renal cell cancer, 90: 254
Repetitive strain injuries (RSI's), 91:
 43-55
Reproductive technology, see Preg-
 nancy and childbirth
Resectoscope, 92: 79
Respirators, 91: 360, 363
Respiratory distress syndrome
 (RDS), 92: 269, 317-318, 368
RESPIRATORY SYSTEM, 92: 316-318,
 91: 315-317, 90: 316-318
 sudden infant death syndrome, 91:
 64
 see also Asthma; Legionnaires' dis-

ease; Lungs; Pneumonia; Smok-
 ing; Tuberculosis
Retin-A, 92: 377
Retina, 92: 264, 279
Reye's syndrome, 91: 195, 301
Rh blood factor, 92: 99-100, 91: 342
Rheumatoid arthritis (RA), 91: 27-41
 ankle brace, 92: 242
 birth control pill, 90: 241
 carpal tunnel syndrome, 91: 49
 fever as symptom, 91: 191
 juvenile, 91: 29, 35, 90: 240-241
 Lyme disease, 91: 240
 metal poisoning, 90: 242 (il.)
Rice bran, 90: 309
Rickettsia, 90: 158
Right to die, 92: 296, 298, 91: 294-295
 see also Suicide
Risk, 92: 57
Rodents, and plague, 92: 168-171,
 174, 176-180
Rogaine, see Minoxidil
'roid rage, 90: 48
Role-playing, and shyness, 92: 194-
 195
RS-61443 (drug), 91: 371
Rubella, 92: 30, 33, 98, 99
Rubeola, see Measles
Running, 91: 278
Rust v. Sullivan, 92: 298

S

Sabin polio vaccine, 90: 368, 372,
 377, 378 (il.)
SAFETY, 92: 318-322, 91: 317-322, 90:
 318-324
 blood supply, 91: 341-351
 falling by elderly, 90: 229
 generic drugs, 91: 268-269
 see also Injuries
Salk polio vaccine, 90: 368, 372, 375,
 377, 379-380
Salmonella, see Salmonellosis
Salmonellosis, 92: 204
Salt, see Sodium
Samples, in science, 92: 60-64
Sanitariums, 90: 96-97, 142-143, 147
 (il.)
Sargramostim, 92: 268-269
Scar tissue, from burns, 90: 224
Schizophrenia, 92: 153-165
 brain structure, 91: 304-305
 drugs, 92: 143, 91: 270-271, 90: 304-
 305
 genetics, 90: 287-288
Sciatica, 90: 202-203
Scientific studies, 92: 55-67
Scrapie, 92: 252-253
Seafood, 92: 321, 90: 312 (il.)
Seat belts, 92: 320, 90: 318-319
Seizures
 caffeine poisoning, 91: 24
 febrile, 91: 188
 sulfites in food, 91: 219
 see also Epilepsy
Selenium, 91: 311
Self-esteem, 92: 187-188, 194, 260-
 261
Seminal vesicles, 92: 76
Sensorineural hearing loss, 90: 271-
 272
Septicemic plague, 92: 171-172
Serotonin, 92: 131

Set point, in fever, 91: 186-191
Sex hormones, 92: 80, 90: 31, 48, 241
 see also Estrogen; Testosterone
Sex-linked disorders, 91: 175
SEXUALLY TRANSMITTED DIS-
 EASES, 92: 210-225, 322-324, 91:
 322-324, 90: 324-325
 cervical cancer, 91: 74-76
 see also AIDS
Shell shock, see Post-traumatic
 stress disorder
Shigellosis, 92: 204
Shock, 90: 349
Shootings, Accidental, 92: 318-319
Shyness, 92: 183-195, 90: 19-20, 260
 see also Social phobia
Sickle cell anemia, 91: 244
SIDS, see Sudden infant death syndrome
SKIN, 92: 324-326, 91: 324-327, 90:
 326-327
 artificial, 90: 223
 burns, 90: 213-225
 leprosy, 91: 196-209
 smoking, 92: 326, 328 (il.)
Skin cancer, 91: 370
 see also Lymphoma; Melanoma
Skin grafting, 91: 324-326, 367-368,
 90: 221-224
Skin test, for tuberculosis, 90: 149,
 151 (il.)
Slap bracelets, 92: 322
Sleep
 back pain, 90: 206-207 (ils.)
 pregnancy, 92: 107
 premenstrual syndrome, 92: 136
 sudden infant death syndrome, 91:
 60, 66
Sleep apnea, 91: 25, 60
Slow viruses, 92: 143
Smallpox vaccination, 90: 370, 372-
 374, 379
Smart needle, 92: 272 (il.)
Smith, Alyssa, 91: 366
SMOKING, 92: 326-329, 91: 328-330,
 90: 328-330
 caffeine, 91: 12
 cancer, 92: 258, 317, 327, 91: 74,
 328, 90: 328-329
 deaths, 92: 326-328, 91: 255, 328,
 90: 316, 328
 gum disease, 92: 263
 heart disease, 92: 327, 91: 245, 297
 passive, 92: 327, 91: 74, 328
 pregnancy, 92: 105, 91: 238 (il.)
 sexually transmitted diseases, 92:
 212
 skin, 92: 326, 328 (il.)
 Soviet Union, 90: 86
 stroke, 91: 331, 90: 65
 students, 92: 234, 91: 235
 sudden infant death syndrome, 91:
 62
 ulcer healing, 90: 75
 vitamin E protection, 90: 309-311
 year 2000, 90: 316-317
Social phobia, 92: 184, 195, 90: 12, 14
 see also Shyness
Sodium, 92: 104, 91: 212, 217, 218,
 225
Sodium fluoride, 91: 247
Soluble CD4, 92: 25
Sonde enteroscope, 92: 266

Sonogram, **92:** 46
Soviet Union
  medicine, **90:** 83-97
  vision test, **91:** 281 (il.)
Speech
  infant development, **91:** 260
  stroke impairment, **90:** 58, 63
Speech therapy, 91: 111, **90:** 58
Spina bifida, 91: 109, 314-315
Spinal column, see **Spine**
Spinal cord injuries, 91: 249-250, 266, 273
Spine
  arthritis, **92:** 241, **91:** 29, 35
  back problems, **90:** 199-211
  fusion surgery, **90:** 209
Spirometer, 92: 317
Spironolactone, 91: 327
Spleen, 90: 134, 139
Splints, 91: 40, 44-46
Spondylolisthesis, 90: 204
Spores, Botulism, 92: 198, 206
Sports, see **Athletics**
Sputum, 92: 88, 90
Stanozolol, 90: 44
Staphylococcus aureus **(bacteria), 91:** 116, 126, 127
STD's, see **Sexually transmitted diseases**
Stendhal syndrome, 90: 307
Steroids, see **Anabolic steroids; Corticosteroids**
Stethoscope, 92: 88
Still's disease, see **Juvenile rheumatoid arthritis**
Stimulants, 90: 53
Stomach acid, 91: 264-265, **90:** 73-74
Stomach cancer, 92: 305, **90:** 264
Stomach ulcers, see **Ulcers**
Strabismus, 92: 208
Strain
  back pain, **90:** 201-202
  repetitive strain injuries, **91:** 43-55
Streptococcus, 91: 303
Streptomycin, 92: 368, 372
Stress
  asthma triggers, **90:** 189-190
  brain aging, **92:** 229
  intensive care nurses, **91:** 361
  students' drug use, **91:** 235
  ulcers, **90:** 75-76
STROKE, 92: 329-331, **91:** 330-331, **90:** 57-69, 330-331
  book, **90:** 248
  drug abuse, **92:** 233
  epileptic seizures, **91:** 150
  fat in diet, **91:** 133
  hypertension, **92:** 229
  Norplant side effects, **91:** 243
Subarachnoid hemorrhage (SAH), 90: 59-61, 270
Substance abuse, see **Alcohol and drug abuse**
Substantia nigra, 92: 142-143
Succimer, 92: 269
Sudafed, 92: 268 (il.)
Sudden infant death syndrome (SIDS), 91: 57-69
Suicide
  doctor-assisted, **91:** 293
  panic disorders, **91:** 306-307
  Prozac users, **92:** 382
  Soviet Union, **90:** 95

  see also **Right to die**
Sulfa drugs, 92: 369, 371
Sulfites, 91: 219
Sun exposure
  cataracts, **90:** 283-284
  skin cancer, **91:** 254-255
Surfactant, 92: 269, 318
Surgeon general of the United States, 91: 295, **90:** 352
Surgery
  back problems, **90:** 209-210
  blood transfusions, **91:** 341, 351
  breast cancer, **90:** 37-40
  epilepsy, **91:** 148 (il.), 154-155
  gall bladder, **92:** 42, 46 (il.), 50-53
  prostate disorders, **92:** 76-80, **91:** 332
  repetitive strain injuries, **91:** 52-53
  rheumatoid arthritis, **91:** 40-41
  Soviet Union, **90:** 84, 91
  see also **Cosmetic surgery; Eye surgery; Fetal surgery; Laser surgery; Transplantation surgery**
Sushi, 90: 312
Synapses, 92: 198-199
Syndrome, 92: 14, 187
Synovectomy, 91: 40
Synovial membrane, 91: 29-31, 40
Syphilis, 92: 212-213, 216-218, 222, 225
  donated blood, **91:** 350
  increase in cases, **92:** 322-323
Systematic desensitization, 90: 24
Systemic lupus erythematosus (SLE), 91: 241

T

T cells
  adenosine deaminase deficiency, **91:** 284-285
  autoimmune diseases, **91:** 238-239, 252
  immune response, **90:** 370
  myasthenia gravis, **92:** 240
  rheumatoid arthritis, **91:** 31
  transplanted immunity, **90:** 240
T-helper cells
  AIDS, **92:** 14, 21, 23
  organ transplant rejection, **91:** 370-373
t-PA, see **Tissue-type plasminogen activator**
Tamoxifen, 90: 35 (il.), 40
Tanning (skin), 92: 325-326
Tardive dyskinesia, 92: 160, **90:** 305
Taspine, 91: 164
Tattoo removal, 92: 324-325
TB, see **Tuberculosis**
Television viewing, 91: 257-258
Tendinitis, 91: 52
Tendons, 91: 29 (il.), 47-48
Tennis elbow, 91: 46
Terminal illness, see **Hospices**
Testicles, 92: 76
Testosterone, 92: 76, 332, **90:** 290
Tetanus, 90: 372, 378-379, 381
Tetracycline, 92: 91, 92, 106, 374, 375, **90:** 262
Tetrahydroaminoacridine (THA), 90: 228-229
Thalidomide, 91: 371-372
Theater Combat Medical System, 92: 346

Therapeutic communities, 92: 118
Thermometer, 91: 190, 334-335
Thoracic outlet syndrome, 91: 52
Thymus gland, 92: 237-239
Thyroid gland, 92: 291, **91:** 274
TIA's, see **Transient ischemic attacks**
Ticlopidine, 90: 330-331
Tics, see **Tourette syndrome**
Timolol, 92: 280
Tinnitus, 92: 271-272
Tissue transplants, see **Skin grafting; Transplantation surgery**
Tissue type, 91: 368
Tissue-type plasminogen activator (t-PA), 91: 330-331, **90:** 62
Tobacco, see **Smoking**
Tolerance (drugs), 92: 112
Toothpaste, 92: 317
Total parenteral nutrition (TPN), 90: 122 (il.), 124
Tourette syndrome, 91: 86-99
Toxic shock syndrome (TSS), 91: 115-127, 303
Toxins
  Parkinson's disease, **92:** 140, 144-147
  plague, **92:** 172
  pneumonia, **92:** 90
  regulations, **90:** 323-324
  see also **Poisoning**
Toxoid vaccines, 90: 376
Toxoplasmosis, 92: 106-107
Toys, and safety, 92: 318, 322
Trachea, 92: 85, 86 (il.)
Tranquilizers
  addiction, **92:** 114, 117
  athletes' use, **90:** 53
  cataract risk, **92:** 282
  deaths, **92:** 234
  premenstrual syndrome, **92:** 137
  shyness, **92:** 195
Transient ischemic attacks (TIA's), 90: 58, 67-69
Transplantation surgery, 91: 365-382
  AIDS risk, **92:** 230-231
  islet cells to liver, **91:** 262
  nondrug methods, **92:** 237-238
  umbilical cord blood, **91:** 245
  see also **Skin grafting** and specific organs
Transurethral resection of the prostate (TURP), 92: 79
Trauma, see **Pediatric trauma centers; Post-traumatic stress disorder**
Travel, vaccines for, 90: 379
Treadmill tests, 92: 279
Tremor, 92: 140
Tretinoin, 92: 377
Trichomonal vaginitis, see **Trichomoniasis**
Trichomoniasis, 92: 218-219
Tricyclic antidepressants, 92: 117, **90:** 20
Trimesters, 92: 104
Trisomy 21, 91: 103
Trocars, 92: 52
TSS, see **Toxic shock syndrome**
Tuberculosis, 92: 368, **90:** 141-153
Tumor-infiltrating lymphocytes (TIL's), 92: 256-257, 287, **91:** 253, 285, **90:** 254, 286

Tumor necrosis factor (TNF), **92:** 257, 287, **91:** 253, 285
Tumor suppressor genes, **92:** 287-288
Tumors, Benign, **90:** 36
 see also **Cancer**
TWAR agent, **92:** 92
Typhoid, **91:** 189

U

Ulcerative keratitis, **90:** 282
Ulcers, **90:** 71-81
 arthritis drug, **90:** 269
 caffeine, **91:** 22
 esophagus, **92:** 267
Ulnar nerve entrapment, **91:** 52
Ultrasonic humidifiers, **90:** 237
Ultrasonography, see **Ultrasound**
Ultrasound
 back pain therapy, **90:** 207
 Doppler, for strokes, **90:** 67-68
 endoscopy, **90:** 264-265
 gallstone detection, **92:** 45-46
 heart imaging, **90:** 299-300
 pregnancy tests, **92:** 101, **91:** 108
 transrectal, **92:** 73
Ultraviolet (UV) radiation, **92:** 325, **90:** 284
Umbilical cord blood transplant, **91:** 245
Umbilical hernia, **91:** 105
Undifferentiated schizophrenia, **92:** 157
United Network for Organ Sharing, **91:** 377
Urethra, **92:** 70, 331-332
Urination, and prostate disorders, **92:** 69, 72, 78
Urine testing, in pregnancy, **92:** 99, 100
Urologists, **92:** 69
UROLOGY, **92:** 331-332, **91:** 331-332, **90:** 330-332
 see also **Prostate gland**
Ursodiol, **92:** 49
Uterine cancer, **92:** 292, **91:** 73 (il.), 288
 see also **Cervical cancer**
Uterus, **92:** 128-129

V

Vaccines, **90:** 368-384
 AIDS, **92:** 22 (il.), 24-25, 232, **91:** 232, **90:** 233, 383
 autoimmune disease, **91:** 238
 birth control, **90:** 243-244
 hepatitis, **92:** 303-305
 influenza, **91:** 301
 leprosy, **91:** 209
 Lyme disease, **92:** 305-306, 332-333
 measles, **92:** 28-39, 95, **91:** 300-302
 plague, **92:** 181
 pneumonia, **92:** 93 (il.), 94-95
 rinderpest, **90:** 332-333
 sexually transmitted diseases, **92:** 213
 tuberculosis, **90:** 151-153

 see also **Allergies and immunology**
Vaginal yeast infections, **92:** 270
Validity, **92:** 62
Valium, **92:** 115
Vancomycin, **92:** 91
Vaporizers, **90:** 237
Vegetarianism, **91:** 217, **90:** 99-111
Venereal disease, see **AIDS; Sexually transmitted diseases**
Ventilators, **92:** 94
Ventricles (brain), **92:** 155 (il.), 159
Vertigo, **92:** 271-272
VETERINARY MEDICINE, **92:** 332-334, **91:** 333-335, **90:** 332-334
Vibrio cholerae (bacteria), **92:** 304
Video display terminals (VDT's), **92:** 314-315
Vietnam War, **92:** 348, 375
Viruses
 book, **92:** 250
 Epstein-Barr, **90:** 127-139
 measles, **92:** 30, 32
 Parkinson's disease, **92:** 143
 pneumonia, **92:** 84, 90
 sexually transmitted diseases, **92:** 213, 220-223
 vaccines, **90:** 369, 371 (il.)
 see also **AIDS**
Vision, see **Eye and vision**
Vitamin A, **91:** 220
Vitamin B, **91:** 220, 315, **90:** 110
Vitamin B$_6$, **92:** 130-131
Vitamin C, **91:** 220, 311, **90:** 108
Vitamin D, **91:** 288, **90:** 110, 142
Vitamin E, **92:** 130, 311-312, **90:** 309-311, 333 (il.)
Vitamin K, **91:** 311
Vitamins
 birth defects, **92:** 315-316, **91:** 314-315
 food labeling, **91:** 214-215, 219-222
 premenstrual syndrome, **92:** 130-131
 Recommended Dietary Allowances, **91:** 309-311
 vegetarian diets, **90:** 110-111

W

Walking, **92:** 277
Walking pneumonia, **92:** 90
Wanglie, Helga, **92:** 298
Warfarin, **92:** 331
Water
 fluoridated, **92:** 262, **91:** 260, 319
 lead pollution, **92:** 276, **90:** 176, 181
WEIGHT CONTROL, **92:** 335-337, **91:** 335-337, **90:** 335-337
 caffeine, **91:** 23
 cholesterol, **90:** 280-281
 food labeling claims, **91:** 210
 genetics, **91:** 286-287
 growth hormone, **91:** 289-290
 L-tryptophan, **91:** 237, 310
 long life factors, **91:** 229-230
 pregnancy, **92:** 102
 weight fluctuations and health, **92:** 312-313, 335-337
 see also **Eating disorders; Obesity**
Western blot, **92:** 20, **91:** 349
White, Ryan, **91:** 233, **90:** 117
White blood cells
 AIDS transmission, **92:** 232

 cancer patients, **92:** 246
 donated blood, **91:** 348
 neutrophils, **90:** 257
 organ transplants, **92:** 307, **91:** 368
 pneumonia, **92:** 88, 90
 see also **B cells; T cells; Tumor-infiltrating lymphocytes**
Whooping cough, see **Pertussis vaccine**
Withdrawal (addiction), **92:** 112, 115-118
Womb, see **Uterus**
Women
 AIDS, **92:** 16, 18-20, 230 (il.)
 bone disorders, **92:** 246-247, **91:** 246-247, 287-289
 books on health, **92:** 250, **91:** 249
 brain structure and sex, **90:** 250
 carpal tunnel syndrome, **91:** 45, 49
 epilepsy, **91:** 150
 estrogen replacement therapy, **92:** 228, **91:** 288-289, **90:** 289-290
 gallstones, **92:** 43
 heart disease, **92:** 64, 278-279, 299-300, **91:** 296-297, 336, **90:** 289-290
 mental health, **92:** 308, 309
 pelvic inflammatory disease, **92:** 212, 214, 216, 323
 self-esteem, **92:** 260-261
 substance abuse, **91:** 236
 vaginal yeast infections, **92:** 270
 weight control, **91:** 336, **90:** 337
 see also **Breast cancer; Estrogen; Menstruation; Pregnancy and childbirth**
Work
 pregnant women, **92:** 316
 students, **92:** 259 (il.), 259-260
 see also **Occupational hazards**
Wound botulism, **92:** 206
Wrist drop, **90:** 179
Wrist injuries, **92:** 247-248, **91:** 43-55

X

X rays
 digital dental, **91:** 261 (il.)
 gallstone detection, **92:** 46-47
 magnetic resonance imaging, **91:** 298
 pregnancy, **92:** 106
 rheumatoid arthritis, **91:** 30 (il.), 36
 tuberculosis, **92:** 149
 see also **Radiation therapy**
Xanax, see **Alprazolam**

Y

Yeast infections, **92:** 270
Yersinia pestis (bacteria), **92:** 168-172, 176-181

Z

Zidovudine, see **AIDS**
Zinc, **90:** 108

Acknowledgments

The publishers of *The World Book Health & Medical Annual* gratefully acknowledge the courtesy of the following artists, photographers, publishers, institutions, agencies, and corporations for the illustrations in this volume. Credits should read from top to bottom, left to right on their respective pages. All entries marked with an asterisk (*) denote illustrations created exclusively for *The World Book Health & Medical Annual*. All maps, charts, and diagrams were prepared by *The World Book Health & Medical Annual* staff unless otherwise noted.

2 Biophoto Associates/SS from Photo Researchers; Alejandro Balauer, Sygma; © Rob Crandall, Picture Group
3 Reuters/Bettmann; National Institute of Mental Health; © Alon Reininger, Contact from Woodfin Camp, Inc.
4 SPL from Photo Researchers; Scott Snow*
5 Tom Herzberg*; AP/Wide World; Burroughs Wellcome Company
10 Good Samaritan Hospital and Health Center; CNRI/SPL from Photo Researchers
11 Bob Dacey*; Lyn Boyer-Pennington*; Michael Medynsky*
12 © J. L. Atlan, Sygma
15-17 JAK Graphics*
22 © Custom Medical; © Hank Morgan and MicroGeneSys, Inc.; © Jackson Hill, Sygma
25 Fujisawa Pharmaceutical Company
26 © Alon Reininger, Contact; Centers for Disease Control
28 © Cheryl Tadin, Chicago Department of Health
33 Centers for Disease Control
34 © Alon Reininger, Contact from Woodfin Camp, Inc.
35 © 1977 20th Century-Fox courtesy Lucasfilm Ltd./Centers for Disease Control; United States Postal Administration, New York
41 Scott Snow*
43 Scott Snow*; Catherine Twomey*
44 © Custom Medical; Catherine Twomey*; Scott Snow*
45 © Lynch Photography from Medical Images; Mayo Clinic
46 Scott Snow*; Joe Rogers*; Catherine Twomey*
49 Siemens Medical System
51 Good Samaritan Hospital and Health Center; Scott Snow*; Catherine Twomey*
54 Marjie Best*; "Study finds..." Copyright © 1991 by The New York Times Company. Reprinted by permission; "Big G..." Reprinted from *Business Week* by special permission. © McGraw-Hill, Inc.; "Hold the Oat..." Copyright 1990 The Time Inc. Magazine Company. Reprinted by permission; Ed Gallucci from *Newsweek*;

Reprinted by special permission from *U.S. News & World Report* (photo: © Louis Psihoyos, Matrix); Reprinted by permission from *In Health* Magazine (photo: Kathryn Kleinman—styling: Amy Nathan)
57-65 Marjie Best*
68 Hal Lose*
71-72 Barbara Cousins*
77 Photos: Gary J. Miller, Department of Pathology, University of Colorado Health Sciences Center—art: Barbara Cousins*
78 Barbara Cousins*
82 SPL from Photo Researchers
86 Sharon Kravs*; CNRI/SPL from Photo Researchers
87 Biophoto Associates/SS from Photo Researchers; © Astrid and Hanns-Frieder Michler, SPL from Photo Researchers
89 CNRI/SPL from Photo Researchers
92 © Philippe Plailly, SPL from Photo Researchers; SPL from Photo Researchers
93 © Diane Rasche; © Doug Plummer, Photo Researchers
96 Bob Dacey*
99-100 © Custom Medical
101 © C. C. Duncan, Medical Images; © Albert Paplialunga, Phototake
103 Adapted from *Food, Pregnancy, and Health*, American College of Obstetricians and Gynecologists Patient Education Pamphlet AP001 © 1982; and *Recommended Dietary Allowances*, 10th edition, © 1989 by the National Academy of Sciences. Published by the National Academy Press
105 © C. C. Duncan, Medical Images
106 © Schleichkorn, Custom Medical
110 © C. C. Duncan, Medical Images
119 © Stephen Shames
120 © Stephen Shames; © Donna Dietrich, *New York Newsday*
121 © James Aronovsky, Picture Group
124-136 Tom Herzberg*
138 Lyn Boyer-Pennington*
141 Barbara Cousins*
142 Rush-Presbyterian-St. Luke's Medical Center
145 © Ken Hayden, Black Star; © M. P. Kahl, Photo Researchers; Blaine L. Beaman, University of California at Davis
146 © Jacques Chenet, Woodfin

Camp, Inc.; © Emilio Mercado; © Emilio Mercado
147 Carolyn Nelson
148 © Emilio Mercado
152 Marjie Best*
155 National Institute of Mental Health
156-157 Marjie Best*
158-159 Artwork provided by Rush North Shore Medical Center, Skokie, Ill., completed in Art Therapy Groups in Acute Psychiatric Unit
161 Artwork provided by Rush-Presbyterian-St. Luke's Medical Center, Chicago, Ill., completed in Art Therapy Groups in Acute Psychiatric Unit
162 Artwork provided by Rush North Shore Medical Center, Skokie, Ill., completed in Art Therapy Groups in Acute Psychiatric Unit
164 Marjie Best*
166 *Triumph of Death* by Pieter Brueghel, oil on panel, 1562; Prado Museum, Madrid (MAS)
169 Adapted from "The Bubonic Plague" by Colin McEvedy. Copyright © 1988 by Scientific American, Inc. All rights reserved.
171 CNRI/SPL from Photo Researchers; © Tom McHugh, Photo Researchers; © John Burbidge, SPL from Photo Researchers
173 Granger Collection
174 *Procession of Gregory the Great for the Cessation of the Plague* from *The Tres Riches Heures du Duc de Berry* by the Limbourg Brothers, illuminated manuscript ca. 1420; Musée Condé, Chantilly, France (Giraudon/Art Resource)
175 Illuminated manuscript from Boccaccio's *Decameron* ca. 1500; Bibliothèque Nationale, Paris (Edimedia)
177 *Procession of the Flagellants* from *Les Belles Heures du Duc de Berry* by the Limbourg Brothers, illuminated manuscript ca. 1410; The Metropolitan Museum of Art, The Cloisters Collection; Granger Collection
179 Granger Collection
182 Guy Wolek*
185 © Rick Friedman, Black Star

186-192 Guy Wolek*
194 © Trapper, Sygma;
© Gamma/Liaison; © V. Shone,
Gamma/Liaison; Barry King,
Gamma/Liaison
196-200 Michael Medynsky*; SPL from
Custom Medical
202-207 Michael Medynsky*
208 Reprinted with permission from
Alan Scott: *Focal Points, Clinical
Modules for Ophthalmologists*
7(2) American Academy of
Ophthalmology, 1989
210-213 Paul Yalowitz*
214 CNRI/SPL/SS from Photo
Researchers
215 National Audiovisual Center
217 NIH from Custom Medical;
National Audiovisual Center
219-220 National Audiovisual Center
222 © Weybridge, SPL from Photo
Researchers; © Custom Medical
223 © Custom Medical; National
Audiovisual Center
224 Paul Yalowitz*
226 Gustav Freedman from U.S.
Department of Agriculture;
© Karen Kasmauski, Woodfin
Camp, Inc.; © Rick Friedman
227 © G. I. Bernard, Animals
Animals; © D. W. Fawcett, SPL
from Photo Researchers; Pet
Love Products, Inc.
228 Iowa State University
229 Gustav Freedman from U.S.
Department of Agriculture;
© Frank Cotham
230 Nancy Andrews, *The
Washington Post*
231 JAK Graphics*
232 University of Texas Health
Science Center
233 Partnership for a Drug-Free
America
235-236 JAK Graphics*
238 Brian Willer
240 © Stephen Dalton, Animals
Animals
241 Joe Rogers*; Van C. Mow, Louis
J. Soslowsky, and Gerard A.
Ateshian
242 Reprinted from the booklet entitled *Exercise & Your Arthritis*,
copyright 1986. Used by permission of the Arthritis Foundation.
243 © Hank Morgan; Joe Rogers*
245 © Rob Crandall, Picture Group;
Mark Lyons
247 Jack Manning, NYT Pictures
249 Ralph Brunke*
251 Hanae Belfar, M.D., Magee-
Women's Hospital
252 Brockton/West Roxbury
Veterans Administration Medical
Center
253 Biomagnetic Technologies

Incorporated
255 © James Keyser, *Time* Magazine
256 JAK Graphics*
259 © Ron Rovtar, FPG
260 © Lawrence Migdale
262 Biophoto Associates/SS from
Photo Researchers
263 Craig Stafford, *Time* Magazine
265 Charles S. Lieber, M.D.
268 AP/Wide World
269 JAK Graphics*
270 Baloo © Cartoon Features
Syndicate, used by permission of
The Wall Street Journal
271 © David Stoecklein, The Stock
Market
272 Allen Balderson, University of
California at San Francisco
274 © Karen Kasmauski, Woodfin
Camp, Inc.
276 Linda L. Creighton, *U.S. News
& World Report*
277 JAK Graphics*
280 Raymond A. Applegate,
University of Texas Health
Science Center at San Antonio
281 David Harbaugh
282 Ralph J. Brunke*
283-284 JAK Graphics*
286 Reuters/Bettmann
288 Joe Rogers*
289 UPI/Bettmann
291 AP/Wide World; Joe Rogers*
292 © Cody, FPG
293 © Rick Friedman
294 JAK Graphics*
295 Boston Children's Hospital
296 © David Burnett, Contact Press
299-301 Joe Rogers*
302 From *The Wall Street Journal* –
Permission, Cartoon Features
Syndicate
304 Alejandro Balaguer, Sygma
305 © G. I. Bernard, Animals
Animals
307 © Joseph Lynch, Medical Images
309 National Institute of Mental
Health; Joe Rogers*
310 Baloo © Cartoon Features
Syndicate, used by permission of
The Wall Street Journal
313 © Douglas Richardson, Medical
Images
314 © J. Barry O'Rourke, The Stock
Market
315 © D. W. Fawcett, SPL from
Photo Researchers
319 JAK Graphics*
324 Current Technology Corporation
326 SPIDER-MAN, STORM,
POWER-MAN: TM &
© 1991 Marvel Entertainment
Group, Inc. All rights reserved.
327 © Richard Elkins,
Gamma/Liaison
328 Joe Rogers*

329 © Richard Laird, FPG
330 Joe Rogers*
331 Technomed International
333 Pet Love Products, Inc.
337 A. Bacall, © Cartoon Features
Syndicate, used by permission
of *The Wall Street Journal*
338 © David Turnley, *Detroit Free
Press* from Black Star; AP/Wide
World; National Hospice
Association
339 © Peter Turnley, Black Star;
The Connecticut Hospice Inc.
340 © David Turnley, *Detroit Free
Press* from Black Star
344 © Peter Turnley, Black Star;
AP/Wide World
345 Joe Rogers*; United States Navy
Military Sealift Command;
© Andrew Skolnick, *Journal of
the American Medical Associa-
tion*, March 27, 1991, Vol. 265,
No. 12, p. 1501. Copyright
1991, American Medical
Association; United States Navy
Military Sealift Command
349 Otis Historical Archives,
National Museum of Health and
Medicine, Armed Forces
Institute of Pathology;
UPI/Bettmann
350 Sygma; AP/Wide World
355 The Connecticut Hospice Inc.
357 Robert Knapp, Northwestern
Memorial Hospital
358 SCALA/Art Resource
359 National Hospice Association;
Robert Knapp, Northwestern
Memorial Hospital; Robert
Knapp, Northwestern Memorial
Hospital
361 Robert Knapp, Northwestern
Memorial Hospital
362 Eddie Adams, Sygma
364 Robert Knapp, Northwestern
Memorial Hospital
366 Burroughs Wellcome Company;
Eli Lilly and Company;
© George E. Jones III, Photo
Researchers
367 © Steven Frink; © Beebe,
Custom Medical
368 © Ken Spencer from *Parents*
Magazine
369 JAK Graphics*
370 University Museums, University
of Pennsylvania;
© George E. Jones III, Photo
Researchers
371 Bettmann
372 David R. Frazier Photolibrary;
© Custom Medical; David R.
Frazier Photolibrary; © Keith,
Custom Medical
373 NIH/SS from Photo Researchers
374 Paul Turnbaugh
376 © Steven Frink; National
Cancer Institute
377 Eli Lilly and Company
378 © Reuters, Sygma; National
Cancer Institute
379 Federal Drug Administration
380 David R. Frazier Photolibrary;
Burroughs Wellcome Company
382 © Beebe, Custom Medical;
© Frank Fournier, Contact
Press from Woodfin Camp, Inc.

World Book Encyclopedia, Inc. provides high-quality educational and reference products for the family and school. They include THE WORLD BOOK MEDICAL ENCYCLOPEDIA,
a 1,040-page fully illustrated family health reference; THE WORLD BOOK OF SPACE
EXPLORATION, a two-volume review of the major developments in space since man first
walked on the moon; and the STUDENT INFORMATION FINDER and the new award-win-
ning HOW TO STUDY, a fast-paced video presentation of key study skills with information students need to succeed in school. For further information, write WORLD BOOK
ENCYCLOPEDIA, INC., P.O. Box 3073, Evanston IL 60204-9974.